Introduction to Global Health

Kathryn H. Jacobsen, MPH, PhD
Assistant Professor of Epidemiology
Department of Global and Community Health
George Mason University
Fairfax, Virginia

JONES AND BARTLETT PUBLISHERS
Sudbury, Massachusetts
BOSTON   TORONTO   LONDON   SINGAPORE

World Headquarters

Jones and Bartlett Publishers	Jones and Bartlett Publishers	Jones and Bartlett Publishers
40 Tall Pine Drive	Canada	International
Sudbury, MA 01776	6339 Ormindale Way	Barb House, Barb Mews
978-443-5000	Mississauga, Ontario L5V 1J2	London W6 7PA
info@jbpub.com	CANADA	UK

Jones and Bartlett's books and products are available through most bookstores and online booksellers. To contact Jones and Bartlett Publishers directly, call 800-832-0034, fax 978-443-8000, or visit our website, www.jbpub.com.

Substantial discounts on bulk quantities of Jones and Bartlett's publications are available to corporations, professional associations, and other qualified organizations. For details and specific discount information, contact the special sales department at Jones and Bartlett via the above contact information or send an email to specialsales@jbpub.com.

Production Credits
Publisher: Michael Brown
Associate Editor: Katey Birtcher
Associate Production Editor: Jennifer M. Ryan
Marketing Manager: Sophie Fleck
Composition: Graphic World
Cover Design: Katherine Ternullo
Cover Images: © Photos.com, © AbleStock
Printing and Binding: Malloy, Inc.
Cover Printing: Malloy, Inc.

Library of Congress Cataloging-in-Publication Data
Jacobsen, Kathryn H.
  Introduction to global health / Kathryn H. Jacobsen.
    p. ; cm.
  Includes bibliographical references and index.
  ISBN-13: 978-0-7637-5159-3
  ISBN-10: 0-7637-5159-6
  1. World health. 2. Public health. 3. Globalization—Health aspects. I. Title.
  [DNLM: 1. World Health. 2. Public Health. WA 530.1 J17i 2008]
  RA441.J33 2008
  362.1—dc22
                                                            2007014257
6048

Printed in the United States of America
11 10 09 08 07   10 9 8 7 6 5 4 3 2 1

CONTENTS

Preface ix

Chapter 1—Global Health 1

    What Is Global Health? 1
    What Is Health? 2
    Medicine and Public Health. 3
    Studying Population Health 7
        Person 7
        Place 7
        Time 8
    Risk Factors 8
        Causal Webs 11
    Prevention 13
        Screening 14
    Selecting Interventions. 16
    References 18

Chapter 2—Health Inequalities 19

    Health Inequalities 20
    Causes of Death 23
        Injuries 24
        Non-communicable Conditions 27
        Infectious Diseases and Other Conditions 30
    Inequalities in Causes of Death 31
    References 36

Chapter 3—Socioeconomic Context of Disease **39**

    Socioeconomic Risk Factors 40
    Poverty 41
    Economic Indicators 43
    Employment and Occupational Status 48
    Literacy and Educational Level 50
    References 54

Chapter 4—Maternal and Child Health **55**

    Causes of Child Death 55
        Pneumonia 58
        Diarrhea 61
        Malaria 62
        Measles 63
        Undernutrition 64
    Child Health Initiatives 65
    Protecting Children 69
    Women's Health 70
        Maternal Health 72
    Family Planning 76
    Population Growth 82
    Demography 83
    Population Planning Policies 88
    References 89

Chapter 5—The Health of Special Populations **91**

    Ethnic, Racial, Religious, and Tribal Minorities 92
    Immigrants, Refugees, and Internally
        Displaced People 94
    Prisoners 96
    Persons with Mental Illness 98
        Measuring the Burden of Disease 101
    Persons with Physical Impairments 101
        Landmines 106
    Older Persons 108
    References 113

Chapter 6—The Spread of Infectious Diseases. **115**

    Infection Transmission. 116
    The Disease Process. 119
    Agent, Host, Environment 122
        Agent 122
        Host 139
        Environment. 140
        Vector 141
    Measuring Disease in Populations. 142
    Disease Control 144
    References 146

Chapter 7—HIV/AIDS, Malaria, and TB **149**

    HIV/AIDS 149
    Malaria. 158
    Tuberculosis (TB) 163
    Comparison of HIV/AIDS, Malaria, and TB. 166
    References 167

Chapter 8—Globalization and Emerging Infectious Diseases. . . . **169**

    "The Epidemiologic Transition"
      and Globalization. 169
    Emerging Infectious Diseases 171
        Influenza. 174
    Bioterrorism. 176
    References 178

Chapter 9—Nutrition **181**

    Essential Nutrients 181
    Undernutrition 189
        Vitamin and Mineral Deficiencies 190
        Vitamin A Deficiency. 193
        Iodine Deficiency Disorders. 194
        Iron Deficiency Anemia 194
        Zinc Deficiency 196
    Measuring Nutritional Status. 196
    Breastfeeding 199

Globalization and Food Safety. 201
Overnutrition 203
Is There Enough Food in the World?. 207
References 209

Chapter 10—Environmental Health **211**
History of Environmental Health. 211
What Is Environmental Health?. 212
The Home Environment. 214
Water 215
Sanitation 222
Fuel and Indoor Air Quality. 225
Conclusion 227
References 228

Chapter 11—Health Effects of Environmental Change. 229
Health Impacts of Local Environmental Change. 229
Urbanization. 234
The Work Environment 237
Community Health Action. 240
Global Environmental Change. 242
References 245

Chapter 12—Global Health Payers and Players **247**
Who Pays for Health? 247
Paying for Personal Health. 247
Paying for Public Health 252
International Funding and Debt Relief. 253
Who Implements Health Programs? 256
National and Local Governments. 256
United Nations Agencies 257
National Governmental Organizations. 259
Non-Governmental Organizations 265
International Businesses. 269
References 270

Chapter 13—Global Health Priorities. **273**

    Health and Human Rights 273
        Trade Agreements, Intellectual Property
            Rights, and Health 277
    Priorities in Global Health 279
        Millennium Development Goals 282
    How Much Will It Cost? 285
    References 288

Chapter 14—Learning More about Global Public Health **291**

    Information Sources. 291
        Reading an Abstract 293
        Finding Reliable Articles 294
    Epidemiologic Study Designs 296
        Ecological Surveys. 296
        Cross-Sectional Surveys. 299
        Case-Control Studies 300
        Cohort Studies 303
        Clinical Trials. 306
    Research Ethics 308
    Interpreting Measures of Association 310
    Bias and Confounding 313
    Validity. 314
    References 319

Appendix I—Countries of the World by WHO Region **321**

Appendix II—Constitution of the World Health Organization. . . **326**

Appendix III—Convention on the Rights of the Child. **329**

Appendix IV—Universal Declaration of Human Rights **331**

Appendix V—Millennium Development Goals, Targets,
   and Indicators **336**

Appendix VI—Preventive and Treatment Interventions for Major Health Issues. 340

Appendix VII—Recommended Childhood Immunizations. 343

Index 345

PREFACE

On June 16, 2006, Bill Gates, founder of Microsoft and the richest man in the world, made headlines when he announced his intention to scale back his work at Microsoft to devote more time to the charitable foundation he co-founded with his wife, Melinda.[1] Ten days later, even bigger headlines were made when Warren Buffett, the second wealthiest man in the world, made a surprising announcement: He was handing over most of his fortune to Bill Gates.[2] More precisely, the bulk of his accumulated wealth was going to the Bill & Melinda Gates Foundation, which focuses primarily on improving global health. As a result, the Bill & Melinda Gates Foundation—the largest philanthropic foundation in the world even prior to Buffett's generous donation—doubled in value to more than $60 billion.

What would inspire the wealthiest men in the world to develop such a passion for one cause? They are dismayed that every year more than 3 million children die of diseases that are completely preventable. They are also concerned about the inequalities between people who live in different parts of the world. In an address to the World Health Assembly, the governing body of the World Health Organization, Bill Gates recalled:

> I first learned about these tragic health inequities some years ago when I was reading an article about diseases in the developing world. It showed that more than half a million children die every year from "rotavirus." I thought, "'Rotavirus?'—I've never even heard of it. How could I never have heard of something that kills half a million children every year!?" Melinda and I had assumed that if there were vaccines and treatments that could save lives, governments would be doing everything they could to get them to the people who needed them. But they weren't. We couldn't

ix

escape the brutal conclusion that—in our world today—some lives are seen as worth saving and others are not. We said to ourselves: "This can't be true. But if it is true, it deserves to be the priority of our giving." [3]

Bill and Melinda Gates have found something that demands their attention. That something is global health, and it is the subject of this book.

In this book you may read about a lot of things you've never heard about that affect the lives and health of millions of people every year. Chapters 2 and 3 focus on the health inequalities that are present in every part of the globe and the socioeconomic factors that contribute to inequalities. Chapters 4 and 5 discuss the special health needs of vulnerable populations, including women and children. In many parts of the world today, pregnancy is a very dangerous time for a woman, and a large percentage of babies do not live to see their fifth birthday. Chapters 6, 7, and 8 focus on infectious diseases, Chapter 9 on nutrition, and Chapters 10 and 11 on environmental health. Three of the most significant global infectious diseases—HIV/AIDS, malaria, and tuberculosis—receive extensive attention, but there are many less studied and less publicized conditions that are equally harmful to the people who have them. Chapter 12 explains how you can find more information about global health issues. The final chapters, Chapters 13 and 14, discuss international health priorities, the key players (and payers) in global public health, and some of the ways that people are working together to improve the health of people around the world.

Why should you care about global health?

First, health is a common human experience. No matter what cultural, social, economic, and other differences may set us apart, all humans know what it is like to be sick, to care for an ill or injured family member or friend, and to mourn the loss of a loved one. That commonality should prompt compassion within us for those whose health is more precarious than our own.

Second, people like Bill and Melinda Gates and activists like physician-anthropologist Paul Farmer have proclaimed that health is a fundamental human right. If health is a human right and a human need—just like water, food, and shelter—then it is an injustice that so many millions of people around the world do not have access to even basic levels of health care because of where they were born, how much their families earn, or a whole host of other circumstances that are often beyond their control. If health is a human right, then basic health care and protection from preventable diseases should be available to all people, regardless of the conditions that have made them vulnerable to illness, disability, and premature death.

Third, we have very valid "selfish" reasons for seeking information about what is going on in other parts of the world. Globalization is changing not just our economies and social structures, but also our health experience. In today's interconnected world, our own health and well-being are literally inseparable from everyone else's. Personal health practices such as eating nutritious food, exercising, frequent hand-washing, and getting vaccinated might help keep you, your family, and your co-workers healthy. But we cannot prevent the birds that may carry influenza, West Nile virus, and other infectious agents from flying over our borders or being carried across national borders on ships or planes, nor can we inspect every imported banana or lettuce leaf for possible contaminants. The complexities of the spread of disease require us all to think beyond our households and communities to regional, national, and global levels.

As the world becomes increasingly interconnected, international health crises will become even more relevant to our own health. Because modern transportation allows infections to cross borders quickly, the need for national governments to work together to track the emergence of new infectious diseases and contain them has become clear. There is also a growing recognition that good sanitation practices and enforcement of environmental laws that keep food products safe cannot be consistently followed when the people who grow produce and raise livestock, live and work in substandard conditions.

For all these reasons and more, educated and informed citizens must take action to protect their own health, respond wisely to infectious disease threats and safety hazards, and advocate for the health of others. This book will give you the vocabulary and knowledge base to understand the language of global health. You will be introduced to the biological and social causes of health and illness and the some of methods used for studying health and implementing programs that promote health. (If you ever find yourself in a conversation with Bill Gates, Bono, or a UN Ambassador like Angelina Jolie, this will come in handy.)

You will also learn how global interconnectedness impacts health. No matter what field you work in—business, politics, education, religion, medicine, relief and development, engineering, social work, agriculture, manufacturing, or anything else—you are likely to be at least peripherally involved in making decisions that impact human and environmental health. In this book you will read about how the health status of people in the most distant parts of the world affects your health and how you, intentionally or unintentionally, affect the health of others around the world.

As you learn about how most people in the world experience life and health, I hope that you will examine your values and consider how the choices you make impact other people's lives. And as your awareness of global health issues enlarges, I hope you will develop a vision for how you can be involved in creating solutions to health problems. You will learn how some individuals and groups are making a difference in the lives of millions of people across the globe and how you can be involved in helping to shape a healthier world.

NOTES

1. Markoff J, Lohr S. Gates to cede software reins. *New York Times*. June 16, 2006.
2. O'Brien TL, Saul S. Buffett to give bulk of his fortune to Gates charity. *New York Times*. June 26, 2006.
3. Gates B. Address to the 2005 World Health Assembly on May 16, 2005. Geneva, Switzerland.

Web links to people, organizations, reports, and other content mentioned in the text are listed on the book's website: http://www.jbpub.com/ catalog/0763751596/

About the Author

Kathryn H. Jacobsen earned an MPH in International Health and a PhD in Epidemiology from the University of Michigan. She is currently an Assistant Professor of Epidemiology in the Department of Global and Community Health at George Mason University in Fairfax, VA.

CHAPTER 1

Global Health

Key Points:
- Global health is the study of the biological, social, and environmental contributors to health and disease in populations around the world.
- Public health focuses on the health of populations. Populations at risk for specific diseases can be described using the person—place—time triad.
- A causal web helps explain the complex interactions between multiple risk factors and a disease outcome.
- Preventive measures can be implemented once risk factors are known.

This chapter begins with an overview of the concepts of health, public health, international health, and global health, then discusses risk factors for disease and methods of disease prevention and health promotion. While the approaches to health and healing may vary across countries and cultures, the pursuit of healthy individuals and communities is a universal goal.

WHAT IS GLOBAL HEALTH?

The term **international health** has traditionally referred to the study of the health of people who live in developing countries. The term *global health* is sometimes used interchangeably with *international health*. In other instances, the term **global health** is used to refer to *transnational health*, health concerns that cross national borders. Global health is an increasing concern because modern transportation allows infectious diseases to spread across the world at an alarming rate. Advances in medical technology and pharmaceuticals are curing diseases that used to be untreatable, but at the same time have created infectious agents (superbugs) that are resistant to current antibiotic therapies. And the threat of bioterrorism requires coordination of public health responses from many nations. The study of global health also arises from concerns about the continued and growing disparities in health

1

between nations and within nations. For example, the main health concerns of a community in rural Zimbabwe are probably HIV/AIDS and malaria, which are very different from the health concerns of urban Canadians, which are most likely heart disease and cancer. Everyone is (or should be) concerned about emerging infections such as multidrug-resistant tuberculosis (MDR-TB), rising cancer rates, and the high prevalence of mental health disorders.

People who want to work in global health need to understand the social and environmental contributors to disease and the biological causes of disease. They must be familiar with the traditional areas of international health, such as infectious disease, nutrition, child health, reproductive health, and water and sanitation. They must also be knowledgeable about global public health concerns, such as aging, mental health, and food safety. An understanding of the impact of poverty, culture, and economic globalization on health is also essential.

WHAT IS HEALTH?

Most people define health as the absence of sickness, injury, infection, pain, tumors, or other physical disorders, or as the ability to conduct normal daily activities. There are several problems with definitions like these. One is that these definitions primarily address physical illnesses and ignore the effects of stress and mental health on overall health. Another problem is that the definition of "normal" health varies from person to person. For example, some people assume that it is normal for an older person to have limited mobility and forgetfulness, but this is not true. Many older people are very active and mentally sharp, and many of those that have joint pain or memory loss could be helped by therapy and medication. If an older person assumes that these limitations are a normal part of aging, he or she may not seek the health care that could increase quality of life.

A more complete definition of health addresses both physical and mental health and the presence of a social support system that facilitates health. The World Health Organization's Constitution (Appendix II), written in 1948, defines **health** as "a state of complete physical, mental, and social well-being and not merely the absence of disease or infirmity." The preamble to the WHO Constitution lists nine health principles (Table 1-1). The boldest claim is that "the enjoyment of the highest attainable standard of health is one of the fundamental rights of every human being." What this means is

Table 1-1. Health Principles from the Preamble to the Constitution of the World Health Organization.

1	Health is a state of complete physical, mental, and social well-being and not merely the absence of disease or infirmity.
2	The enjoyment of the highest attainable standard of health is one of the fundamental rights of every human being without distinction of race, religion, political belief, economic, or social condition.
3	The health of all peoples is fundamental to the attainment of peace and security and is dependent upon the fullest cooperation of individuals and States.
4	The achievement of any State in the promotion and protection of health is of value to all.
5	Unequal development in different countries in the promotion of health and control of disease, especially communicable disease, is a common danger.
6	Healthy development of the child is of basic importance; the ability to live harmoniously in a changing total environment is essential to such development.
7	The extension to all peoples of the benefits of medical, psychological, and related knowledge is essential to the fullest attainment of health.
8	Informed opinion and active cooperation on the part of the public are of the utmost importance in the improvement of the health of the people.
9	Governments have a responsibility for the health of their peoples which can be fulfilled only by the provision of adequate health and social measures.

that the *standard* of health should be raised so that everyone has access to at least basic medical and psychological care (principle 7), especially people in at-risk population groups (principles 2 and 6). The preamble also notes that health is linked with peace (principles 3, 4, and 5), that areas with poor health standards put everyone at risk of pandemic outbreaks of infectious disease (principle 5), and that both the public (principle 8) and governments (principle 9) must take active responsibility for public health.

MEDICINE AND PUBLIC HEALTH

Medicine is concerned with the health of individuals, and medical professionals are instrumental to creating and maintaining healthy populations. Doctors and nurses diagnose and treat nutritional problems, heart conditions, infections, and other diseases. Dentists treat tooth and gum diseases and help individuals maintain good oral hygiene. Yet, individual health is not something that exists in isolation but as part of a broader social context; medicine is a limited approach to health. Although medical practitioners play a key role in helping people reach and maintain health, other health workers, counselors, spiritual advisors, elected officials and government workers, and many people in many other professions make important contributions to the health of individuals, communities, and nations. The public health system, which works at local, state and provincial, national, and international levels, also works to keep people safe and healthy. The different domains of medicine and public health are listed in Figure 1-1.

Public health is concerned with the health of populations. Public health workers aim to prevent illness, injury, and death at the population level by identifying and mitigating health hazards, responding to population health needs, and providing health education (Table 1-2).

A variety of professionals work in the area of public health. The five core disciplines of public health include health education (and the social sciences that relate to health and health behavior), health services administration (which includes health economics and health policy), environmental health, biostatistics, and epidemiology. Epidemiologists measure health status in populations defined by age, sex, national boundaries, or other categories, and determine what conditions are key causes of **mortality** (death), **morbidity** (illness), and disability in a given population. When physicians make diagnoses, they often rely on public health data to help them figure out what illnesses are most likely to affect a person of a particular age and sex who

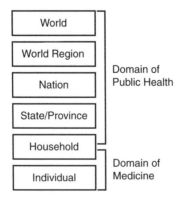

Figure 1-1. The Domains of Medicine and Public Health.

Table 1-2. Essential Public Health Services.

1	Monitor health status to identify community health problems.
2	Diagnose and investigate health problems and health hazards in the community.
3	Inform, educate, and empower people about health issues.
4	Mobilize community partnerships to identify and solve health problems.
5	Develop policies and plans that support individual and community health efforts.
6	Enforce laws and regulations that protect health and ensure safety.
7	Link people to needed personal health services and assure the provision of health care when otherwise unavailable.
8	Assure a competent public health and personal health care workforce.
9	Evaluate effectiveness, accessibility, and quality of personal and population-based health services.
10	Research for new insights and innovative solutions to health problems.

Source: American Public Health Association.

lives in a particular place. Epidemiologists also determine the risk factors for acquiring disease and use this information to make suggestions about how populations can become healthier.[1]

Public health professionals work in a variety of ways to promote population health. Among other roles, public health workers track outbreaks of infectious diseases, develop new vaccines, monitor the safety of pharmaceutical agents, assess environmental risk factors for disease, educate communities about diabetes care, and promote AIDS awareness and prevention. Public health geneticists determine which genes are associated with an increased risk of cancer. Public health educators and nutritionists work with schools and communities to reduce risky behaviors, such as unsafe sex, drug use, and reckless driving, and to promote healthy behaviors such as wearing bicycle helmets, getting screened for hypertension, and eating vegetables. Environmental public health experts develop plans for communities that want to reduce the spread of infections caused by mosquito bites. Public health professionals work with hospitals and physicians, elected officials and lawyers, biomedical researchers, the pharmaceutical industry, and others to promote health.

Public policies have a direct impact on individual and household health (Figure 1-2). Family, workplace, and hobbies contribute to the kinds of health

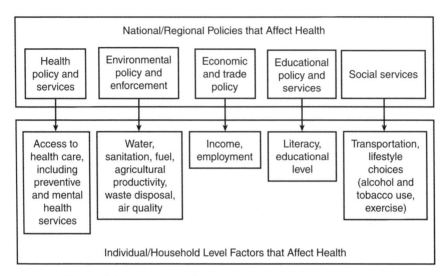

Figure 1-2. Framework for Understanding Population Health.

problems an individual is likely to encounter, whether that is an increased risk of knee injuries in an avid basketball player or an increased risk of high blood pressure in a person with a family history of hypertension. Individual health is not only the result of personal choices. Age, ethnicity, and genetic tendencies for certain diseases are examples of **unmodifiable risk factors** that cannot be changed. **Behavioral risk factors**, which include the lifestyle choices a person makes, such as whether or not to smoke or to engage in exercise, can be modified. That is not to say that it is easy to change these habits. Personal decisions are influenced by family and friends, and it is difficult to change a habit if change requires engaging in behavior that runs counter to an individual's social group. On the other hand, if an entire family or community decides to work together to eat healthier and to increase exercise, the individual is likely to feel more positive about making changes. Other groups, such as businesses and governments, also influence individual health. An individual's job may put him or her at risk of certain types of exposures or injuries, and government agencies may force an employer to reduce or to eliminate these risks in a work environment. Whether or not an individual has health insurance may influence the kind of treatment that person receives. The type of health insurance may influence how quickly that person can see a specialist, and how much of the cost of health care has to be paid out of pocket. Many societal factors influence public health;

solutions to global health often must begin at the regional and national levels rather than at the individual or household levels.

STUDYING POPULATION HEALTH

Epidemiology is the study of the distribution and causes of health and illness in populations. While the words *epidemic* and *epidemiology* have the same root, the subjects studied by epidemiologists go far beyond simply tracking outbreaks. Epidemiology helps categorize which populations or groups within a population are at increased risk of morbidity, mortality, and disability from specific diseases. The two main subfields of epidemiology are **descriptive epidemiology**, the study of disease distribution, and **analytic epidemiology**, the study disease determinants (risk factors).

Descriptive studies categorize illnesses according to three primary characteristics: person, place, and time. A descriptive epidemiology study aims to answer the questions who, where, and when.

Person

Who is the person who usually develops a certain disease? Does the disease primarily affect people from one sex or a particular age group, genetically similar people, or people with a certain occupation or income level? A descriptive study of lung cancer would note that lung cancer affects both men and women who are long-term smokers and that the risk increases with increasing duration of tobacco use and intensity of tobacco exposure. A descriptive study of bone fractures would indicate that fractures in older women with low or average body weight are likely to be related to osteoporosis whereas fractures in active adolescents and young adults are frequently the result of sports-related injuries. Understanding who is at greatest risk for a particular illness or injury is important for developing targeted prevention methods.

Place

Where are the geographic or spatial links between people who contract an illness? Are most cases in a specific state, province, nation, or region of the world? Do most cases occur near a woodland area, by a body of water, in the tropics, in the mountains, or in the arctic? Do the people who are sick share an activity in common, such as working in the same building or profession, eating at the same restaurants, shopping at the same stores, attending the same school, living in the same neighborhood or village, worshiping together, playing on the same sports team, or riding the same bus? Has a sick person recently traveled or hosted out-of-town visitors who could have exposed the person to an infection not usually found where the sick person lives?

Time

When do the cases typically occur? Does the disease occur more often during certain months of the year or during special holiday seasons? Some diseases occur in epidemics every several years; others (like influenza) occur seasonally. Are symptoms worse during the night than the day? Do most people become ill after eating a meal or following a certain medical procedure? How long do the symptoms last? On what day did symptoms appear? Community outbreaks often follow a predictable epidemic curve and tracking the number of new cases each day can provide information about whether the epidemic is ending or getting worse.

RISK FACTORS

Analytic epidemiologic studies seek to answer the question—why? A main goal of analytic epidemiology is to assess the relationship between an exposure and an outcome. An **exposure** might be a particular infectious agent, an on-the-job chemical solvent or cleaning agent, participation in a recreational football league, consumption of a dietary supplement, or years of education. An **outcome** could be death, illness, disability, pregnancy, or some other health state. John Snow, one of the founders of modern epidemiology, determined in the late 1800s that cholera was a waterborne infection by using epidemiologic methods to trace the source of an outbreak in London back to one water pump. In Snow's case, the exposure was drinking from the Broad Street pump and the outcome was cholera.

A **risk factor** is an exposure that increases the likelihood of contracting an infection, sustaining an injury, or developing a chronic disease condition. There are three criteria for an exposure being classified as a risk factor: (1) the exposure must precede the onset of the disease; (2) the frequency of the disease should vary according to the value of exposure. For example, if exposure to coal dust is a risk factor for lung disease, then people who have worked in mines for 20 years should have more lung disease than people who have been miners for only 10 years; (3) the observed association should not be due to bias or measurement error.

In John Snow's investigation of cholera, the contaminated water was proven to be the cause of the cholera outbreak. However, it is easy to make incorrect conclusions about risk factors. William Farr, one of John Snow's contemporaries, who is highly regarded for developing methods for collecting and classifying population health statistics, found that there was an association between elevation above sea level (an exposure) and the risk of death from cholera (an outcome). It turned out that elevation had an association with cholera because people living in the lower areas near rivers were more likely to be supplied with contaminated water. Studies of other London neighborhoods might have found no association between elevation and cholera or that living at higher elevations was riskier than living at low elevations. A public health program forcing people to move to higher ground might not have had any effect on reducing cholera and may even have put additional households at risk.

Technically there is a distinction between showing an **association** between an exposure and an outcome and proving **causation**. An association is a statistically significant relationship between an exposure and an outcome. This association may be a true causal association or it may be due to random variation, bias, poor study design, confounding, or some other exposure. A causal factor is an exposure that occurs before the disease outcome and directly contributes to its occurrence (Table 1-3).

Medical science depends on making distinctions between association and causation, but global health practitioners also make educated guesses about whether changing an exposure will have an impact on the frequency of disease. There may be an association between hot weather and the number of shark attacks, but that does not prove that hot weather causes shark attacks. A more likely explanation is that hot weather increases the number of humans in the water, which increases the number of humans attacked. For that matter, there may be an association between ice cream sales and shark attacks. Removing the "exposure" by banning ice cream sales at the beach would probably not do much to prevent shark attacks, unless people stopped going to beaches because of the absence of ice cream.

It is important to keep in mind that most conditions are **multifactorial**, that is, they have many different causes. Type 2 diabetes mellitus is due to

Table 1-3. Criteria for Causation.

Criterion	Explanations / Examples
Is the association strong?	If smokers are 15 times more likely to develop lung cancer than non-smokers that is stronger evidence of causality than if smokers are 1.1 times more likely to develop lung cancer. Prevalence of the disease (the total amount of disease in a population) should be significantly higher in those exposed to the risk factor than those not. In studies that follow people over time (prospective studies), the incidence of the disease (number of new cases in a population) should be significantly higher in those exposed to the risk factor than those not exposed.
Is there clear temporality (time sequence)?	Exposure to the agent or risk factor must precede development of the disease, and the disease should follow exposure to the risk factor within a predictable time frame.
Is there a dose-response effect?	If exercising for 3 hours a week is slightly protective against breast cancer and exercising for 6 hours a week is more protective, it is more likely that exercise is protective than if the extra hours of exercise are not associated with increased protection. If exposure to radiation is harmful, then people with higher radiation exposure should be sicker than people with minimal exposure.
If an experiment removes the risk factor does that reduce the risk of the disease?	People who are exposed to the risk factor should get the disease more frequently than those who do not have the exposure, and exposure to the risk factor should be more frequent among those with the disease than those without. Reducing or eliminating the risk factor should reduce the risk of the disease.
Other criteria	Is the link between the exposure and the outcome specific, biologically plausible, and consistent with existing knowledge? Have alternate explanations for the apparent causation been considered? Have different studies in different populations made consistent conclusions?

Source: This table was developed from the criteria developed by Hill and Evans. Hill AB. The environment and disease: association or causation? *Proc R Soc Med*. 1965;58:295–300. Evans AS. Causation and disease: the Henle-Koch postulates revisited. *Yale J Biol Med*. 1976;49:175–195.

the body's loss of response to the hormone insulin, which is produced by the pancreas, but obesity is often an underlying or contributing cause, genetics may play a role in the development of type 2 diabetes, and a history of gestational diabetes during a pregnancy increases the risk of type 2 diabetes in women. Heart disease is caused by atherosclerosis (the build-up of plaque in the walls of blood vessels) of the arteries that supply blood to the heart, but this build-up is possibly associated with high cholesterol levels in the blood, inflammation, infection, and genetics. Diet, stress, and physical inactivity also contribute to the development of cardiovascular disease. A broken hip may directly result from a fall, but the underlying cause of the fracture might be osteoporosis (loss of bone density) caused by genetics, inactivity, lack of calcium in the diet during childhood, endocrine disorders, or many other medical conditions. The fall may have been the result of a loss of balance due to nervous system disorders like Parkinson's disease or multiple sclerosis, or due to vision problems. Furthermore, not living in a barrier-free home or with someone who can assist with tasks that require reaching or balancing may increase the likelihood of a fall. Addressing any one of the contributing factors may prevent a negative health outcome.

Causal Webs

A *causal web* displays the relationships among the many different behavioral, social, environmental, and biological exposures that could possibly have a causal relationship with a certain health outcome. Causal webs indicate the immediate biological causes of disease and may also show more distant causes like hygiene behavior, nutritional status, educational level, and poverty status.

Interrupting any of the causal pathways shown on a causal diagram may prevent the disease outcome for at least some members of a population. For example, Figure 1-3 shows the relationships between both direct and less direct causes of diarrheal disease. Most diarrheal diseases are transmitted through fecal-oral spread (when human excrement is ingested through contact with contaminated food, water, or hands) or ingestion of contaminated food or water. An intervention that removes any one of the arrows on the diagram could be successful in reducing the amount of diarrhea in a population.

Once it has been shown that an exposure is a likely contributor to disease, the type of causal contribution can be described using the terms necessary and sufficient. An exposure is **necessary** if it must be present for a person

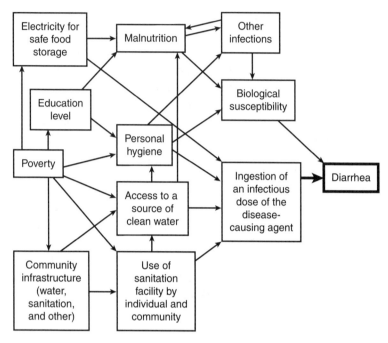

Figure 1-3. Sample Causal Web for Diarrhea.

to develop a disease. An exposure is **sufficient** if it alone can cause disease. Some exposures are necessary but not sufficient, which means that a person must have a specific exposure to develop a disease, but that exposure alone does not mean that the exposed person will develop disease. You cannot develop hepatitis A disease without first being infected with hepatitis A virus, but most hepatitis A virus infections do not cause illness. Some exposures are sufficient but not necessary. You may have a gene that increases the likelihood that you develop a particular type of cancer, but some people without that gene may also develop the same type of cancer. Women who have the BRCA1 (breast cancer 1) gene have a higher risk of developing both breast and ovarian cancer than women who do not carry this gene, but according to the American Cancer Society only about 5% of women with breast cancer in the United States have BRCA1 mutations.[2] On rare occasions a cause is both necessary and sufficient, and that one exposure alone can cause disease. It is necessary to have the gene that causes Huntington Disease to develop the neurological disease, and anyone with the gene will develop the degenerative brain disease.

In global health, few of the risk factors that contribute to disease are likely to be necessary and sufficient. However, when several risk factors are present they together they create a situation in which disease can occur. As you read the chapters on infectious disease, nutrition, and environmental health, keep in mind the socioeconomic, political, behavioral, and environmental risk factors that contribute to creating the context in which disease occurs.

PREVENTION

When a complex set of socioeconomic, biological, and environmental characteristics contribute to causing disease, there are also multiple paths to a solution, whether it is developing drug therapies for cancer that target specific cellular structures and functions or working to improve the water and sanitation facilities in a community. One of the big challenges of public health is trying to determine those risk factors that are the most influential to the disease process and the most modifiable.

There are three levels of prevention (Table 1-4). When we understand the causes of a disease or disability, or at least some of the exposures that we know are related to a particular health outcome, we can work toward **primary prevention** and keep the disease or disability from occurring. Primary prevention methods include immunizations, improved nutrition, safety devices, health education, and any interventions that reduce susceptibility to infection, injury, or disease. In some cases, we do not have the knowledge or ability to prevent a person from becoming sick or injured. Once a person develops a disease condition, the goal of **secondary prevention** is to reduce severity and to minimize the extent of disability and the risk of premature death. Early detection and prompt intervention are key components of secondary prevention. For people who have already sustained an injury or disease that has led to impairment or chronic pain, the goal of **tertiary prevention** is rehabilitation that seeks to maximize function and palliative care that works to minimize pain.

Given the three levels of prevention, there is almost always some intervention that could improve the health status of a sick or injured person. Appendix VI lists some examples of primary prevention and secondary prevention interventions for some of the major global health concerns, including child mortality, maternal mortality, undernutrition, HIV/AIDS, and TB. Most of these preventive interventions focus on changing health behavior through promotion of hand washing, breastfeeding, latrine use, mosquito net

Table 1-4. Levels of Prevention.

Level	Also called . . .	Goal	Examples
Primary Prevention	Prevention	Prevent disease from ever occurring	Give vitamin A capsules to at-risk children to prevent blindness. Give tetanus shots to pregnant women to prevent tetanus.
Secondary Prevention	Treatment	Reduce severity of disease and prevent disability and death	Detect cases of acute respiratory infections of children early so they can be treated with antibiotics. Give ORT (oral rehydration therapy) to children with diarrhea.
Tertiary Prevention	Rehabilitation	Reduce impairment and minimize suffering	Provide rehabilitation services to people who have been in a motor vehicle accident. Provide palliative (pain-relieving) care to people with advanced cases of cancer.

use, family planning methods, and immunizations. Some focus on changing the health environment by spraying insecticides, implementing clean delivery room practices, and having access to improved sanitation facilities. Others focus on improving access to health care, to drugs, to micronutrient supplements, and to healthy foods.

Screening

Screening is a type of secondary prevention in which an entire population is encouraged to be tested for a disease based on evidence that early intervention improves health outcomes. The goal of screening is to diagnose cases of the disease at an early, more treatable stage and to identify people who have risk factors for the disease (Figure 1-4).

A good screening test maximizes the number of correct results and minimizes the number test errors. Diseases that are part of screening programs

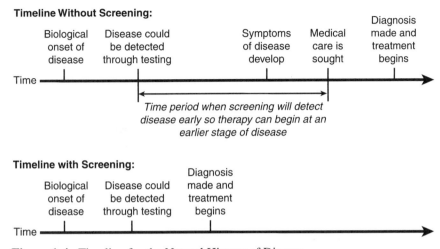

Figure 1-4. Timeline for the Natural History of Disease.

are usually severe and relatively common, so screening is considered a cost-effective way to diagnose people in early, asymptomatic stages of disease when treatment is easier and cheaper (Table 1-5).

Decisions about whether to implement a screening program are made by health professionals after considering the scope of local health conditions. Pap smears for cervical cancer, PSA (prostate-specific antigen) tests for prostate cancer, mole checks for skin cancer, mammograms for early detection of breast cancer or pre-cancerous lesions, and blood pressure checks

Table 1-5. Questions to Ask Before Starting a Screening Program.

Is the disease of public health importance?

Is the disease severe?

Is the disease relatively common in the population?

Is there an acceptable treatment for individuals found to have disease?

Are facilities for further testing and for treatment available to the screening population?

Is there an early asymptomatic stage of the disease that could be detected through screening?

Is the test acceptable to the population?

Is the test valid?

at community centers and shopping centers are all examples of screening programs that are common in developed countries. Screening in developing countries is more often geared at children and pregnant women, who are regularly weighed and examined. Researchers, practitioners, policy-makers, and communities work together to use screening to maximize the health of specific populations.

SELECTING INTERVENTIONS

Implementation of public health interventions often requires public health workers to partner with social workers, business owners, religious leaders, and other community members. All people working in public health (whether as educators, policy makers, or in another field) must always be aware of the cultural dimensions of health. Health interventions must target behavior change in a manner that is appropriate and acceptable to the populations in which they are implemented.

In some communities, blending conventional (also called Western or allopathic) medicine and traditional medicine may be appropriate. **Traditional medicine (TM)** uses natural remedies (often made from plants, animals, and minerals), manual techniques, and spiritual therapies based on traditional cultural practices and beliefs for treating particular illnesses and promoting general well-being. The majority of Africans use traditional healers for at least some of their health care, and some governments are encouraging the integration of traditional medicine into conventional health care systems.[3] TM is used extensively in Asia, and is gaining popularity in other parts of the world.

Complementary / alternative medicine (CAM) refers to the use of health care practices outside of a person's own tradition or that are not part of conventional medical practice. More than half of all North Americans and Europeans have used herbal medicines, acupuncture, or other forms of CAM at least once.[4] The distinction between TM/CAM and conventional therapies is blurring. About one in four modern medicines are made from plants first used in traditional treatments, such as Artemisia (used for treating malaria), Taxol (a drug made from the Pacific Yew tree and used to treat breast cancer), and Digitalis (used to treat congestive heart failure). TM/CAM therapies, such as acupuncture, are increasingly used in conventional medical practice.[5]

Approaches to global health must also consider how health and illness are understood in various cultural systems, and how to make use of appropriate technology and care practices. Many people agree that modern science proves that most disease is caused by "germs" (in the case of infectious diseases) or "genes" (in the case of cancers and other non-communicable conditions). But we also have other beliefs about what causes disease.

Many people take a mechanistic approach to health that sees illness as a dysfunction or breakdown of the human body, which is supposed to function like a well-oiled machine. Some people add an ethical component by saying that health results from following a good, clean, moral lifestyle and illness is a type of punishment for sin. Others see health in terms of maintaining the equilibrium of the body. The Chinese idea of yin and yang, the Ayurvedic medicine practiced on the Indian subcontinent, and Hippocrates' belief that disease is the result of imbalance between the four "humors" (which forms the basis of Unani, also called Arabic medicine) are all equilibrium theories.[6] Personalistic systems like the voodoo practiced in Haiti interpret sicknesses supernaturally. These beliefs about health and illness may be an important part of understanding the disease process. They can influence the way people interpret symptoms and diagnoses, the timeline for seeking treatment, and the type of therapy that will be effective.

Think about your own health practices. When you are sick, who do you consult? A physician? A chiropractor? A massage therapist? An acupuncturist? A spiritual leader? What kinds of remedies do you take? Prescription medications? Over-the-counter drugs? Herbal or homeopathic remedies? Vitamins? How do you decide what is appropriate for helping you become healthy and stay healthy? How do you measure effectiveness? Your answers to these questions are based on both availability (perhaps limited by an insurance policy that only covers certain health care providers and only pays for certain drugs and physical therapies) and your belief system.

If you believe that disease has a supernatural origin like a god, spirit, ancestor, sin, or lack of faith, then you might seek to be cured through religious ritual like prayer, confession, or making sacrifices. If you believe that disease is caused by imbalances in the body, you might get a massage, sweat in a sauna, or change your eating, drinking, or sleeping habits. While holistic medicine may have a limited ability to cure infections and cancers when compared to conventional medicine, holistic approaches may be very valuable for prevention of illness and for psychological well-being. Social and spiritual components of health programs may be crucial for their success.

REFERENCES

1. The Morbidity and Mortality Weekly Report (MMWR) published by the CDC (Centers for Disease Control and Prevention) and the Weekly Epidemiological Record (WER) from the World Health Organization, both available online, cover current health issues around the world. For quick links to these and other global health sites, visit the website for this book: http://www.jbpub.com/.
2. The American Cancer Society provides cancer statistics and information about cancer prevention, screening, and support for patients.
3. World Health Organization, WHO Traditional Medicine Strategy 2002–2005, Geneva, Switzerland: World Health Organization, 2002 (WHO/EDM/TRM/2002.1). World Health Organization, Traditional Practitioners as Primary Health Care Workers, Geneva, Switzerland: World Health Organization, 1995 (WHO/SHS/DHS/TRM/95.6).
4. World Health Organization, WHO Traditional Medicine Strategy 2002-2005, 2002.
5. World Health Organization, Guidelines on Developing Consumer Information on Proper Use of Traditional, Complementary and Alternative Medicine, Geneva, Switzerland: World Health Organization, January 2004.
6. World Health Organization, Legal Status of Traditional Medicine and Complementary/Alternative Medicine: A Worldwide Review, Geneva, Switzerland: World Health Organization, 2001.

CHAPTER 2

Health Inequalities

Key Points:
- Health inequalities between the richest and poorest segments of the population exist between countries and within countries.
- Injuries occur in all populations and may be unintentional (like road traffic injuries, falls, drowning, poisoning, and burns) or intentional (violence that is self-directed, interpersonal, or collective).
- Non-communicable conditions such as heart disease and cancer are the most common causes of death in higher-income populations and are becoming more common in low-income populations.
- Infectious diseases and nutritional deficiencies are common causes of death in lower-income populations.

Kofi Annan, former Secretary-General of the United Nations, spoke hopefully at an African summit in 2001: "There has been a worldwide revolt of public opinion. People no longer accept that the sick and dying, simply because they are poor, should be denied drugs that have transformed the lives of others who are better off."[1] If we truly have accepted that no one should die from easily preventable and treatable illnesses, then why are so many people still suffering and dying?

Bill Gates was moved to become involved in global health work after learning that preventable diseases killed millions of children every year and that few organizations were working to alleviate this injustice. Gates recalled that he "couldn't escape the brutal conclusion that—in our world today—some lives are seen as worth saving and others are not."[2] Other world leaders in politics and business, entertainment stars, and other influential people have begun to speak often and openly about their belief that health inequalities are wrong and about their commitment to do something to mitigate them. Entertainers, for example, have supported fundraisers for AIDS and other causes, and the television series *e.r.* has raised awareness about global health issues by featuring several episodes set in central Africa. This chapter provides an overview of some of the most common causes of illness, death, and disability in the world, and highlights some of the health inequalities that have spurred people to take action.

HEALTH INEQUALITIES

The constitution of the World Health Organization (Appendix II) states that health is a fundamental right of all people regardless of "race, religion, political belief, economic, or social condition." We could add to that list other categories like age, sex, nationality, immigration status, educational level, occupation, ethnicity, health insurance type, and marital status. Yet significant differences in health continue to exist between groups. Black Americans are much more likely than white Americans to have strokes, hypertension, congestive heart failure, and diabetes.[3] Married British and American men live longer and are healthier than unmarried men.[4,5] A baby born in Sierra Leone in 2005 has a life expectancy of 38 years, while a baby born in Japan can expect to live more than twice as long, to 82 years.[6] These differences are largely a function of social, political, and economic environments, and not innate biological differences.

Inequalities in health, differences in health experience and health status, exist at many levels. Some of these differences are avoidable, unfair, and unjust and are referred to as **inequities**.[7] The poor are often more susceptible to illness and injury because of a limited diet, existing infections, and dangerous work and home environments. They are less likely to have the means to prevent illness by, for example, being screened for early-stage cancer or buying a bednet to prevent the mosquito bites that cause malaria infections. Limited money or insurance coverage, inability to take time off from work and home responsibilities, and lack of access to transportation may delay diagnosis and treatment, so by the time poor people see a doctor, their disease conditions tend to be at an advanced stage that is harder to treat. People from marginalized populations may receive inadequate explanations of their health conditions due to language barriers, and often cannot afford referrals for second medical opinions or specialized care.

Each year the World Health Organization publishes updated population and health statistics by country and region and uses those indicators to highlight a particular global health concern.[8] The 1995 World Health Report focused on poverty and health inequalities. The authors noted that advances in modern medicine have created some of the longest-living and healthiest populations in history, yet the benefits of these discoveries are not available globally:

> Beneath the heartening facts about decreased mortality and increasing life expectancy, and many other undoubted health

advances, lie unacceptable disparities in health. The gaps between rich and poor, between one population group and another, between ages and between sexes, are widening. For most people in the world today every step of life, from infancy to old age, is taken under the twin shadows of poverty and inequity, and under the double burden of suffering and disease.[9]

Consider the disparities in the deaths of children during their first five years of life, what health workers call "under-5 mortality." In high-income countries, 6 of every 1000 children die before their 5th birthday, while in developing countries about 88 of every 1000 children die before reaching this age. In the poorest countries, 120 of every 1000 under-5 children die.[10] The gap in child death rates between income groups has been increasing. Between 1970 and 2000, under-5 mortality rates decreased by 71% in high income countries but by only 40% in low-income countries.[11] Figure 2-1 is a world map of life expectancy at birth and Figure 2-2 is a bar graph of life expectancy at birth in each of the six regions of the World Health Organization. (The countries in each region are listed in Appendix I.) The average baby born in the African region can expect to live less than 50 years (and has a high risk of dying in infancy or childhood), while the average baby born in the European, American, or Western Pacific regions can expect to live more than 70 years.

If we look at individual countries, life expectancies are even more disparate. Babies born in 2005 had a life expectancy of less than 40 years in several countries, all in Africa—Swaziland (35 years), Botswana (36), Zimbabwe (37), Lesotho (38), Sierra Leone (38), and Zambia (39).[12] They face a high risk of death during infancy and childhood, and those who survive to adulthood face a high risk of contracting HIV infection and dying prematurely from AIDS. In contrast, babies born in 2005 in more than a dozen European nations and Japan have a life expectancy of 80 years or more.

Survival rates are low in developing countries in part because of limited access to life-saving and life-extending drugs and therapies. Figure 2-3 shows that although North America (the United States and Canada), Europe, and Japan represent only about 18% of the world's population, these regions account for nearly 88% of drug sales. Although Asia, Africa, the Middle East, and Oceania make up nearly 73% of the world's population, only about 8% of drug sales are to these regions.

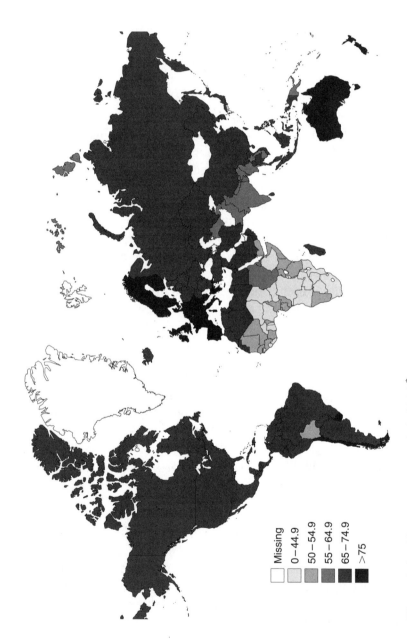

Figure 2-1. Life Expectancy at Birth, 2004.*

Data Source: World Bank, World Development Indicators Database, 2006.

*Map projections may not reflect true differences in land areas between countries.

Missing
0 – 44.9
50 – 54.9
55 – 64.9
65 – 74.9
>75

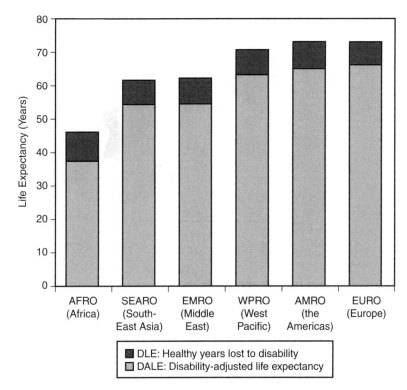

Figure 2-2. Life Expectancy and Healthy Life Expectancy in Each WHO Region, 1999.

The total height of each bar represents total life expectancy at birth. The lighter portion of the bar represents the number of years the average person in the region is expected to live a healthy life and the darker portion of the bar represents years the average person is expected to live with disability.

Data Source: Mathers CD, Sadana R, Salomon JA, Murray CJL, Lopez AD. Estimates of DALE for 191 countries: methods and results. WHO Health Systems Performance Report, Global Programme on Evidence for Health Policy Working Paper No. 16. Geneva: World Health Organization, June 2000.

CAUSES OF DEATH

Pathogenesis is the study of the process of disease. Many different processes can lead to disease, including infectious agents, injuries, malnutrition, and genetics. These exposures are called etiologic agents, or causal agents, and **etiology** is study of the origin of disease. Some diseases

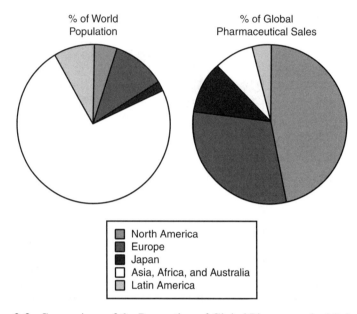

Figure 2-3. Comparison of the Proportion of Global Pharmaceutical Sales by Region to the Proportion of the World Population that Lives in Each Region.

Data Sources: Population Reference Bureau, "Population, Mid-2006." IMS Health, "Global pharmaceutical sales by region, 2005."

are classified as **idiopathic**, which means that we do not (at least not yet) know what causes them. The etiology of many neurological conditions like Parkinson's Disease and epilepsy are unknown in most cases, as are the causes of many mental illnesses, autoimmune diseases, and other conditions.

The World Health Organization uses three main classifications for causes of death and disability: (1) injuries, (2) non-communicable conditions, and (3) communicable (infectious) diseases, maternal (pregnancy-related) conditions, perinatal conditions (diseases of newborns), and nutritional deficiencies.

Injuries

An **injury** is physical damage to the body. An injury may be a fracture of a bone, a strain or sprain of a joint, a brain or spinal cord injury, wounds to the skin, or damage to internal organs. Injuries may be unintentional, such as a traffic accident, fall, burn, or drowning, or intentional, whether self-inflicted or suffered during an act of violence or war. Intentional acts are further classified as self-directed violence (self-mutilation or suicide), interpersonal violence against family members, intimate partners, or community members, or collective violence such as war, mob violence, gang violence, or terrorist acts (Table 2-1).[13]

Figure 2-4 shows the proportion of deaths due to various types of injuries. About 68% of injury deaths worldwide in 2005 were from unintentional injuries (road traffic accidents, poisoning, falls, fires, drowning, and other unintentional injuries) and 32% from intentional injuries (self-inflicted injuries, violence, and war).

Poor people are at increased risk of injury because they more often live, work, and go to school in unsafe environments. They use overcrowded and poorly maintained vehicles for transportation, are pedestrians on crowded streets, live in homes that are vulnerable to fire, do not have access to preventive tools, and have less access to treatment and rehabilitative services.[14] Environmental exposures to chemicals, like poisons, alcohol, smoke, and heavy metals, or to physical trauma, radiation, heat, cold, or allergens can also cause illness and injury. In addition to immediate health problems that can be caused by exposure, these exposures may cause

Table 2-1. Examples of Types of Injuries.

Unintentional Injuries	Intentional Injuries
• Road traffic injuries	*Self-directed violence*
• Falls	• Suicide
• Burns	• Cutting
• Drowning	*Interpersonal violence*
• Poisoning	• Spousal / intimate partner abuse
	• Child abuse
	• Elder abuse
	Collective violence
	• War
	• Terrorist acts
	• Gang violence

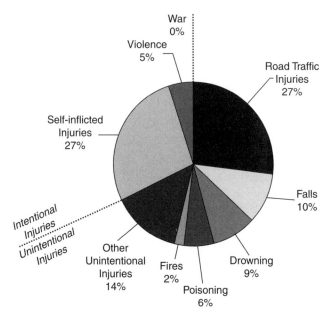

Figure 2-4. Proportion of Various Causes of Death Worldwide due to Injury, 2005 Estimates.

Data Source: WHO, Global Burden of Disease database, 2006 update.

long-term disability and lead to the development of other chronic conditions. For example, radiation exposure can cause cancer and repeated alcohol exposure can cause cirrhosis of the liver. Harmful exposures are a common problem in low-income nations where there is limited access to clean water and trash removal, where food must be prepared over an indoor fire, and where enforcement of safety laws is minimal. (Chapters 10 and 11 explain the environmental context of health.)

Males are significantly more likely than females to die from all types of injuries other than burns and self-inflicted injuries (Figure 2-5). Men are at greater risk of injury because they are more likely than women to work in hazardous occupations, to participate in dangerous recreational activities, to spend time on the road, to use alcohol, and to be involved armed conflict. Because women spend more time cooking, they are more likely to fall into fires or scald themselves by dropping a pot of boiling liquid. Females are also more likely than males to be abused by intimate partners and family members, and the rate of injuries due to physical and sexual violence is probably under-reported.

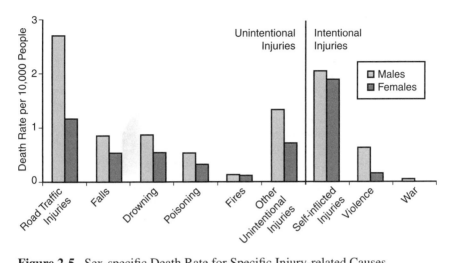

Figure 2-5. Sex-specific Death Rate for Specific Injury-related Causes Worldwide, 2005 Estimates.

Data Source: WHO, Global Burden of Disease database, 2006 update.

Most people who are injured survive their injuries, but many are left with permanent disabilities. Although some injuries are the result of accidents, many injuries could have been prevented by the use of safety belts in motor vehicles, child car seats, helmets, designated drivers who have not consumed alcohol, flame-resistant clothing, smoke detectors, fencing around water bodies, swimming lessons, protective eyewear, use of safety harnesses when working at dangerous heights, and locked storage of weapons and ammunition.[15]

Non-communicable Conditions

Non-communicable conditions are diseases that are not contagious (Table 2-2), such as cancers (sometimes called "neoplasms" in health reports), endocrine disorders, neurological and psychiatric disorders, heart disease and other cardiovascular disorders, chronic respiratory diseases, digestive diseases, kidney diseases, and musculoskeletal and skin diseases. Non-communicable conditions may be caused by genetic disorders or congenital abnormalities or may be related to aging processes or autoimmune disorders. The causes of many non-communicable diseases are not yet

Table 2-2. Examples of Non-communicable Conditions.

Cancers (Neoplasms)	• Lung cancer • Stomach cancer • Colorectal cancer • Liver cancer • Breast cancer • Esophageal cancer	• Lymphoma • Mouth and throat cancer • Prostate cancer • Leukemia • Cervical cancer • Pancreatic cancer • Bladder cancer	• Ovarian cancer • Uterine cancer • Melanoma and other skin cancers
Endocrine and nutritional / metabolic disorders	• Diabetes mellitus	• Thyroid disease • Disorders of the pituitary gland	• Adrenal disorders (Addison Disease, Cushing's Syndrome)
Neuropsychiatric disorders	• Alzheimer's and other dementias • Epilepsy • Parkinson's disease • Multiple sclerosis • Migraine • Cerebral palsy • Schizophrenia	• Depressive disorder • Bipolar disorder • Panic disorder • Obsessive-compulsive disorder • Huntington Disease • Alcoholism	• Drug addiction • Eating disorders • Insomnia • Post-traumatic stress disorder • Tourette Syndrome • Autism
Sense organ disorders	• Blindness • Cataracts	• Glaucoma • Pterygium	• Deafness

clear. Non-communicable conditions are sometimes called chronic diseases because many of them develop gradually and then last for a long time.

Some non-communicable conditions are caused by immune system dysfunctions. The immune system helps the body to fight disease by recognizing and attacking invaders like infectious agents and allergens. Autoimmune disorders occur when the body has trouble distinguishing between "self" and "non-self" and begins to attack its own cells. Lupus (systemic lupus erythematosus) and rheumatoid arthritis are autoimmune diseases. Allergies are another type of immune dysfunction in which the body is hypersensitive to substances that are usually not harmful. Another "internal" disease process is inflammation. Although the process is not yet well understood, it appears that inflammation plays a role not just in arthritis and other conditions in

Table 2-2. Examples of Non-Communicable Conditions—cont'd.

Cardiovascular diseases and blood disorders	• Ischemic heart disease (heart attacks) • Cerebrovascular disease (strokes) • Hypertension	• Inflammatory heart disease • Congestive heart failure • Hemophilia • Anemia	• Hemochromatosis • Sickle cell • Thalassemia
Respiratory diseases	• Chronic obstructive pulmonary disease (COPD)—emphysema, chronic bronchitis, and chronic asthma		• Asthma • Cystic fibrosis
Digestive diseases	• Appendicitis • Liver cirrhosis • Gallstones	• Hernias • Peptic ulcer disease	• Hemorrhoids • Inflammatory Bowel Disease
Oral diseases	• Dental caries (cavities)	• Periodontal disease	• Edentulism (toothlessness)
Genitourinary diseases	• Nephritis (kidney disease)	• Benign prostatic hypertrophy (BPH—enlarged prostate)	• Pelvic inflammatory disease (PID)
Skin diseases	• Albinism • Acne	• Eczema	• Psoriasis
Musculoskeletal diseases	• Muscular dystrophy • Osteoarthritis	• Rheumatoid arthritis	• Osteoporosis

which swelling is easily observed, but also in heart disease and possibly in diabetes, cognitive disorders, and many other conditions. Poor nutrition and some infections (like HIV) can also cause immune system suppression and lead to other illnesses.

Genetic make-up also plays a key role in health.[16] Many genetic disorders are present at birth, and some of the symptoms caused by these genetic disorders can be avoided through early testing and lifestyle adjustments. A person with cystic fibrosis can receive percussion therapy, which involves "drumming" the chest to help clear out mucus. A boy known to have hemophilia can be treated with injections of blood clotting factors. Blood tests at birth can identify metabolic disorders, so that potentially harmful foods can be avoided. For example, infants can be tested for phenylketonuria

(PKU), a metabolic disorder in which infants and children with a particular version of a gene found on the 12th chromosome do not make an enzyme that is needed to metabolize phenylalanine, an amino acid that is found in some proteins. A blood test done just after the baby is born can let parents know if their child has PKU, so they can help the child avoid phenylalanine and develop normally. If parents do not know that their child has the genetic disorder and feed their children foods that contain phenylalanine, the children can develop mental retardation. A simple blood test for PKU is mandated for newborns in many high-income countries, but is not available in most low-income countries.

Other conditions are caused by genetic **mutations** (permanent changes in the sequence of bases that make up DNA) that occur after birth. These mutations may result from exposure to radiation, chemicals, pollutants, or other substances. Cancers generally involve a series of mutations that can lead to tumor development. A chemical that can cause a mutation and lead to cancer is called a **carcinogen**, and the process of cancer development is **carcinogenesis**.

Birth defects, developmental disabilities, and other disabilities are common in both high- and low-income areas, but the challenges for disabled individuals and their families are greater in resource-poor settings. Furthermore, as the global population ages, the burden of non-communicable diseases such as heart disease, stroke, vision and hearing loss, and cancer will increase. When a person in a developing country develops a non-communicable disease like cancer, it is often diagnosed at an advanced stage and the treatment options that are available are limited. As a result, the survival rate following diagnosis is significantly lower in developing countries than in developed countries. (These inequalities are discussed in more detail later in the chapter.)

Infectious Diseases and Other Conditions

The third WHO category for causes of death is a broad one, and includes infectious diseases, pregnancy-related conditions, diseases of newborns, and nutritional deficiencies.

Communicable diseases are caused by infectious agents such as bacteria, viruses, fungi, and helminths (worms), and can be passed from an infected person to a susceptible person. Deaths from infectious diseases like tuberculosis, sexually transmitted infections, diarrheal diseases, meningitis, malaria, and respiratory infections are all in this category. In the early and middle part of the twentieth century, the use of microscopes and the development of new laboratory techniques led to the identification of many specific microbes and the development of vaccines and antibiotics like penicillin. These discoveries generated a great deal of optimism and confidence in our ability as humans to control and eradicate communicable diseases, leading the U.S. Surgeon General to declare in 1967 that "the war against infectious diseases has been won!" Unfortunately, this declaration was premature. Although modern science has given us a good understanding of the infectious disease process and allowed us to develop therapies and cures for many types of infection, we now know that microbes continue to adapt, to develop, and to emerge. Even with improved prevention and therapeutic techniques, infectious diseases continue to be a health risk in all populations. Developing new vaccines, treatments, and prevention methods remains an important part of global health. (Infectious diseases are discussed in detail in Chapters 6, 7, and 8.)

Maternal deaths are those related to pregnancy, childbirth, and the hours after giving birth. Perinatal conditions include low birthweight, premature (early) birth, birth asphyxia, and birth trauma. (Maternal health and infant health are discussed in Chapter 4.)

Malnutrition may result when a person does not consume nutrients in the right quantities and combination. Taking in too few, or too many, calories or nutrients can be a cause of poor health. Common nutritional deficiencies include protein-energy malnutrition and diseases related to particular vitamins and minerals such as iron, vitamin A, zinc, and iodine. Undernutrition, deficiencies in energy or nutrients, contributes to more than half of child deaths worldwide each year.[17] (Nutrition is discussed in more detail in Chapter 9.)

INEQUALITIES IN CAUSES OF DEATH

Figure 2-6 shows the breakdown of deaths by cause in each of the WHO regions. The proportion of deaths due to injuries is roughly equal across groups, but less developed regions like Africa have a very high proportion of deaths due to infectious disease and undernutrition while the large majority of deaths in Europe are due to non-communicable conditions like heart disease and cancers. Everyone will eventually die of something, but because infectious diseases are usually associated with premature death and noncommunicable

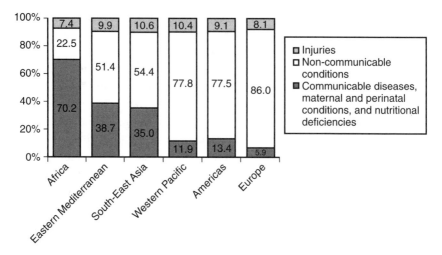

Figure 2-6. Percent of Deaths due to Injury, Non-communicable Disease, and Communicable Disease by WHO Region (2005 Estimates).

Data Source: WHO, Global Burden of Disease database, 2006 update.

conditions are associated with aging, a region with a large proportion of non-communicable deaths is generally considered to be healthier than a region with a majority of deaths from infectious diseases. There are also proven ways to prevent and cure many infectious diseases, so a large portion of infectious disease deaths could have been averted. (Immunization and the boiling of contaminated water are specific and immediate methods of preventing some infectious diseases. Some cases of cancer and other chronic conditions can be prevented, too, by avoiding tobacco products, eating a healthier diet, and exercising, but these are inexact and long-term methods of staying healthy.)

Figure 2-6 makes it look like less developed regions of the world (Africa, the Middle East, and South-East Asia) bear the burden of infectious disease, while industrialized regions (Europe, the Americas, and the western Pacific) bear the burden of non-communicable conditions. This is a bit misleading, because most of the world's population lives in less developed countries.

Figure 2-7 presents the same data as Figure 2-6, but shows the *number* of deaths by region and cause rather than the *percent* of deaths. A comparison of these graphs shows, for example, that although the percent of deaths from non-communicable diseases is lower in South-East Asia (54.4%) than

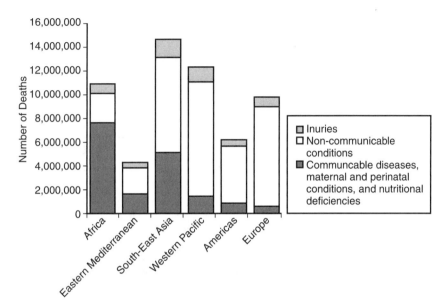

Figure 2-7. Number of Deaths due to Injury, Non-communicable Disease, and Communicable Disease by WHO Region.

Data Source: WHO, Global Burden of Disease database, 2006 update.

in the Americas (77.5%) many more people who live in South-East Asia (7.9 million) die from non-communicable diseases each year than people who live in the Americas (4.8 million). In fact, nearly 80% of the deaths from chronic disease[18] worldwide each year are in low- and middle-income countries, including more than 50% of cancers.[19] Cardiovascular (heart) disease, a non-communicable condition, is already the leading cause of death in developing countries.[20]

The difference between the incidence rates of various types of cancer (the percent of people in a population who are diagnosed with cancer in one year) and the number of deaths from these cancers in low-income and high-income regions is particularly striking. The percentage of people who live in high-income countries who develop cancer is higher than the percentage of people who live in low- and middle-income countries who develop cancer (Figure 2-8), partly because cancer is more common in older adults and more people in high-income countries reach older ages. But the number of cancer deaths in low- and middle-income countries is higher than the number

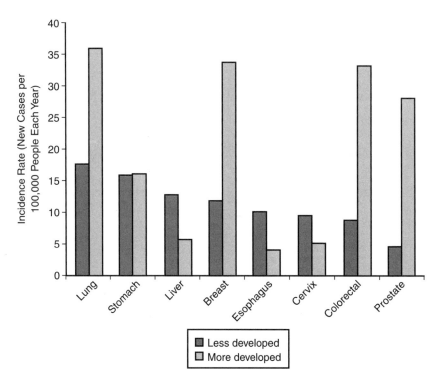

Figure 2-8. Cancer Incidence Rates (Number of New People in a Year Who Are Diagnosed with the Disease per 100,000 People in the Population) in 2002 in Less Developed and More Developed Countries.

For most types of cancer, the incidence rate is higher in more developed countries.

Data Source: Kamangar F, Dores GM, Anderson WF. Patterns of cancer incidence, mortality, and prevalence across five continents: defining priorities to reduce cancer disparities in different geographic regions of the world. *J Clin Oncol* 2006;24:2137–2150.

of deaths in high-income countries (Figure 2-9). This means, for example, that although a person who lives in a more developed country is more likely to be diagnosed with lung cancer or breast cancer than a person who lives in a less developed country (Figure 2-8), the total number of deaths each from these cancers is very similar in less developed and more developed regions (Figure 2-9).[21]

If cancer patients in low-income countries had access to the same screening and diagnostic tests (which allow for detection of cancer at an earlier,

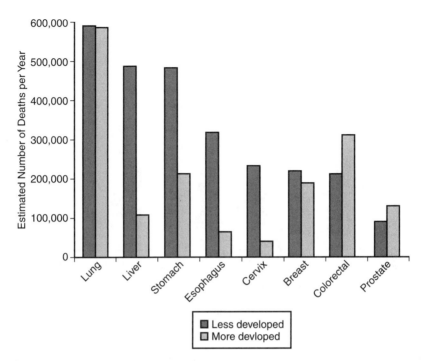

Figure 2-9. Estimated Average Number of Cancer Deaths in 2002 in Less Developed and More Developed Countries.

For most types of cancer, more deaths each year occur in less developed countries than in more developed countries.

Data Source: Kamangar F, Dores GM, Anderson WF. Patterns of cancer incidence, mortality, and prevalence across five continents: defining priorities to reduce cancer disparities in different geographic regions of the world. *J Clin Oncol* 2006;24:2137–2150.

more treatable stage) and advanced therapies (like chemotherapeutic drugs, surgical techniques, and radiology regimens) as cancer patients in high-income nations, many more people with cancer would survive. At present, the survival rate for people diagnosed with cancer in developing countries is much lower than the survival rate in industrialized nations (Figure 2-10).

Life expectancy will increase when more people gain access to technologies that allow for early diagnosis and effective treatment. One of the goals of global health is to increase healthy life expectancy, so it is important to make technology more widely available in all countries.

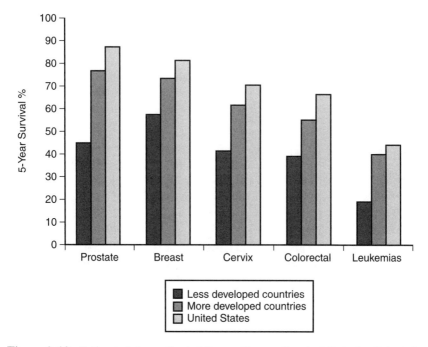

Figure 2-10. Estimated Age-adjusted 5-year Cancer Survival Rate for Selected Cancers.

Data Source: Parkin DM, Bray F, Ferlay J, & Pisani P. Global cancer statistics, 2002. *CA Cancer J Clin* 2005;55:74-108.

Global cancer statistics are compiled by IARC, the International Agency for Research on Cancer. Cancer statistics from the United States are compiled by the SEER (Surveillance, Epidemiology, and End Results) registry sponsored by the National Cancer Institute of the National Institutes of Health.

REFERENCES

1. From an address given to the African Summit on HIV/AIDS, Tuberculosis, and Other Infectious Diseases in Abuja, Nigeria, 2001. In this speech Secretary-General Annan proposed the creation of the Global Fund to Fight AIDS, TB, and Malaria.
2. Address to the 2005 World Health Assembly on May 16, 2005.
3. American Heart Association. "Heart Disease and Stroke Statistics—2005 Update."
4. Goldman N, Koernman S, Weinstein R. Marital status and health among the elderly. *Soc Sci Med.* 1995;40:1717–1730.
5. Murphy M, Glaser K, Grundy E. Marital status and long-term illness in Great Britain. *J Marriage Fam* 1997;59:156–164.
6. World Health Organization. World Health Report 2005.

7. Gwatkin DR. Health inequalities and the health of the poor: What do we know? What can we do? *Bull World Health Organ.* 2000;78:3–18.
8. The United Nations agencies are some of the few organizations that collect global data, so United Nations statistics will be used extensively throughout the book.
9. World Health Organization. World Health Report 1995.
10. Victora CG, Wagstaff A, Armstrong Schellenberg J, Gwatkin D, Claeson M, Habicht JP. Applying an equity lens to child health and mortality: more of the same is not enough. *Lancet.* 2003;362:233–241.
11. Ibid.
12. World Health Organization. World Health Report 2005.
13. Krug EG, Dahlberg LL, Mercy JA, Zwi AB, Lozano R, eds. *World report on violence and health.* Geneva: World Health Organization, 2002.
14. World Health Organization. "How can injuries be prevented?" Online Q&A, 28 March 2006.
15. World Health Organization. "Facts about Injuries: Preventing Global Injuries." 2001.
16. Supplemental information on genetics and genetic disorders:
Genes are sequences of nucleic acids that are part of the chromosomes that are found in the nucleus of every cell in our bodies. This genetic material directs every function of the body, including cell replication, which is important for healing as well as for growth and development. Each cell contains identical DNA (deoxyribonucleic acid), although only parts of the code are active in certain cells, which is why cells in your heart form different kinds of tissue than the cells that line your intestine. Your genotype is the version of a gene you carry and your phenotype is the way a characteristic that results from having a particular allele, or version of a gene, is expressed. Phenotype can refer to physical appearance, the way a person develops or functions physiologically, or disease status.

   Some alleles are dominant, which means that inheriting a copy of that allele from either parent will cause you to display the phenotype associated with that allele. Huntington Disease, which causes a progressive degeneration of brain cells, is the result of inheriting a copy of a defective gene found on chromosome 4 from one parent. Some alleles are recessive, which means that a person must inherit a copy of the allele from both parents to display the phenotype associated with the allele. Cystic fibrosis is a recessive disorder carried on the 7th chromosome that causes excessive mucus production in the lungs and digestive tract. Sickle cell and thalassemia are genetic blood disorders that may confer some protection against malaria but can cause death if not treated. A person who inherits the sickle cell allele from both parents develops sickle cell anemia because the red blood cells, which carry oxygen to all the cells in the body, become misshapen and impede blood flow. A person in sickle cell crisis experiences extreme pain and possible organ damage due to oxygen deprivation.

   Some conditions are caused by the presence of an extra chromosome or a missing part of a chromosome. Down Syndrome (trisomy 21) is the result of an extra 21st chromosome. Most humans have 23 pairs of chromosomes: 22 pairs of autosomal chromosomes and one pair of sex chromosomes, usually XX for females and XY for males. Sometimes there are extra copies of an X or Y chromosome or a missing X. Males may have an extra X (Klinefelter Syndrome) and develop female characteristics or have an extra Y (Jacob Syndrome), which may cause speech and reading problems. Females may have an extra X (Poly-X Syndrome) or a missing X (Turner Syndrome) and have developmental delays.

Some sex-linked genetic disorders are carried by healthy women who can pass the trait on to their sons. Hemophilia, a blood clotting disorder, and Duchenne muscular dystrophy, which causes progressive muscle weakness, are examples of X-linked recessive disorders. Some genetic disorders are caused by deletions, duplications, translocations, or inversions of parts of chromosomes. Cri du Chat Syndrome is the result of missing a portion of the 5th chromosome and causes a malformed larynx and mental retardation.

17. Pelletier DL, Frongillo EA Jr, Schroeder DG, Habicht JP. The effects of malnutrition on child mortality in developing countries. *Bull World Health Organ.* 1995;73:443–448.
18. Strong K, Mathers C, Leeder S, Beaglehole R. Chronic diseases 1: Preventing chronic diseases: how many lives can we save? *Lancet.* 2005;366:1578–1582.
19. Parkin DM, Pisani P, & Ferlay J. Global cancers statistics. *CA Cancer J Clin.* 1999;49:33–64.
20. The World Health Report 2003 focused on emerging health concerns like chronic diseases. Yach D, Hawkes C, Gould CL, Hofman KJ. The global burden of chronic diseases: overcoming impediments to prevention and control. *JAMA.* 2004;291:2616–2622.
21. Kamangar F, Dores GM, Anderson WF. Patterns of cancer incidence, mortality, and prevalence across five continents: defining priorities to reduce cancer disparities in different geographic regions of the world. *J of Clin Oncol.* 2006;24:2137–2150.

CHAPTER 3

Socioeconomic Context
of Disease

Key Points:
- Socioeconomic status (SES) is a strong predictor of health status.
- Poor households have limited resources for preventing and treating illnesses and injuries.
- Manual workers have greater all-cause mortality than skilled workers and professionals.
- Literacy allows individuals to acquire health information and navigate health systems. Mothers who can read generally have fewer children and healthier children than mothers who are not functionally literate.

Thabo Mbeki, who became the president of South Africa in 1999, has raised questions about the link between HIV and AIDS in Africa in numerous venues over many years.[1] One of Mbeki's first public critiques of HIV and AIDS was an open letter to world leaders that was released on April 3, 2000, in which he wrote that "It is obvious that whatever lessons we have to and may draw from the West about the grave issue of HIV-AIDS, a simple superimposition of Western experience on African reality would be absurd and illogical."[2] He noted key differences between AIDS in Africa and AIDS in Western countries—the primary mode of sexual transmission (heterosexual versus homosexual), the prevalence of the disease (millions of deaths versus relatively few deaths), and the population trends (more cases versus declining cases)—and asked what might account for the difference. His conclusion was that poverty was the main cause of health problems in South Africa.

In response, more than 5000 scientists and physicians signed the "Durban Declaration," released just prior to the 2000 International AIDS Conference that was held in South Africa, which stated that the evidence that AIDS is caused by HIV is "clear-cut, exhaustive, and unambiguous."[3] The Declaration further stated that "As with any other chronic infection, various

39

co-factors play a role in determining the risk of disease. Persons who are malnourished, who already suffer from other infections, or who are older, tend
to be more susceptible to the rapid development of AIDS following HIV infection. However, none of these factors weaken the scientific evidence that
HIV is the sole cause of AIDS."

Although the amount of scientific evidence supporting HIV as the cause
of AIDS is overwhelming, Mbeki's point that AIDS is also related to
poverty and development is valid, and has been recognized by doctors and
researchers working with AIDS since the start of the epidemic in Africa.
There is a clear relationship between health and many aspects of development, such as access to adequate nutrition, clean drinking water, and necessary drugs. Consider this observation by Kofi Annan, former Secretary-
General of the United Nations:

> The incidence of HIV/AIDS, tuberculosis and other infectious
> diseases is higher on this continent [Africa] than on any other.
> Of course, this fact is connected to Africa's other problems.
> Africans are vulnerable to these diseases because they are poor,
> undernourished, and too often uninformed of basic precautions,
> or unwilling to take them. Many are vulnerable because they have
> neither safe drinking water nor access to basic health care. They
> are vulnerable, in short, because their countries are underdevel-
> oped. And, therefore, the best cure for all these diseases is eco-
> nomic growth and broad-based development.[4]

SOCIOECONOMIC RISK FACTORS

Socioeconomic Status (SES) indicates a person's (or family's) position
in a society based on social, economic, and educational characteristics.
There is no one measure of SES, but proxies such as ownership of various
assets (like a house, car, bicycle, television, radio, or livestock), occupation,
amount and type of education, residential area, and other social and economic
characteristics can be used to estimate a person's relative position in a
community or larger population group. Health is inextricably linked with
socioeconomic status, and measures of national development consider both
economic data and health data as important markers of development. For
example, the **Human Development Index (HDI)** is an estimate of national development based on composite data on longevity (life expectancy

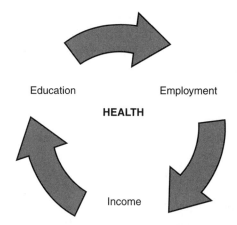

Figure 3-1. Income, Education, Employment, and Health.

at birth), knowledge (adult literacy rate and mean years of schooling), and income (real GDP per capita in purchasing power parity dollars). The remainder of this chapter highlights three components that contribute to the socioeconomic status of an individual or household—economic status, occupational status, and educational status—which are inextricably linked to each other and to health status. Figure 3-1 illustrates the interrelationship of these three components.

POVERTY

Poverty creates conditions where diseases are more likely to occur and less likely to be treated. More than one billion people in the world, about 1 in 6 people, survive on less than $1 per person per day[5], usually by "subsistence farming"—trying to grow enough food on a small plot to feed the household (Figure 3-2). Drought, flood, or other disaster can cause crop failure and push the household into starvation. The 1995 World Health Report opened with a shocking analysis of "the world's biggest killer and the greatest cause of ill-health and suffering across the globe"—extreme poverty. It continued:

> Poverty is the main reason why babies are not vaccinated, why clean water and sanitation are not provided, why curative drugs

and other treatments are unavailable, and why mothers die in childbirth. It is the underlying cause of reduced life expectancy, handicap, disability, and starvation. Poverty is a major contributor to mental illness, stress, suicide, family disintegration, and substance abuse.

The two most common ways of measuring the economic status of a household are income and wealth. **Income** is the amount of take-home pay earned by household members in a given time period. **Wealth** is the accumulated worth of the household and can include a house, car, television or radio, livestock, and other consumer goods. In parts of the world where trade exists mostly in the form of bartering, a household may have very little income to spend on health costs. These households are also likely to have very little wealth, so they have few resources to draw on if someone in the household develops a severe illness.

Poverty impacts the type of dwelling a household lives in (which can be unstable, unventilated, and/or built with harmful materials), how crowded it is (which can facilitate spread of infectious diseases like tuberculosis), and where it is located (such as proximity to schools, transportation, waste facilities, and clean water sources). Many poor communities do not have a source of consistently safe drinking water, properly installed latrines, or enough water to practice good hygiene, so the risk of contracting an infection is

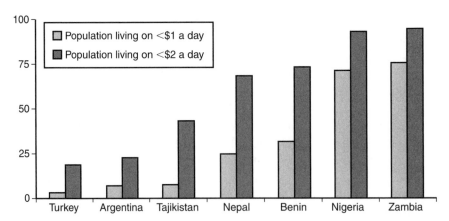

Figure 3-2. Percentage of the Population Living on Less than $2 a Day for Selected Countries, 2003.

Data Source: World Development Report 2007.

greatly increased. In others, dwindling availability of wood for fuel limits the ability of households to boil water and cook food. And without electricity for refrigeration there is no way to store food safely or to keep vaccines viable. In rural areas, the lack of infrastructure for communication (such as telephones and radios) and transportation makes it difficult to access health providers and health education. Furthermore, poor households may be unable to spend money on disease prevention, such as the purchase of insecticide-treated bed-nets for malaria, because they must dedicate all income to immediate survival needs like food, housing, clothing, and emergency medical care.

Low-resource households must make health care decisions very carefully and consider all the costs of health care, including transportation to a health care facility, food for the sick person and caregivers (since many hospitals do not provide food for inpatients), fees for seeing clinicians, the price of medications and supplies like bandages, and lost wages for the patient and caregiver. When people from poor households do decide to seek medical attention they may receive sub-standard care because they have to seek care at an under-funded, under-stocked, and under-staffed clinic. Hospitals that serve the poor rarely have highly-trained specialists on staff and may not have the support staff and technology to offer advanced care.

A difference in health is seen both when we compare countries and when we compare population groups within one country. No matter where you live, there is probably a significant and visible difference in the health of the poorest residents and the richest residents. Wealthier people generally have better access to advanced health care when they are sick. They can afford the best diagnostic tests and the best therapies, and they have the resources to seek care for relatively mild conditions (that, if untreated, could develop into severe problems). And because wealthier people have better access to good nutrition, work jobs that are less dangerous, and have probably had previous injuries and infections treated, they are usually in better overall health than poorer people. Figure 3-3 shows that babies born to relatively rich families have a much higher chance of survival than babies born to relatively poor families.

ECONOMIC INDICATORS

Health economists seek to understand the relationships between health spending, health resources, and health outcomes for individuals, families, companies, and states and nations. Macroeconomic indicators measure the

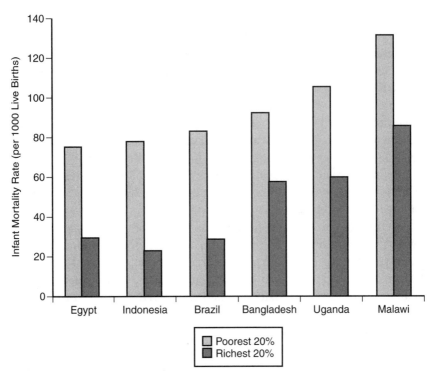

Figure 3-3. Comparison of Infant Mortality Rate (per 1000 Live Births) Between the Poorest 20% and Richest 20% of the Population in Several Countries.

Richer babies have a significantly greater chance of survival than poorer babies.

Data Source: Human Development Report 2005.

amount of economic activity in a country. The GDP and GNP are two of the most common measures. To make the distinction between these two measures clear, consider the way the GDP and GNP of Canada would be calculated. The **gross domestic product (GDP)** is the total amount of goods and services produced in Canada by both Canadian corporations and foreign corporations. It includes consumer spending, investment, government spending, and exports. The **gross national income (GNI)** is similar to the GDP, but puts the focus on the total income from the selling of goods and services produced in the country. The **gross national product (GNP)** is the total amount of goods and services produced by Canadian companies in Canada and by Canadian corporations working in other countries.

Because the amount of goods and services that can be purchased with a given amount of money varies from place to place, these values are often recorded in terms of **purchasing power parity (PPP)**, which measures how much "stuff" (goods, services, and other products) can be purchased in each country with a fixed amount of money (say, USD $1000). A popular example of PPP is the "Big Mac Index" that determines the relative price of a McDonald's burger in two different countries and uses that exchange rate to determine the relative value of other items. If a Big Mac costs $2 in one country and $3.50 in another, it is likely that the costs of living are much higher in the $3.50-per-hamburger country and workers in the higher-priced country will have to earn a much higher salary to stay above the poverty line than workers in the $2-per-burger country.

GDP, GNI, and GNP can also be recorded in "per capita" (per person) terms by dividing the total gross product by the population of the country. The GNI per capita of a country is about equal to the average income of an individual. Although these numbers are only a rough guide to the average economic picture in a country, they do allow for comparisons between countries. Figure 3-4 shows where the richest and poorest countries are located.

The economic status of a country can be used to estimate average health status of its residents just as the economic status of a household is an indicator of the likely health status of its members.[6] High income countries generally have high life expectancies and low income countries generally have low life expectancies (Figure 3-5).

Summary values like the GDP and GNP have some major limitations if they are being used to estimate health and development. They don't count unpaid labor like work caring for children and growing food to feed a family. They ignore issues of sustainability, environmental damage, and the distribution of wealth and quality of life (standard of living) in a country. These values show the economic experience of the "average" person living in each country, but the "average" economic measure may be misleading if most people in a given country are very poor and some are extremely rich and there is almost no middle class. Even when a large proportion of the population experiences something near the average reported for the country, there will still be variability in the experiences of individuals. There are millionaires in every country, even the countries with the poorest "average" person. And there are people in every country, even the wealthiest ones, who live on almost nothing.

The **Gini Index** is a measure of the inequality in the distribution of incomes within a particular country. A country in which everyone has exactly

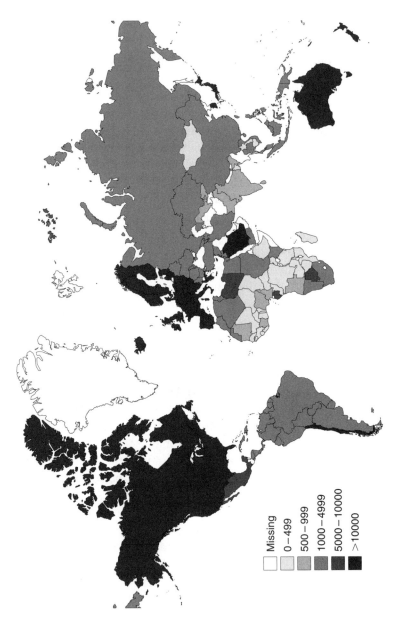

Figure 3-4. Gross National Income (GNI) per Capita, 2005.

Data Source: World Bank, World Development Indicators Database.

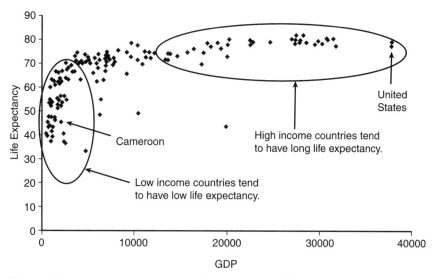

Figure 3-5. Gross Domestic Product (GDP) and Life Expectancy.

Each point represents the data for one United Nations member state. For example, the point for the United States shows a GDP (in 2003) of $37,738 and a life expectancy at birth of 77.3 years while Cameroon, a country in west Africa, shows a GDP of $2,118 and a life expectancy of 45.8 years.

Data Source: Human Development Report 2005.

the same income has an index of 0 (perfect equality) and a country in which one person has all the income and everyone else has zero income has an index of 100 (perfect inequality). For example, Namibia has a Gini Index of 70.7 and a very unequal distribution of income. The richest 10% of the population makes 128.8 times more than the poorest 10%.[7] In contrast, Denmark has a Gini Index of 24.7 and a very equal income distribution. The richest 10% make only 8.1 times more than the poorest 10%. The United States has a Gini Index of 40.8. In general, European countries have the greatest income equality and countries in Africa and the Americas have the greatest income inequalities. Several research groups are studying the relationship between income inequalities and health inequalities and suspect that populations with greater income inequalities will also tend to have worse health outcomes.[8]

EMPLOYMENT AND OCCUPATIONAL STATUS

Employment of at least one wage-earner is generally critical for keeping a household out of poverty. In addition to income, employment often provides benefits, including health insurance and compensation for on-the-job injuries. In some cases, employers provide housing, food allowances, and schooling for children of employees. However, these benefits are not available to all workers. Low-skilled people work the most dangerous jobs, get little compensation, and have little or no job security. This is true in every country, even in the United States, where, for example, many meat-processing plants employ foreign workers who do not hold work visas to do the most hazardous tasks.

In most countries there are significant differences in health based on occupational status. Unemployed people have worse health than employed people, and for employed people the type of job is strongly related to health outcomes. Manual workers have a higher probability of dying from job-related illnesses and injuries, but also have a higher all-cause mortality rate, even for diseases not related to the work environment.[9] For example, Figure 3-6 shows the relative risk of death for men in five different job classes in the United Kingdom over time. Unskilled workers consistently have the highest death rate, professional workers the lowest death rate, and skilled workers an intermediate rate. The graph shows that these inequalities appear to be increasing over time.

Given the increased risk of all-cause mortality, it is no surprise that low-skilled workers have an increased risk of death and illness from many specific causes. Compared to professional workers (like engineers and teachers), unskilled workers (like security guards and janitors) have a significantly higher risk of death from coronary heart disease, stroke, lung cancer, respiratory disease, and suicide.[10] The lower job classes in Europe also report higher rates of chronic illness, obesity, high blood pressure, and mental health disorders.

In less formal class systems, like the British system shown in Figure 3-6, it is possible, though often difficult, to move to a higher social class through education. In more formal class systems, it can be nearly impossible for an individual to improve his or her occupational status. For example, Hindus in India are born into a caste that, at least traditionally, determines occupation, social interaction, and power. A Brahmin will be a teacher or religious person, a Kshatriya a soldier, a Vaisya a merchant, trader, or craftsman, and a Sudra a laborer or farmer. Within each of these ranks, called varnas, are hundreds of ranked subcastes. A person born into the Untouchables class is

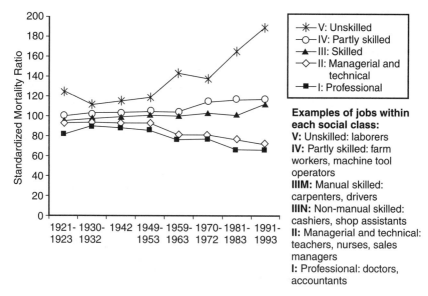

Figure 3-6. The Standardized Mortality Ratio (SMR) for Deaths of Men Aged 20 to 64 in Five Social Classes in England and Wales.

The SMR compares the death rate in one subpopulation (one social class) to the total population death rate (all five social classes). If a subpopulation has an SMR greater than 100, people in that group have an increased risk of death compared to the national rate. If a subpopulation has an SMR less than 100, people in that group have a decreased risk of death compared to the national rate. A greater deviation from SMR = 100 indicates greater health inequalities. This graph shows that health inequalities between social (occupational) classes are growing in the United Kingdom.

Data Source: The Wales NHS Resource Allocation Review: Independent Report of the Research Team (David Gordon, Elizabeth Lloyd, Martyn Senior, Jan Rigby, Mary Shaw, and Yaov Ben Shlomo), June 2001.

typically only allowed to work the least desirable jobs, which include butchery, leather work, and cremation of the dead, that involve contact with blood, excrement, and other impurities. Although discrimination based on caste is illegal, and Untouchability has been legally abolished, Untouchables may be denied access to education, water wells, temples, and other basic rights, especially in rural areas. While a person may be able to change status within his or her caste, no amount of achievement will allow a person to change to a different caste.

LITERACY AND EDUCATIONAL LEVEL

Literacy is usually defined as functional literacy, the ability to understand written words well enough to complete normal daily tasks. Educational level is usually measured in terms of years of education completed and diplomas, certificates, or degrees earned. Both literacy and educational level can have a significant impact on health.

People with higher educational levels generally have higher incomes and, therefore, a less crowded home, access to adequate calories and nutritious food, the ability to seek medical treatment for conditions before they become severe, and a safer work environment. They may also have been raised in a wealthier home with increased nutrition, literate parents who could help with schoolwork, and social connections that increase the likelihood of further educational and occupational success. Increased personal educational level is associated with an increase in reported overall health and life expectancy and a decrease in chronic conditions, long-term disabilities, use of prescribed medications, and hospital admissions.

Literacy allows readers to acquire health information and navigate health systems. Readers can learn about food preparation and exercise programs in newspapers and magazines, comprehend health and safety warnings on medicines and consumer products, access air and water quality reports, read posters advertising immunization and screening campaigns, follow directions on medication bottles and hospital discharge orders, understand health benefits packages offered by employers and the government and apply for benefits, read brochures about their health conditions, use signs to navigate hospitals, and seek out additional information online or at libraries. People who cannot read or write will have difficulty with all of these health-related activities. They may delay seeking a diagnosis or treatment for a health problem because they worry about being unable to complete paperwork at the doctor's office or being ridiculed for not knowing how to read or write. They may have difficulty taking their prescribed medications properly if their doctors have not fully explained dosage and timing and they cannot read the instructions on the label. They may not be able to read the safety information provided by a pharmacist or know when to return for a follow-up examination.

Female literacy has been shown to be particularly important for family health.[11] Maternal literacy and educational level are associated with improved child growth and nutritional status, improved ability of mothers to provide appropriate care for family members (Figure 3-7), and decreased child mortality (Figure 3-8). Maternal education is also associated with increased

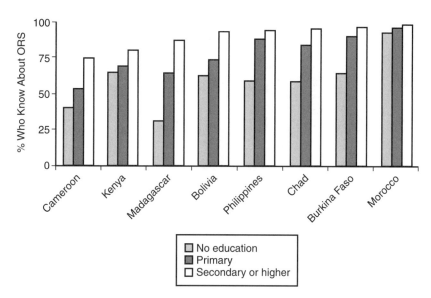

Figure 3-7. Percent of Women Who Know about Using Oral Rehydration Solution (ORS) for Treating Their Children's Diarrhea, by Mother's Educational Level.

Data Source: National Demographic and Health Surveys, 2003–2004.[12]

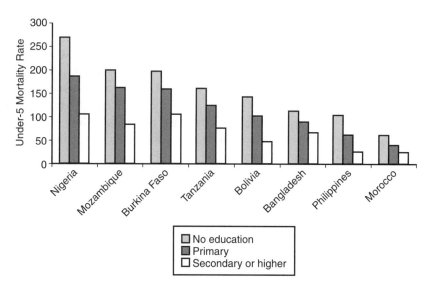

Figure 3-8. Under-5 Child Mortality Rates by Mother's Educational Level in 1993–2003.

Data Source: National Demographic and Health Surveys, 2003–2004.

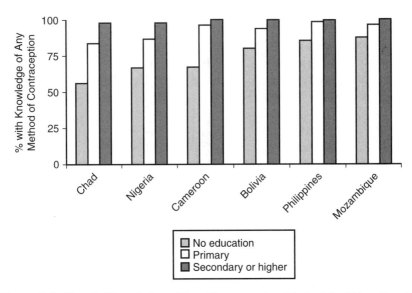

Figure 3-9. Female Knowledge of Any Contraception Method, by Educational Level.

Data Source: National Demographic and Health Surveys, 2003–2004.

contraceptive knowledge (Figure 3-9) and use, and women who give birth to fewer children generally have healthier children.

Furthermore, educated women have better and more frequent interactions with the health care system. Less educated women are more likely to report problems with accessing health care, such as not knowing where to go for treatment, not being able to get permission to go for treatment, not getting money to go for treatment, being too distant from the health facility, having to take transportation, not wanting to go alone, or having a concern that there might not be a female health care provider available (Figure 3-10).

Even though the economic and health benefits of education are well established, in many countries girls are much less likely to be in school than boys (Figure 3-11). Some health intervention programs focus on helping girls to enroll in primary school and complete their basic education, which is usually considered to be about seven years of classroom learning. Other health-related programs focus on female adult literacy and sponsor reading classes for mothers and other adult women.

Because health status is closely related to income, employment, and education—and these three components are always linked (Figure 3-1)—

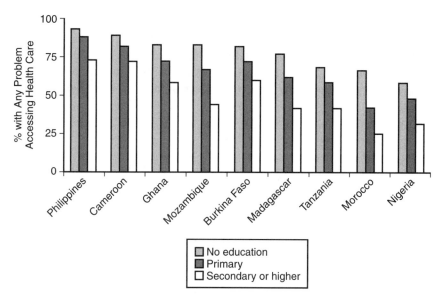

Figure 3-10. Percent of Women Who Have Experienced Any Problem in Accessing Health Care, by Educational Level.

Data Source: National Demographic and Health Surveys, 2003–2004.

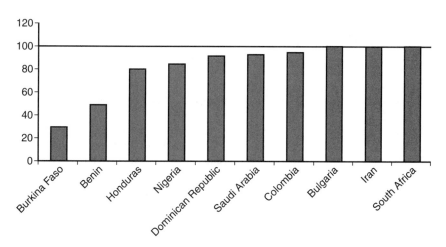

Figure 3-11. Number of Girls Enrolled in Primary and Secondary School for Every 100 Boys Enrolled, 2004.

Data Source: World Development Report 2007.

an intervention that is aimed at increasing income or occupational skills or educational level will impact other aspects of SES. New reading skills may lead to a better job. Increased job skills may lead to a higher hourly wage. Extra income may be used to pay for additional training. And any one of these improvements can lead to increased health.

REFERENCES

1. Mbeki appointed several prominent AIDS deniers (AIDS dissidents), who deny that HIV is the agent that causes AIDS and that the symptoms that are attributed to HIV/AIDS are caused by poverty, to his AIDS Advisory Panel and followed their advice when making policy decisions. For a while he declared that anti-HIV drugs were "too toxic" to be used in South Africa even for prevention of mother-to-child transmission.
2. Gellman B. South African president escalates AIDS feud: Mbeki challenges Western remedies, *Washington Post*, 19 April 2000.
3. The Durban Declaration. *Nature.* 2000;406:15–16.
4. From an address given to the African Summit on HIV/AIDS, Tuberculosis, and Other Infectious Diseases in Abuja, Nigeria, 2001.
5. United Nations Development Programme. 2005 Human Development Report.
6. Bloom DE & Canning D. The health and wealth of nations. *Science.* 2000;207: 1207–1209.
7. All Gini Index statistics are from the 2005 Human Development Report.
8. Wilkinson RG, Pickett KE. Income inequality and population health: a review and explanation of the evidence. *Soc Sci Med.* 2006;62:1768–1784.
9. An example of this is from a study of occupational class and health in European men ages 45 through 65 that found that manual workers in each of the eleven countries studied had a higher probability of dying than non-manual workers. Kunst AE, Groenhof F, Mackenbach JP, EU Working Group on Socioeconomic Inequalities in Health. *BMJ* 1998;316:1636–1642.
10. Independent Inquiry into Inequalities in Health Report. Chairman: Sir Donald Acheson. Prepared 26 November 1998 and published by The Stationery Office as ISBN: 0113221738.
11. King EH, Hill MA. Women's Education in Developing Countries: Barriers, Benefits, and Policies. Baltimore, MD: Johns Hopkins University Press, 1993.
12. DHS surveys are sponsored by USAID, and their results are available through STATcompiler (www.measuredhs.com).

CHAPTER 4

Maternal and Child Health

Key Points:

- The most common causes of death in children under 5 years of age are birth-related conditions, acute respiratory infections (ARIs), diarrhea, malaria, and measles. Undernutrition is a contributing factor in about half of all child deaths.
- Pregnancy is the most common cause of death of women of reproductive age in low-income countries.
- Family planning programs seek to reduce the number of unwanted pregnancies and to improve the health of mothers and babies.
- Demography, the measurement of population health characteristics, is important for understanding the current and future health needs of a population.

Maternal and child health (sometimes shortened to MCH) is one of the major sub-fields of public health. Child health workers pay special attention to "under 5s," children in their first 5 years of life, who are the children most vulnerable to illness and death. Maternal health workers focus on the reproductive health of women by educating women about contraceptives and child spacing, increasing access to prenatal care and to assistance by trained health workers at deliveries, and fostering conditions in which women can make good health decisions for themselves.

CAUSES OF CHILD DEATH

In 2005, more than 10 million children died.[1] Most of these children were in their first five years of life. Figures 4-1 and 4-2 show the global distribution of deaths in children in their first five years of life. Some regions bear a particularly high burden; 42% of children who died lived in the WHO Africa region and 29% in the South-East Asia region.[2]

Most child deaths were due to neonatal conditions (preterm birth, birth asphyxia, and birth-related infections such as tetanus), pneumonia, diarrhea,

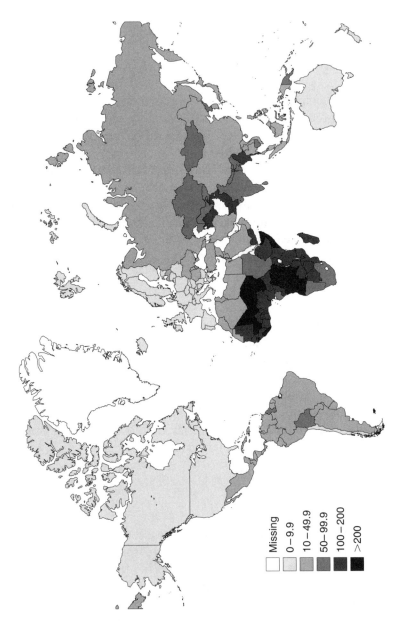

Figure 4-1. Child Mortality During the First Five Years of Life per 1000 Live Births, 2004.

Data Source: World Bank, World Development Indicators Database.

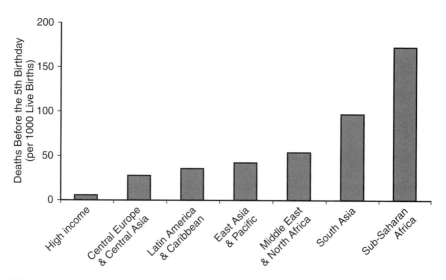

Figure 4-2. Child Mortality During the First Five Years of Life per 1000 Live Births, by Region for 2001.

Data Source: Lopez AD, Mathers CD, Ezzati M, Jamison DT, Murray CJL. Global and regional burden of disease and risk factors, 2001: systematic analysis of population health data. *Lancet,* 27 May 2006;367:1747–1757. Webtable 1: World bank regions, composition, and demographic characteristics, 2001.

malaria, and measles. Table 4-1 shows the percent of deaths by cause in children under five years of age.

It is disgraceful that so many newborn babies die, especially since so many of these deaths could be prevented. The implementation of several proven interventions before birth, during delivery, and in the minutes, hours, and days after birth could significantly improve the likelihood of survival for millions of newborns (Table 4-2).

Babies who survive their first month of life remain vulnerable to a variety of infectious diseases and other conditions. Figure 4-3 shows the distribution of cause of death for under 5s who survived for at least one month after birth. More than 7 in 10 of these deaths occurred as a result of preventable and treatable conditions: pneumonia, diarrhea, malaria, and measles. If malnutrition, which contributes to more than half of all deaths in under 5s, is also considered, then the percent of preventable child deaths is even higher.[3]

Table 4-1. Causes of Mortality in Children under Five Years of Age. Undernutrition is not listed separately but is a contributing factor in more than 50% of deaths of children under 5 years of age.

Cause	Estimated Annual Number of Deaths Worldwide, 2000–2003	Estimated % of Deaths
Neonatal causes (deaths in the first 28 days after birth), includes preterm birth, infection, birth asphyxia, and other conditions	3,910,000	37%
Acute respiratory infections (ARIs), including pneumonia	2,027,000	19%
Diarrheal diseases	1,762,000	17%
Malaria	853,000	8%
Measles	395,000	4%
HIV/AIDS	321,000	3%
Injuries	305,000	3%
All other causes	1,022,000	10%

Data Source: World Health Report 2005.

Pneumonia

Pneumonia, which is an infection of the lungs, and other acute respiratory infections (ARIs) cause about 19% of under-5 child deaths worldwide each year. **Pneumonia** occurs when part of the lung fills with fluid.

The main function of the body's respiratory system is the exchange of gases, which mostly means taking in oxygen and getting rid of carbon dioxide (Figure 4-4). When you take a breath, the air enters your lungs and fills little air sacs called alveoli. Each alveolus is wrapped in tiny blood vessels called capillaries and has a very thin surface so that gas exchange can take place. When you inhale, oxygen is absorbed into the blood in those capillaries. This oxygenated blood is then pumped to the rest of the body so that all of your cells can receive the oxygen they need to function properly. When the cells take in oxygen from nearby capillaries, they can also get rid carbon dioxide and other waste products by dumping them into the blood. Carbon dioxide and other waste products can then be released from the blood into the alveoli. When you exhale, these wastes are expelled from your body.

Table 4-2. Examples of Effective Interventions for Infant Health.

Time	Intervention
Preconception	• Folic acid supplementation to prevent neural tube defects • Birth spacing
Antenatal / prenatal (before birth)	• Tetanus toxoid immunization • Syphilis screening and treatment • Intermittent presumptive treatment for malaria (in endemic areas) • Maternal supplementation with iron, zinc, and iodine • Maternal antihelminthic (de-worming) treatment • Prevention of mother-to-child HIV transmission
Intranatal / intraparturm (during delivery)	• Detection and management of breech births (by Caesarian section, if required) • Antibiotics for preterm premature rupture of membranes • Corticosteroids for preterm labor • Early diagnosis of complications during labor
Postnatal (after birth)	• Resuscitation of newborns • Delayed umbilical cord clamping • Breastfeeding • Kangaroo mother care (keeping low birthweight babies in an upright position on a parent's bare chest so they have skin-to-skin contact and the baby's ear is near the parent's heart) • Prevention and management of hypothermia • Pneumonia case management • Neonatal vitamin A supplementation • Insecticide-treated bednets for malaria prevention

Source: Darmstadt GL, Bhutta ZA, Cousens S, Adam T, Walker N, Bernis L, for the Lancet Neonatal Survival Steering Team. Evidence-based, cost-effective interventions: how many newborn babies can we save? *Lancet*. 2005;365:977–985.

If the alveoli are filled with fluid, they cannot efficiently exchange oxygen and carbon dioxide. People with pneumonia can feel like they are drowning as fluid fills their lungs and they develop hypoxia (lack of oxygen). The symptoms of an acute respiratory illness (ARI) usually include a cough accompanied by difficult or short, rapid breathing. A child with severe infection may turn bluish in color due to hypoxia.

ARIs can be caused by a variety of infectious agents, including bacteria and viruses. Bacterial infections can often be cured by inexpensive oral

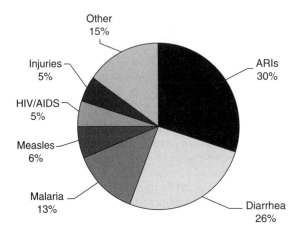

Figure 4-3. Causes of Death in Children Ages 29 Days Through 5 Years Old. *Data Source:* World Health Report 2005.

antibiotics if treatment is sought soon after the onset of symptoms. One component of improving child survival is educating caregivers about the importance of seeking medical care as soon as the symptoms of pneumonia appear so that a course of antibiotics can be started. UNICEF estimates that only about half of the world's children are taken to a health-care provider when they have an acute respiratory infection (Figure 4-5).[4] Antibiotics are effective against most bacterial infections, but will not speed recovery from colds and other upper respiratory infections like bronchitis that are

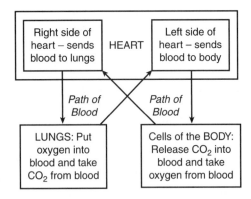

Figure 4-4. Path of Blood Through the Heart, Lungs, and Body.

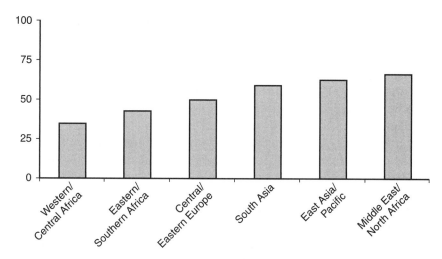

Figure 4-5. Percent of Under-5 Children with Suspected Pneumonia Taken to a Health Care Provider, 2005.

Data Source: UNICEF, State of the World's Children 2007.

usually caused by viruses. However, there are some types of viral pneumonia that can be prevented through vaccination. If every child received the *Haemophilus influenzae* type b (Hib) vaccine, approximately half a million child deaths could be averted each year.

Diarrhea

About 17% of child deaths each year are due to diarrhea. **Diarrhea** is an increase in the volume of stool or the frequency of defecation and can quickly cause dehydration and death. Diarrhea causes the loss of excessive amounts of water and the loss of electrolytes like sodium, potassium, and bicarbonate. Severe dehydration can cause low blood pressure (because fluid loss decreases blood volume), a fast and weak pulse, rapid breathing (but insufficient oxygen intake), sunken dry eyes, loss of skin elasticity, muscle contractions and convulsions, and delirium. Electrolyte imbalances can lead to kidney and heart failure.

Diarrhea is usually caused by an infection like rotavirus, *E. coli*, or cholera. (It can also be caused by conditions like lactose intolerance that cause poor absorption of water, and by food allergies, some antibiotics and other medications, and some chemicals, such as caffeine and toxins.) The infectious agents that cause diarrhea are transmitted through contaminated food and water, by physical contact with people who have an infection that causes diarrhea, and by contact with feces. It is estimated that unsafe water, inadequate availability of water for hygiene, and lack of access to sanitation (such as a toilet or latrine) together contribute to about 88% of deaths from diarrhea each year.[5] Prevention of diarrhea requires access to clean water for drinking, food preparation, hand washing, and bathing, and safe disposal of feces.

Once a child has diarrhea, the most important method for preventing death is the administration of **oral rehydration therapy (ORT)**. Sometimes called oral rehydration solution or salts (ORS), ORT is a solution of sugar, salt, and clean drinking water that replaces lost fluids and restores the balance of electrolytes in the blood. ORS salts are sometimes distributed in packets at clinics. Parents can also make their own ORS solution by mixing 8 teaspoons of sugar and one-half teaspoon of salt into one liter of boiled water. Potassium can be added to the solution through fruit juice, coconut water, or mashed bananas. Children with diarrhea need to drink ORT every time they pass watery stool for a total of at least one liter each day. If they also have vomiting they need to drink more ORT and take smaller sips of the solution.

Adequate nutrition is also important because malnutrition increases the risk of death from diarrhea. Children with diarrhea should be encouraged to eat the same foods that they normally consume, as long as they are not vomiting, and breastfed children should continue to breastfeed during their illness. After children recover from diarrhea they should be encouraged to eat more food than normal to regain lost weight and lost nutrients.

ORT combined with continued feeding leads to the best health outcomes for children with diarrhea,[6] but not all children with diarrhea receive this care (Figure 4-6). Additional health education for parents is needed to increase the use of ORT and continued feeding.

Malaria

Malaria, which causes about 8% of under-5 child deaths annually, is a parasitic infection spread by the bites of infected mosquitoes. Malaria usually presents with a fever and flu-like symptoms, but children with malaria can

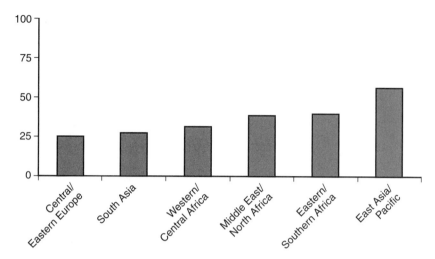

Figure 4-6. Percent of Under-5 Children with Diarrhea Who Receive Both ORT and Continued Feeding, 2005.
Data Source: UNICEF, State of the World's Children 2007.

deteriorate quickly and enter into a coma (cerebral malaria) or shock. In many cases, children with malaria can be successfully treated with inexpensive anti-malarial tablets, but malaria can cause weeks or even months of illness due to relapses and anemia. Reinfection with malaria is common, and in some areas the average child may have six or more bouts of malaria each year. Furthermore, when pregnant women contract malaria, their babies have an increased risk of low birth weight, birth complications, and stillbirths. One of the most effective ways to prevent infection is the use of insecticide-treated bednets (ITNs) that shield sleeping people from the bites of mosquitoes, yet many households in regions where malaria is common do not have ITNs or fail to use them consistently. (Chapter 7 has a more complete description of malaria.)

Measles

Measles is a highly contagious viral infection that is spread from one person to another through the air or by contact with body secretions from the nose or throat of people with the infection. Symptoms include a fever, runny nose, cough, and sore eyes, followed by a rash that starts on the face and spreads down the body. Measles can also cause severe complications such as diarrhea, ear infections, pneumonia, encephalitis (brain swelling), and permanent disabilities, such as blindness. The case fatality rate in developing countries is usually 1% to 5% but may be as high as 25% in populations with high levels of nutrition deficiencies, especially vitamin A deficiency.[7] Although an effective vaccine is available, more than a half million children die from measles each year, approximately 4% of deaths in children less than 5 years old. (Appendix VII lists all currently recommended childhood vaccinations.) There is no treatment available for measles, so prevention through immunization is crucial.

Undernutrition

Undernutrition occurs when children do not consume enough calories or do not take in adequate amounts of specific nutrients like proteins, fats, vitamins, and minerals. In addition to deaths directly caused by undernutrition, being malnourished increases the risk of death from infectious diseases. Undernutrition causes or contributes to more than half of all deaths in children under five years of age. New mothers should be encouraged to breastfeed their babies, preferably for at least six months, so that they can pass both nutrients and disease-fighting antibodies to their children. Older infants and children need a variety of nutrient-rich age-appropriate foods.

While most child hunger stems from a lack of food at the household level, it may be possible in some cases to improve the nutritional status of children by changing social eating practices. In cultures where tradition holds that when food is served men should eat first and children should eat last, children may not get an adequate amount of high-quality proteins. In cultures where everyone at the meal eats from a common pot, small children may not eat quickly enough to secure adequate calories. New serving practices, such as giving children their own plate or bowl of food, may help children to consume the food they need to be healthier.

Vitamin and mineral supplements can also have a drastic impact on child health. An estimated 25% of child deaths in the countries with the highest child mortality rates could be prevented by a simple set of nutritional interventions that include breastfeeding (exclusive breastfeeding for the first six months of life), complementary feeding (introducing solid foods with continued breastfeeding after six months), and vitamin A and zinc supplementation.[8] (Chapter 9 focuses on nutrition and explains the importance of vitamins and minerals.)

CHILD HEALTH INITIATIVES

Several multinational initiatives have sought to standardize efforts to improve global child health (Table 4-3).[9] One of the first was primary health care (PHC), a system of community-based health that employs community health workers and focuses as much on prevention as on cures. PHC became the focus of most international health work following the Alma-Ata Conference in 1978, which developed the goal of "Health for All by 2000" through the reduction of barriers to health care access, especially in poor and rural areas. PHC prioritizes prevention of common local infectious diseases, promotion of nutrition, provision of essential drugs and treatments for common diseases and injuries, coordination of health services with traditional health practitioners, and programming for maternal and child health (including immunization and family planning).

A hallmark of PHC is regularly scheduled health clinics for children under 5 years of age, which monitor child growth and provide necessary immunizations for children from birth through their fifth birthdays. Since all children, whether sick or healthy, are encouraged to have frequent interactions with the health care system through these "under-5" health clinics, warning signs for potentially life-threatening conditions in relatively healthy children can be detected early and treated. For example, growth monitoring tracks child weight so that caregivers will know if a child has lost weight or is failing to gain weight. Weight loss or stagnation can be a sign of serious illness, and early detection means that a nutritional intervention can be implemented before a health crisis occurs.

The Expanded Program on Immunization (EPI), was started in the mid-1970s by the World Health Organization and expanded the number and types of

Table 4-3. Acronyms for Global Child Health Programs.

Acronym	Program
EPI	Expanded Program on Immunization
GOBI	Growth monitoring, Oral rehydration therapy, Breastfeeding, and Immunization
GOBI/FFF	Growth monitoring, Oral rehydration therapy, Breastfeeding, and Immunization + Family planning, Food production, and Female education
IMCI	Integrated Management of Childhood Illness
PHC	Primary Health Care

vaccines typically given to children. (The currently recommended immunizations for children are listed in Appendix VII.) EPI succeeded in significantly increasing the percentage of children receiving essential immunizations. GOBI, a program started in the 1980s by UNICEF, focused on increasing child survival through promotion of four components: Growth monitoring, Oral rehydration therapy for diarrhea, Breastfeeding, and Immunization. Later, a partnership between UNICEF, WHO, and the World Bank added the new community-focused components of Family planning, Food production, and Female education to the GOBI program, creating a program called GOBI/FFF.

Integrated Management of Childhood Illness (IMCI) is a package of simple, affordable, and effective interventions for major childhood illnesses and undernutrition that was first developed in the 1990s by UNICEF and

Table 4-4. Key Family Practices Under IMCI.

	#	Practice
Physical and Mental Growth	1	Breastfeed infants exclusively for at least six months (if the mother does not have HIV infection).
	2	Starting at about 6 months of age, feed children freshly prepared energy and nutrient rich complementary foods, while continuing to breastfeed up to two years or longer.
	3	Ensure that children receive adequate amounts of micronutrients (especially vitamin A and iron) either in their diet or through supplementation.
	4	Promote mental and social development by responding to a child's needs for care and through talking, playing, and providing a stimulating environment.
Disease Prevention	5	Take children as scheduled to complete a full course of immunizations before their first birthday.
	6	Dispose of feces safely and wash hands after defecation, after contact children's feces, before preparing meals, before feeding children.
	7	Protect children in malaria-endemic areas from mosquito bites by ensuring that they sleep under insecticide-treated bednets.
	8	Adopt and sustain appropriate behavior regarding prevention and care for HIV-infected people, including orphans.
Appropriate Home Care	9	Continue to feed and offer more fluids, including breastmilk, to children when they are sick.

WHO.[10] The term "integrated" has several layers of meaning. One aspect of integration is the emphasis on the interrelatedness of children's health conditions. A child with malaria is more vulnerable to diarrhea. A child with vitamin A deficiency is more vulnerable to death from measles. Clinicians working under an IMCI framework complete a series of medical assessments on each sick child that allow for diagnosis of underlying conditions in addition to the primary illness. Integration also emphasizes families and communities working together with the staff of various levels of health care facilities to care for sick children, and clinicians at out-patient clinics knowing when to refer patients to in-patient hospital departments or specialty clinics.

IMCI provides guidelines for families with young children (Table 4-4) and designs decision charts for clinicians to use when assessing children and

Table 4-4. Key Family Practices Under IMCI—cont'd.

	#	Practice—cont'd
Appropriate Home Care—cont'd	10	Give sick children appropriate home treatment for infections. For example, give ORT for diarrhea and first aid for injuries.
	11	Take appropriate actions to prevent and manage child injuries and accidents.
	12	Prevent child abuse and neglect and take appropriate action when it has occurred.
	13	Ensure that men actively participate in the provision of childcare and are involved in reproductive health initiatives.
Care Seeking and Compliance	14	Recognize when sick children need treatment outside the home and seek care from appropriate providers.
	15	Ensure that every pregnant woman has adequate antenatal care. This includes at least four antenatal visits with an appropriate health care provider and having the recommended dose of the tetanus toxoid vaccination. The mother also needs support from her family and community in seeking care at the time of delivery and during the postpartum and lactation period.
	16	Follow recommendations given by health worker and nutritionists about treatment, follow-up, and referral.

Source: Vincent Orinda for UNICEF. Community IMCI: a strategy for accelerating child survival and development interventions. Discussion paper. New York: UNICEF, September 2001.

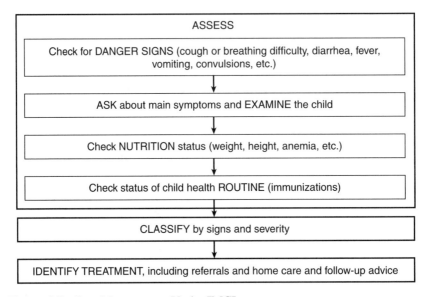

Figure 4-7. Case Management Under IMCI.

treating common illnesses (Figure 4-7). The main strategy of IMCI is to improve family and community health practices and to improve case management skills of health care staff. For example, consider the ideal integrated response to a child who has diarrhea. The family of the child should know how to prepare ORT correctly and know what symptoms require the child to be taken to the local clinic or hospital. The clinic should support community health education programs and be prepared to provide care for advanced cases of dehydration and to make referrals for hospital-based treatment if necessary. Or, perhaps a family is concerned about its children contracting malaria. In an integrated response, the parents would be instructed to install and consistently use insecticide-treated bednets and to monitor their children for fevers and other symptoms of malaria. The local clinic should support community health education efforts, be prepared to effectively treat cases of malaria that do occur, and make referrals for advanced treatment if needed.

Each of these programs had some success in improving child health, but infant and child health statistics show that there is still a great deal of work to be done. If we want as many children as possible to have a healthy start in life, we need to continue to work to increase access to essential drugs and immunizations, to educate parents about the use of ORT and insecticide-treated bednets, to promote breastfeeding, to improve access to safe drinking water, and to implement other important public health measures.

PROTECTING CHILDREN

In addition to infectious disease and malnutrition, children may be at risk of injury and abuse. Both boys and girls may be subject to physical, emotional, and sexual abuse by family members or other adults or children. In 1989, the General Assembly of the United Nations adopted the Convention on the Rights of the Child. (Appendix III contains an excerpt from this Convention.) Several of the Articles are related to child health and survival. The rights of the child include freedom from all forms of exploitation, the right to an adequate standard of living, protection from all forms of violence, access to education and appropriate information, the right to be heard, and the right to rest, leisure, and play. Acknowledging the right of every child in the world to these basic protections is a start, but must be acted on to be meaningful. The sad reality is that millions of children are denied these protections.

Many children are sent to work at an early age. Some types of work, such as when rural children work alongside their parents on the family farm, can be a positive experience. But some children develop lasting physical and psychological scars from long hours doing domestic labor, agricultural work, or factory work. The International Labor Organization (ILO) makes a distinction between children participating in economic activity—working for a few hours or full time, whether for pay or not, doing activities other than household chores or schooling—and children who are involved in "child labor." It is permissible for children 12 years old and older to spend a few hours a week in light work that is not hazardous. But it is a child labor violation when a child has an excessive workload, unsafe work conditions, or extreme work intensity, because any of these conditions may harm a child's physical health, mental health, or moral development. At worst, a child may be sold by his or her family into bonded labor, forced into sex work, or forced into armed conflict. The ILO estimates that more than 125 million children between the ages of 5 and 14 conducted hazardous work in 2004 and more than 215 million children were laborers.[11]

Girls are especially vulnerable. In some parts of the world, they are subject to infanticide, heavy domestic responsibilities at a very early age, female genital mutilation (FGM), violence, and sexual abuse. When a family has limited resources, girls may face discrimination in food allocation, may not be allowed to attend school, and may be forced into early marriage, sometimes even before reaching puberty. In 1995, the United Nations adopted the Beijing Declaration that affirms several strategic objectives for promoting the rights of the "girl-child," including eliminating discrimination in education, eliminating the economic exploitation of child labor, and eradicating violence against the girl-child.[12] Although some improvements have been achieved, such as increasing school enrollment, significant inequalities between boys and girls remain.

Several groups are dedicated to protecting children. The most prominent is UNICEF. UNICEF (initially called the United Nations International Children's Emergency Fund but now shortened to the United Nations Children's Fund) has a mandate to advocate for the protection of children's rights, to help meet their basic needs, and to expand opportunities to reach their full potential. UNICEF advocates for children by promoting prenatal health care, girls' education, childhood immunizations and nutrition, HIV/AIDS prevention among young people, and protective environments free of violence, abuse, and exploitation. UNICEF also responds to emergencies in order to protect the rights of children and to relieve the suffering of children and their caregivers. About two-thirds of the UNICEF budget comes from governments, but the rest must be obtained from non-governmental organizations, partnerships, and private donations.

WOMEN'S HEALTH

Men and women face different health challenges because of both biological characteristics related to sex and social structures related to gender. **Sex** refers to the biological classification of people as male or female based on genetics (the presence of XX or XY sex chromosomes) and reproductive anatomy. **Gender** refers to social, cultural, and psychological aspects of being male or female, and is shaped by the social and cultural environment and experience as well as biology. There is tremendous variability in the way individual women and individual men express their gender and in the way cultures define gender roles.

Gender roles describe how a culture believes men and women should behave. Gender roles may indicate what tasks women must do, such as cooking, cleaning, and taking care of children. They also define what tasks women cannot do, which might include working with heavy machinery, being in religious leadership, or driving cars. Traditional cultures often consider women to be under the authority of their fathers (or other male relatives) until marriage and of their husbands after marriage, and they may limit the ability of a woman to own property or manage her own finances. Some cultures have strict rules about what women can wear in public and whether they can be in public spaces unaccompanied by a male. This can limit the ability of women to participate in the marketplace and government, to attend school and religious meetings, and to acquire medical attention and information.

Women may have little power over their own bodies both because of gender norms that give men authority over women and because women tend to be smaller and physically weaker than men. For example, women may not have the ability to choose when to have children or how many children to have. Women may also be subject to domestic violence (violence by intimate partners and family members) and other acts of physical aggression, including rape. In a multi-country study of violence against women, 23% to 49% of women in most study sites reported being physically abused by an intimate partner.[13] A large number of women in the study indicated that they believe that a man has good reason to beat his wife if she does not complete housework, disobeys her husband, is unfaithful, or if the husband suspects infidelity. Many women reported that they did not think it acceptable for a woman to refuse sex with her husband even if she does not want to have sex, he is drunk or mistreats her, or she is sick. The immediate health consequences of violence against women include serious injuries, death, damage caused to fetuses when injured women are pregnant, and psychological trauma. Sexually abused women may also have an unwanted pregnancy or contract sexually transmitted infections (STIs) such as HIV. Violence against females may occur at any stage of their lives (Table 4-5).

The standard of medical care for women has historically been less than that of men. Until recently, Western medicine treated women as "small men." It is now recognized that women's bodies differ from those of small males. For example, for a long time no one realized that the prevalence of heart disease is similar in both sexes and that heart disease is the most common cause of death in both men and women in the United States. Because men are more likely to have "dramatic" heart attacks with crushing chest pain while women often have subtle symptoms like feeling more tired than normal, doctors do not as easily recognize heart attacks in women. As a result, heart disease in women has traditionally been under-diagnosed. Some other differences are listed in Table 4-6. For example, because women have longer life expectancies than men, women are more likely to develop some age-related disease like Alzheimer's disease and adult-onset blindness.[14]

Table 4-5. Violence Against Women Throughout the Life Cycle.

Phase	Type of Violence
Pre-birth	Sex-selective abortion; effects of battering during pregnancy on birth outcomes
Infancy	Female infanticide; physical, sexual, and psychological abuse
Girlhood	Child marriage; female genital mutilation (FGM); physical, sexual, and psychological abuse; incest; child prostitution and pornography
Adolescence and adulthood	Dating and courtship violence (e.g., acid throwing and date rape); economically coerced sex (e.g., school girls having sex with "sugar daddies" in return for school fees); incest; sexual abuse in the workplace; rape; sexual harassment; forced prostitution and pornography; trafficking in women; partner violence; marital rape; dowry abuse and murders; partner homicide; psychological abuse; abuse of women with disabilities; forced pregnancy
Elderly	Forced "suicide" or homicide of widows for economic reasons; sexual, physical, and psychological abuse

Source: WHO, "Violence Against Women," FRH/WDH/97.8.

Men and women have different hormones and different brain function, and that means that they have different symptoms and different pathways to recovery. Because of differences in body chemistry, finding medications that work for women involves more than merely cutting the dosage to account for the differences in mass between the average man and woman. Because of differences in brain function, women are more likely to recover language ability after a stroke than men. (Women typically use the whole cerebrum of the brain for language, while men rely primarily on the left frontal lobe of the cerebrum.) There are many other significant differences between the sexes, and it may be important to develop sex-specific approaches to health education and other preventive, diagnostic, and therapeutic health services.

Maternal Health

The hours of labor and delivery during childbirth are extremely dangerous for many women. Pregnancy and childbirth and their consequences are still the leading cause of death, disease, and disability among women of

Table 4-6. Comparison of Burden of Disease in Women and Men.
Although all of these conditions occur in both females and males, the risk of developing these conditions varies by sex.

Women are more likely than men to . . .	Men are more likely than women to . . .
. . . have cancers of the reproductive system	. . . have lung, bladder, mouth, esophageal, and stomach cancer
. . . have complications from sexually-transmitted infections like chlamydia and gonorrhea	. . . become infected with trypano-somiasis, schistosomiasis, leish-maniasis, lymphatic filariasis and other tropical infections
. . . die from burns	
. . . have depressive disorder, post traumatic stress disorder, panic disorder, and migraines	. . . die from traffic accidents, poisonings, falls, drowning, violence, and war
. . . develop vision problems related to glaucoma, cataracts, and trachoma	. . . commit suicide and have drug use disorders
. . . have Alzheimer's and other dementias	. . . develop liver disorders such as cirrhosis, hepatitis B, and hepatitis C
. . . die from diabetes	. . . have lung diseases like TB and COPD (chronic obstructive pulmonary disease)
. . . develop musculoskeletal disorders like rheumatoid arthritis and osteoarthritis	
. . . develop autoimmune disease like lupus	
. . . develop iron-deficiency anemia	

Data Source: World Health Report 2004.

reproductive age in developing countries. More than 500,000 women die each year as a result of pregnancy and childbirth, which is about one death every minute.[15] Nearly 40% of women worldwide give birth without the assistance of a skilled birth attendant, such as a nurse or midwife, who is trained to manage complications. The most common cause of maternal death, which is a death during pregnancy, childbirth, or soon after, is severe postpartum bleeding (Figure 4-8). Other common causes include infections, unsafe abortions, eclampsia, and obstructed labor.[16,17,18] (Pre-eclampsia is characterized by high blood pressure and protein in the urine and can develop into eclampsia, which is characterized by convulsions and possible organ failure.)

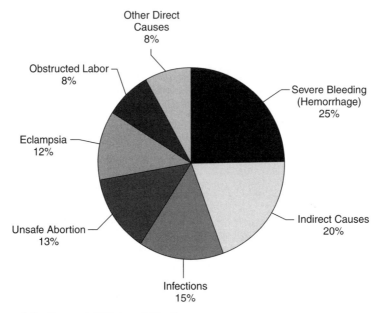

Figure 4-8. Causes of Maternal Death.
Data Source: World Health Report 2005, Figure 4.1.

The difference in risk of maternal death between high-income and low-income regions is huge. In Africa, about 830 mothers die for every 100,000 births, compared to about 24 maternal deaths for every 100,000 births in high-income regions. Women in Africa tend to have several pregnancies, so the lifetime risk of maternal death is 1 in 16. In high-income countries, women usually have only one or two pregnancies, so the lifetime risk of maternal death is about 1 in 2800. This means that women in Africa are 175 times more likely to die while giving birth than women in the United States, Canada, and Europe. Table 4-7 compares maternal health indicators for several countries.

Women who survive pregnancy and delivery may be left with permanent disabilities. For example, some women who are small, as is often the case with girls who become pregnant in their pre-teen or early teenage years, develop a condition called obstructed labor, which is when the unborn baby is wedged so tightly into the birth canal that blood flow to surrounding tissues is cut off and the tissue starts to die. Women who are able to get to a hospital can have surgery (a Cesarean section) to deliver the baby before too

Table 4-7. Maternal and Neonatal Health Indicators in Selected Countries, 2000.

Country	Afghanistan	Kenya	Senegal	Peru	Philippines	United States	Canada
Births attended by skilled health personnel	14%	42%	58%	59%	60%	99%	98%
Maternal mortality ratio (deaths per 100,000 live births)	1900	1000	690	410	200	14	5
Neonatal mortality rate (deaths within 28 days of birth per 1000 live births)	60	29	31	16	15	5	4

Data Source: World Health Report 2005.

much damage is done. Women who do not have access to a surgeon may be in labor for several days. The outcome, if the woman survives, is often the formation of a fistula—a hole between the rectum or bladder and the vagina— that constantly leaks urine or feces. Because of the odor, most women with an obstetric fistula are ostracized by their communities. Some women are left paralyzed because of nerve damage, and some are left infertile. In nearly all of these cases the baby is stillborn. The World Health Organization estimates that there are nearly two million women living with an obstetric fistula and more than 50,000 new cases occur every year.[19] Fistulas can be surgically corrected, but the best scenario is to delay pregnancy until women are fully grown and to have access to medical professionals during delivery.

Women who have been circumcised (also called female genital cutting, female genital mutilation, or FGM), a common practice in some parts of Africa and the Middle East, have particularly high risks of adverse reproductive health outcomes, such as bacterial vaginosis and herpes (HSV-2), anemia, and obstetric complications during delivery, such as tears and the need for episiotomies.[20,21,22,23]

Safe motherhood programs need to address issues from prior to conception through the time after delivery.[24] All women and men of reproductive age need to have access to information about reproduction and contraception so they are better prepared to make decisions about sex and are able to prevent unwanted pregnancies, unsafe abortions, and sexually transmitted infections. During pregnancy women need information about how to stay healthy, eat well, and recognize potential complications so they can be addressed as soon as possible. All deliveries should be attended by a trained health professional, the woman and her baby should be observed after delivery, and both should be examined several weeks later to be sure that they are recovering and healthy.

FAMILY PLANNING

Contraception is the intentional prevention of pregnancy. Contraceptive methods include abstinence, barriers, medications, and surgery (Table 4-8). Complete sexual abstinence is the only absolute guaranteed way to avoid pregnancy. Some couples practice periodic abstinence and avoid intercourse during the days after ovulation (when an egg is released from an ovary), the time when a woman is most fertile. Some forms of contraception, like condoms and diaphragms, are used as a barrier during sexual intercourse to prevent sperm from coming into contact with an egg.

The method by which other forms of contraception work is not as clear. Oral contraceptives (birth control pills) generally prevent ovulation, so no eggs are released from the ovaries and a pregnancy cannot occur. Oral contraceptives must be taken at the same time every day, without skipping any doses, for this method to be effective. In many parts of the world, oral contraceptives are called the "family planning pill" in recognition of the importance of birth spacing. IUDs (intrauterine devices) prevent fertilization of an egg by creating an environment that is hostile to sperm or prevent implantation of a fertilized egg in the endometrium that lines the uterus.

Some women and men prefer a longer-term method of pregnancy prevention. Norplant is a female contraceptive that is placed under the skin of the upper arm and works in the same was as oral contraceptives, but lasts for up to five years. Contraceptive hormones may also be delivered through a weekly patch or monthly injections. For permanent sterilization, a woman may have tubal ligation or a man may have a vasectomy. Only condoms help to prevent the transmission of sexually transmitted infections, so sexually active people who are sterile or infertile need to consider what methods they will use to prevent sexually-transmitted infections.

Abortion is the termination or loss of a pregnancy. Miscarriages are called spontaneous abortions by medical professionals. Induced abortions are chemically-induced or surgically terminated pregnancies and are not a form of contraception, since they end a pregnancy rather than prevent it. Increased access to contraception reduces the number of induced abortions by preventing unplanned and unwanted pregnancies.

There are a number of different ways to report a woman's reproductive history. **Gravidity** refers to the total number of times a woman has been pregnant, and includes miscarriages, abortions, stillbirths, and live births. **Fertility** is the total number of births, whether the result was a stillbirth or a live birth. Figure 4-9 shows the average number of births per woman by country. African countries have the highest fertility rates, while most European countries have a very low fertility rate. **Parity** refers to the total number of live births. Because very few miscarriages and abortions are reported to health care professionals, most reports use fertility to measure pregnancies in a population. The goal of family planning is to minimize unwanted pregnancies (minimize gravidity) but maximize the health of babies from pregnancies that do occur (so that parity is as close as possible to gravidity).

One of the best predictors of decreased fertility is increased female education (Figure 4-10), so many population planning campaigns focus not just on education about contraception but also on general literacy. Educated

Table 4-8. Contraceptive Methods.

Type	Approach	Approximate 1-Year Pregnancy Rate	STD Protection	Note
Complete abstinence	Abstinence	0%	Yes	No intercourse
Sterilization (tubal ligation or vasectomy)	Surgery	Nearly 0%	No	Permanent
Subdermal implants (Norplant)	Hormones	1%	No	Effective for about 5 years after implantation
Injection (Depo-Provera)	Hormones	1%	No	One injection every 3 months
Oral contraceptives	Hormones	1–2%	No	Pill must be taken daily to be effective
Transdermal (patch) contraceptives (Ortho Evra)	Hormones	1–2%	No	The patch must be replaced weekly
Intravaginal contraceptives (NuvaRing)	Hormones	1–2%	No	The vaginal ring must be replaced monthly

Emergency contraception ("morning after pill" / Plan B)	Hormones	—	No	Reduces pregnancy rate after unprotected sex from about 8% to about 2% if used within 72 hours of intercourse
Male Condom	Barrier	11%	Yes	Apply just before intercourse
Diaphragm with spermicide	Barrier + spermicide	6–20%	No	Inserted before intercourse
Sponge	Barrier	14–28%	No	Can be inserted hours before intercourse
Periodic abstinence	Timing	20%	No	Requires daily monitoring of body functions and periods of abstinence
Female condom	Barrier	21%	Some	Use just before intercourse
Spermicides	Spermicide	20–50%	No	Apply just before intercourse
No contraceptive method used	None	85%	No	

Data Sources: Estimates of risk of pregnancy during one year of consistent use in sexually active American women from the U.S. FDA, "Birth Control Guide," December 2003. "Contraception," In: *The Merck Manual of Diagnosis and Therapy.* 18th ed., Whitehouse Station, NJ: Merck Research Laboratory, 2006.

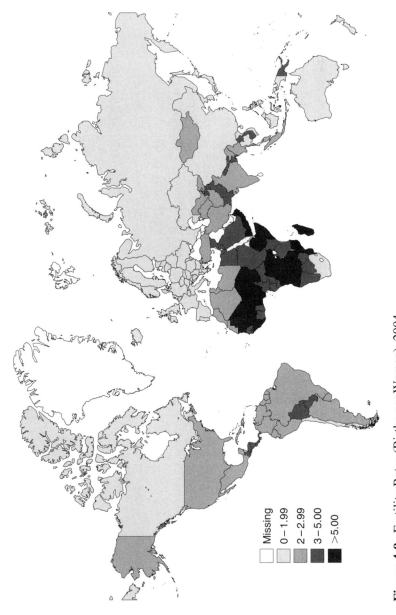

Figure 4-9. Fertility Rates (Births per Woman), 2004.

Data Source: World Bank, World Development Indicators Database.

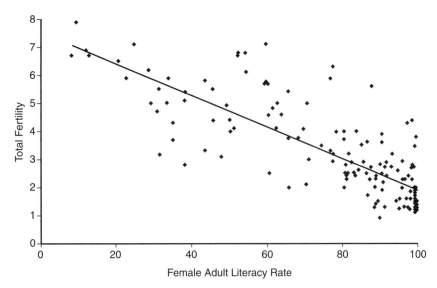

Figure 4-10. Female Education (% of Females Ages 15 and Higher Who Are Literate, 2003) and Fertility (Total Births Per Woman, Estimated from 2000–2005 Data).

Each point represents data for one country. Lower literacy rates are associated with higher fertility rates.

Data Source: Human Development Report 2005.

women have smaller families for many reasons. One is that work outside the home that is made possible by literacy may delay marriage and first pregnancy. Another reason is that educated women can make better decisions about contraception and childbearing with their partners because they have the ability to read and act on information about good health practices, nutrition, disease prevention, and child rearing strategies.

It is generally agreed that women and their babies are healthier when women have fewer pregnancies. Each pregnancy carries risks, but it is especially risky when a woman has existing health problems, has had a high risk pregnancy in the past, is having twins or other multiple children, or will not have access to a trained birth attendant. And when the birth spacing between one baby and the next is short, the older baby is at risk of malnutrition because of being weaned from breastmilk at a young age and losing the extra attention of his or her parents. When women have fewer babies, it also helps to control global population growth.

POPULATION GROWTH

Picture a small island in the middle of an ocean. It is arable (can grow food) and has a variety of plant and animal species. Say that at first 10 people settle on the island. They build homes, develop a system for collecting fresh water (since ocean water is too salty to drink or to use for irrigation), and begin to farm the land. They also begin to have children, and eventually those children have children. Soon the population has reached 100, and then it grows to 1000. The amount of land available for farming decreases as more homes are built, yet the need for food is greater because there are more people to feed. Getting rid of waste and finding energy sources are growing problems. The amount of fresh water available is becoming a source of stress, as the demand for water is greater, but water quality is decreasing because waste is polluting water sources. Some plants and animals are threatened and at risk of extinction. Crime is increasing as resources become scarce. What would happen if the population increased to 10,000, or to a million? Is there a limit to the number of people a small island could support?

Many people have similar concerns about the growth of the worldwide human population. For a long time the size of the global population was relatively steady, but recent population growth has been exponential. Figure 4-11 is a plot of world population over time that shows a "J-shaped" growth pattern. After many years of relatively limited population growth there has been a very steep increase in the total world population in recent centuries. The doubling time, the number of years it takes for the world's population to double, is getting shorter. It took only forty years—from 1950 until 1990—for the number of humans to double from 2.5 billion to 5 billion.

Carrying capacity is the maximum human population the Earth can sustain. The ecological footprint is the per capita area of land needed to meet consumption needs. There is no easy way to calculate carrying capacity because it depends on the assumed standard of living and cultural factors in addition to the land and natural resources that are available. (We can be fairly certain that the world could not support 6 billion or more people who aspired to the North American standard of living.) It is definitely related to population density (either as land area per person or arable land area per person) but must also consider climate, natural resources, and other criteria.

What will happen if the world population continues to grow? One famous scenario was proposed in 1798 by Thomas Malthus. In "An Essay on the

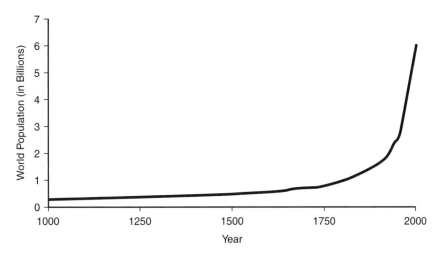

Figure 4-11. World Population Growth over Time.

Data Source: United Nations, "The World at Six Billion," Table 1: World Population from Year 0 to Stabilization, 1999.

Principle of Population," Malthus predicted that at some point the population would exceed food supply, and the result would be mass famine, epidemics, and war. These "Malthusian catastrophes" have not occurred, and at present global food production is growing faster than the population. However, food and other resources are not distributed equally. Fertility rates are highest in the poorest parts of the world where food production is often low. There are valid reasons to be concerned about the unequal distribution of food and natural resources, the risks of increased pollution and congestion with continued population growth, and the possibility of increased crime and war as resources in some regions of the world become scarce. One check on exponential growth is that fertility rates generally decrease when economic conditions in a region improve. Another check is the increased use of family planning methods.

DEMOGRAPHY

Demography is the study of the size and composition of human populations. Most countries maintain **vital statistics** on their residents, which are collected from birth and death certificates, from marriage and divorce certificates, and from census records. Demographers use these statistics to understand the current population distribution and to predict the size and characteristics of the population in future years.

The **birth rate** is the annual number of births per 1000 people in the total population and the **death rate** (or **mortality rate**) is the annual number of deaths per 1000 total population. (The death rate is usually higher in populations with a large percentage of older adults than in populations with lots of children, so an "age-adjusted" rate that accounts for differences in the age structures of populations is usually used to compare death rates in two or more populations.)

The **fertility rate** is the average number of children a woman gives birth to during her childbearing years (Figure 4-12). If each woman has, on average, about 2 children, then each couple will produce only a "replacement population" and over the generations the population size will remain about the same. If the number is higher than 2, then the size of the population will

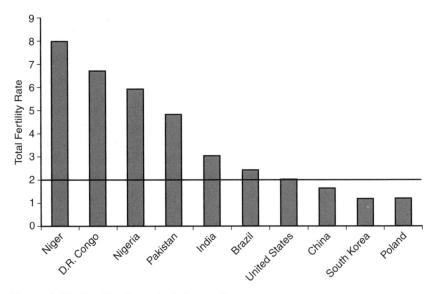

Figure 4-12. Fertility Rates in Selected Countries.

The horizontal line represents the threshold for a replacement population. The population size of countries with fertility rates below this line will over time decrease (unless immigration increases the number of people living within the borders of the country), while the population size of countries above the line will increase.

Data Source: Population Reference Bureau, "2005 World Population Data Sheet."

increase over time. If the number is lower is lower than 2, then the average age of the population will increase and the number of people in the total population will begin to decrease.

Other population statistics measure various aspects of the age structure. The **aging index** is usually calculated as the number of people age 65 or older for every 100 children under the age of 15. Social support ratios like the **dependency ratio** indicate the number of dependent children and older people for every person of working age, usually defined as people ages 20 through 64 (Figure 4-13). The **elderly support ratio** is usually defined as the number of people aged 65 or older for every 100 people ages 20 through 64 in a population. Because many older people remain active and economically independent, alternate measurements may include only dependent older people.

A **population pyramid** that shows the number of males and females by age group in a population is an effective way to visually display the population age structure. Less developed countries usually have a population pyramid with a wide base (many children) that gradually narrows in older age groups (Figure 4-14). More developed countries have lower fertility rates and the population "pyramid" may look more like a "cube" (Figure 4-15).

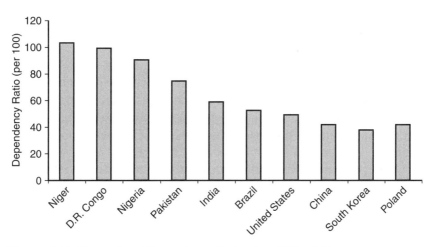

Figure 4-13. Examples of Dependency Ratios (per 100), 2004.

The same countries shown in Figure 4-12 are displayed here. Note the relationship between high fertility rates and high dependency ratios.

Data Source: World Health Report 2006.

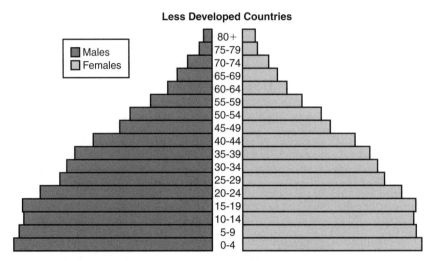

Figure 4-14. Population Pyramid for Less Developed Countries, 2006.
Data Source: U.S. Census Bureau, International Data Base, Table 094.

A population with a narrow base (few children) and a wider adult population is probably facing a dependency crisis because in a few decades there will be few young adults working to support a large population of older adults in addition to raising their own children.

Measuring population characteristics is important for understanding the current needs of the population and making policies that will help the population prepare for the future. Many countries are concerned about population growth and are taking measures to encourage a decrease in the fertility rate. At the same time, some countries, especially in Europe, face a shrinking population and are concerned about who will care for the population as it ages.

Demographers call these different patterns of birth and death rates the **demographic transition** (Figure 4-16). Pre-transition populations have high birth rates and high death rates, and the population maintains a stable, but small, number of people. During the demographic transition, increased food security and health care reduce the death rate but the birth rate stays high and the population size increases, possibly drastically. At some point, education, technology, family planning, and other factors reduce the birth rates and the population begins to stabilize at its larger size. Eventually, prolonged low birth rates may lead to a slow decline in population size.

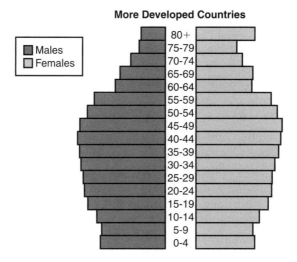

Figure 4-15. Population Pyramid for More Developed Countries, 2006.

Data Source: U.S. Census Bureau, International Data Base, Table 094.

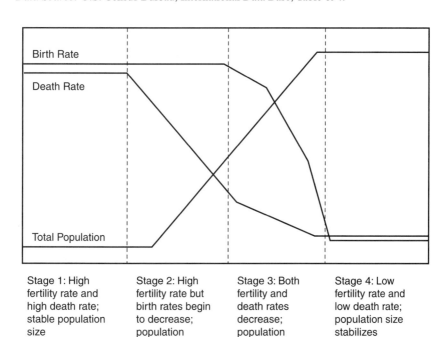

Figure 4-16. The Demographic Transition.

POPULATION PLANNING POLICY

Reproductive rights have been a controversial topic on the global health agenda. For example, when the Cairo Conference on Population and Development in 1994 focused on women's empowerment and reproductive rights, in particular the ability of a woman or couple to decide how many children they want without interference from governments or other groups, it sparked concern by religious groups. The Roman Catholic Church was particularly concerned about the use of contraceptives and possible increases in the number of induced abortions.

China has been one of the most aggressive countries in limiting population growth. The "late, long, few" policy of the 1970s encouraged later child-bearing, longer spacing between children, and fewer children, and cut the total fertility rate in half. The goal of China's one-child policy, which was adopted in 1979, is to use economic and educational incentives to promote one-child families, especially in urban areas. Because there are exemptions to the policy for rural residents, for highly educated or wealthy parents, for parents who are both only children, and for certain minority groups, the actual fertility rate in China is currently 1.7 children per couple and not 1 child per couple.[25] The program has been controversial since its inception because of reports that, despite official policy, there are instances of forced abortions and sterilizations, infanticide (especially of females in rural areas), and other human rights abuses. Another concern is that the preference for male children may have made sex-selective abortions common enough to skew male-female birth ratios.[26] Within China, the main concern is that there are now many families with a "one-two-four" structure—only one grandchild to support two parents and four grandparents.

China is not the only country that supports population planning. Nearly all countries in Africa provide direct government support for the distribution of family planning information and contraceptives,[27] as do most Asian, Latin American, and Caribbean countries.[28] Still, millions of people who would like to use contraception do not have access to family planning services. Organizations like the United Nations Population Fund (UNFPA, formerly the United Nations Fund for Population Activities) and Planned Parenthood seek to bring information and supplies to these men and women. UNFPA helps developing countries that request assistance to improve access to quality reproductive health care, including voluntary family planning, safe motherhood programs, and prevention of sexually transmitted infections. One of UNFPA's goals is "to ensure that every pregnancy is wanted, every birth is safe, and every girl and woman is treated with dignity and respect."[29] The most common criticism of UNFPA is that it does not take a strong enough stance against abortion, even though it does not fund abortions. In recent years, the United States has cut its UNFPA budget in response to this concern.

Population planning programs need to target both women and men because men often make the decisions in a household, and a woman whose partner does not want her to use contraception will often follow her partner's wishes. Effective population planning policies may increase a woman's ability to choose how many children she wants to have and how she wants to space them. It is important for all adults and adolescents, both males and females, to understand their options for contraception and family spacing.

REFERENCES

1. Unless otherwise noted, statistics in this section are from World Health Organization (WHO), "Make Every Mother and Child Count." World Health Report 2005, Geneva: WHO Press, 2005.
2. Bryce J, Boschi-Pinto C, Shibuya K, Black RE, World Health Organization Child Health Epidemiology Reference Group. WHO estimates the causes of death in children. *Lancet.* 2005;365:1147–1152. The countries in each WHO region are listed in Appendix I.
3. WHO/UNICEF Joint Statement on Clinical Management of Acute Diarrhea, 2004 (WHO/FCH/CAH/04.7).
4. UNICEF, State of the World's Children 2007: Women and Children—The Double Dividend of Gender Equality, New York: UNICEF, 2007.
5. Black RE, Morris SS, Bryce J. Where and why are 10 million children dying each year? *Lancet.* 2003;361:2226–2234.
6. Victora CG, Bryce J, Fontaine O, Monasch R. Reducing deaths from diarrhoea through oral rehydration therapy. *Bull World Health Organ.* 2000;78:1246–1255.
7. World Health Organization (WHO). "Measles," Fact sheet 286, January 2007.
8. Jones G, Steketee RW, Black RE, Bhutta ZA, Morris SS, & the Bellagio Child Survival Study Group. How many child deaths can we prevent this year? *Lancet.* 2003;362:65–71.
9. Claeson M, Waldman RJ. The evolution of child health programmes in developing countries: from targeting diseases to targeting people. *Bull World Health Organ.* 2000;78:1234–1245.
10. Lambrechts T, Bryce J, Orinda V. Integrated management of childhood illness: a summary of first experiences. *Bull World Health Organ.* 1999;77:582–594.
11. International Labour Organization (ILO), 2006 ILO Global Report: "The End of Child Labour: Within Reach." Geneva: ILO Publications, 2006.
12. The Platform for Action, UN Fourth World Conference on Women, 1995. Available online at http://www.un.org/womenwatch/daw/beijing/platform/.

13. García-Moreno C, Jansen HAFM, Ellsberg M, Heise L, Watts C. WHO Multi-country Study on Women's Health and Domestic Violence against Women: Initial results on prevalence, health outcomes and women's responses. Geneva: World Health Organization, 2005.

14. The Institute of Medicine's Committee on Understanding the Biology of Sex and Gender Differences. Exploring the Biological Contributions to Human Health: Does Sex Matter? Wizemann TM and Pardue M-L, eds, Washington, D.C.: The National Academy Press, 2001.

15. Unless otherwise noted, statistics in this section are from the World Health Report 2005.

16. World Health Organization. World Health Report 2005.

17. AbouZahr C. Global burden of maternal death and disability. *Br Med Bull.* 2003; 67:1–11.

18. Khan KS, Wojdyla D, Say Lm, Gülmezoglu AM, Van Look PFA. World Health Organization analysis of causes of maternal death: a systematic review. *Lancet.* 2006;367:1066–1074.

19. UNFPA, "Obstetric Fistula: A Tragic Failure to Deliver Maternal Care."

20. Jones H, Diop N, Askew I, Kabore I. Female genital cutting practices in Burkina Faso and Mali and their negative health outcomes. *Stud Fam Plann.* 1999;30:219–230.

21. Morison L, Scherf C, Ekpo G, Paine K, West B, Coleman R, Walraven G. The long-term reproductive health consequences of female genital cutting in rural Gambia: a community-based survey. *Trop Med Int Health.* 2001;6:643–653.

22. Makhlouf Obermeyer C. The health consequences of female circumcision: science, advocacy, and standards of evidence. *Med Anthropol Q* 2003;17:394–412.

23. Snow RC. Female genital cutting: distinguishing the rights from the health agenda. *Trop Med Int Health.* 2001;6:89–91.

24. AbouZahr C. Safe Motherhood: a brief history of the global movement 1947–2002. *Br Med Bull.* 2003;67:13–25.

25. Hesketh T, Lu L, Xing ZW. The effect of China's one-child family policy after 25 years. *N Engl J Med.* 2005;353:1171–1177.

26. UNFPA, State of the World Population, 2005: The Promise of Equality: Gender Equity, Reproductive Health and the Millenium Development Goals. New York: UNFPA, 2005.

27. The Arusha Conference (the Second African Population Conference which met in Arusha, Tanzania, in 1984) adopted the Kilimanjaro Programme of Action, which provided a framework for population policies on the African continent. Recommendations said that governments should acknowledge that family planning and child spacing strengthen families, that family planning services should be incorporated into maternal health care services, that governments should ensure access to family planning for all individuals seeking it and should offer services at free or subsidized prices, and that a variety of family planning methods should be made available to users.

28. United Nations. *Fertility, Contraception, and Population Policies.* 25 April 2003 (ESA/WP.182).

29. UNFPA also supports broader UN goals like universal primary education for both boys and girls, reducing maternal and infant mortality, increasing life expectancy, and reducing HIV infection rates.

CHAPTER 5

The Health of Special Populations

Key Points:
- Racial, ethnic, religious, and tribal minorities may face intentional or unintentional health care discrimination.
- Immigrants, refugees, and displaced populations have special health needs during the cycle of displacement.
- Prisoners have a high risk of contracting infectious diseases and sustaining injuries caused by violence.
- People with mental illnesses or physical impairments need specialty care and support from their families and communities.
- Aging is a growing global concern.

Access to health care is obviously correlated with wealth, prestige, and education, but it is also related to power. Power is conferred in some cases by political position and in some cases by economic position. Government officials may have the authority to demand certain services, and business leaders may have the money and connections to access care that is denied to others. Sometimes power is conferred by cultural systems. A tribal or religious leader may have the power to mobilize people and resources at will. A husband may have power to control his wife's movements and activities.

Powerful people can choose to limit or grant access to goods like property, technology, social networks, and health care. In a given population, some people may have the power to secure health for themselves and their families while others without power will have limited or no access to the resources they need to be safe and healthy. This chapter highlights several population groups that often do not have the power to demand access to an equitable level of health: ethnic, racial, religious, and tribal minorities, immigrants, refugees, and internally displaced populations, prisoners, people with mental illness, people with physical impairments, and older persons.

ETHNIC, RACIAL, RELIGIOUS, AND TRIBAL MINORITIES

Ethnicity is based on many dimensions of cultural heritage, tribal affiliation, nationality, race, religion, and language. **Race** refers to artificial categories that group individuals based primarily on physical attributes like skin color. Race is a less important factor for health than ethnicity since there is great cultural and genetic diversity present within "racial" groups.

At best, celebrating one's own cultural traditions and the cultural traditions of others can be a bridge between people with diverse backgrounds. At worst, ethnicity can be used to divide people and can lead to abuse, violence, hate crimes, war, and genocide.

In medical practice, a patient's ethnic identity may give doctors important clues about dietary, behavioral, and genetic risk factors for disease. Many genetic disorders have a higher prevalence in specific population groups. Tay-Sachs disease, a fatal neurological disease that presents in young children, is mostly found among people whose ancestors were Jews from Eastern Europe. Sickle cell anemia is more common in people of African, African-American, and Mediterranean heritage. A variety of rare genetic diseases are only known to exist among the Amish, a Christian sect that has lived in isolation from outsiders for centuries and whose members only marry other members. Response to drug therapy may also vary based on genetics, so some new treatments are now being targeted to specific population groups. In 2004, the FDA approved BiDil, a heart drug that is particularly effective in patients who self-identify as black. BiDil became the first drug targeted to a particular racial group to be approved by the FDA (U.S. Food and Drug Administration) for use in the United States.[1]

In some cases, however, people who belong to racial, ethnic, tribal, or religious minority groups may also face health care discrimination along with language, cultural, and belief barriers. The lower standard of care given to members of minority groups can be unintentional. Medical practitioners may be unfamiliar with the special health needs of patients from other backgrounds, and patients may be uncomfortable discussing health concerns and being examined by a doctor who is not a member of their group. For example, women from traditional cultural and religious sects may be uncomfortable being examined by a male doctor. In some cases, however, barriers to health care access are legally sanctioned, as when proof of legal residency is required before health care can be offered.

Because of these barriers to accessing health care, the health status of minority populations tends to be worse than that of the majority populations.

Indigenous peoples—the more than 300 million people who are descendents of the peoples who lived in a geographic area prior to colonization and who have maintained their own cultural institutions—tend to have especially low health status compared to other residents of their countries. They are more likely to be poor than their non-indigenous neighbors, to have higher rates of death and disease, and to have a lower life expectancy at birth (Table 5-1).[2]

The corollary to this, of course, is that some ethnic groups experience significantly better health than others. For example, a study of tribal health in Africa identified several groups with significantly better child health outcomes than the general population, such as a greatly reduced under-5 child mortality rate.[3] These tribes also generally had a higher percent of women attending school, a higher percent of husbands with a modern (professional, technical, managerial, clerical, or skilled manual) occupation, a higher percent of dwellings with electricity, and a higher percent of completely immunized children.

Minority populations may also unintentionally receive sub-standard care because medical research focuses on common conditions rather than diseases that affect smaller population groups. For example, in the United States African-American women diagnosed with breast cancer are more likely than

Table 5-1. Life Expectancy at Birth for Indigenous and Non-Indigenous Populations in Selected Countries.

Country (Year)	Population	Male	Female
Australia (2001)	Indigenous (Aborigine)	59.4	64.8
	Non-Indigenous	76.6	82.0
Canada (2000)	First Nations	68.9	76.6
	All Canadians	76.3	81.8
New Zealand (2002)	Māori	69.0	73.2
	non-Māori	77.2	81.9
United States (2001)	American Indian / Alaskan Native	67.4	74.2
	White	74.8	80.0

Data Sources: Australian Bureau of Statistics and Australian Institute of Health and Welfare, The Health and Welfare of Australia's Aboriginal and Torres Strait Islander Peoples 2005, 2005. Health Canada, A Statistical Profile on the Health of First Nations in Canada for the Year 2000. Statistics New Zealand, New Zealand Life Tables 2000–2002, July 2004. Bramley D, Hebert P, Tuzzio L, Chassin M. Disparities in indigenous health: a cross-country comparison between New Zealand and the United States. *Am J Public Health.* 2005;95:844–850.

white women with breast cancer to have estrogen-receptor negative (ER−) tumors.[4] ER− tumors are associated with a higher death rate than ER+ tumors because ER− tumors do not respond to standard breast cancer chemotherapies. But because ER− tumors occur in relatively few women they have not been the focus of the same level of research as ER+ tumors.

Some members of minority groups, however, may be cautious about participating in medical research because of a history of unethical research in marginalized populations. One of the worst examples from the United States is the Tuskegee Syphilis Experiment, which was conducted by the U.S. Public Health Service in Alabama for forty years beginning in 1932. Nearly 400 African-American men with late-stage syphilis were offered "free medical care" by doctors who were conducting a study on the progression of the disease; the men were not told that they had syphilis and were denied antibiotics even after penicillin became the standard treatment for the disease in 1947. Treatment was provided only after a major newspaper reported on the study in 1972; by this time, many of the men had died of syphilis and many of their wives had been infected. Studies today require extensive oversight by an ethics committee, and participants must be made fully aware of the risks of participation before providing an *informed consent* to participate. The tragic legacy of the Tuskegee syphilis study is a resulting distrust of the health system by many African-Americans, which contributes to the propagation of health inequities by reducing the number of African-Americans willing to participate in clinical trials.

IMMIGRANTS, REFUGEES, AND INTERNALLY DISPLACED PEOPLE

People move from one community or country to another for a variety of reasons. Some move voluntarily to be closer to family, to start a new job, or to pursue educational opportunities, while others are forced to move because of violence, persecution, or natural disasters. Some migrants intend to permanently settle in their new host country, while others are temporary guest workers and expatriates. Thus, it is impossible to speak generically about the health effects of migration. Some immigrants may experience an increase in access to health when they move from a country with a poor health infrastructure to a country with an easily accessible health care system. Others immigrants may experience reduced access to health care in their new community because of low incomes, the need to work long hours, language barriers, or lack of health insurance.[5]

Some immigrants have special refugee status. A **refugee** is a person who has been forced to involuntarily move because of security concerns like war, civil conflict, political strife, or persecution based on race, tribe, religion, political affiliation, or membership in some other group. At the beginning of a refugee migration, UNHCR, the office of the United Nations High Commissioner for Refugees, and other humanitarian organizations, both governmental and private, attempt to provide for the basic needs of refugees including shelter, food, water, sanitation, and medical care. The long-term goal is to find durable (lasting) solutions by helping refugees to repatriate if possible, or to integrate into their countries of asylum or resettlement. UNHCR reported 9.4 million refugees worldwide at the end of 2005, the lowest number since 1980.[6]

To be classified as a refugee by the United Nations, a person must have crossed an international border. An **internally displaced person (IDP)** who fled his or her home community because of civil war, famine, natural disaster, or another crisis, but did not cross into another country is not afforded the same protection and assistance. IDPs may have the same health needs as refugees, but these special needs cannot be addressed by groups like UNHCR because of their classification status. There were estimated to be nearly 24 million IDPs worldwide at the end of 2005; 70% to 80% of the IDPs were women and children.[7]

Refugees, IDPs, and people who have survived a natural disaster such as an earthquake, hurricane, tsunami, tornado, mudslide, or flood, or have fled from an area of drought, famine, or war, all share the experience of having lost their homes, jobs, social support networks, and some of their independence and sense of security. Special health concerns are associated with different stages of the *cycle of displacement*, which begins at the onset of a complex emergency and continues until a lasting solution is implemented. Emergency interventions focus on the provision of water, food, sanitation, shelter, fuel, and health care for sick, pregnant, and vulnerable individuals. Acute malnutrition tends to be higher among refugees than nationals[8] and displaced populations may have mortality rates up to ten times higher than those of the local population.[9] Violence and lack of security may also be key concerns, and involuntary migrants may develop mental health disorders as a result of their traumatic experience.

Communities that are hosting displaced people or migrants may also have special health concerns related to having new members in their population. One risk is that infectious disease outbreaks might occur as the host community is exposed for the first time to infectious agents carried by the migrant population. Smallpox and other infectious diseases were carried by European explorers to the Americas starting in the fifteenth century and ended up causing the death of a huge percentage of the indigenous American population. Another concern is that when a large number of displaced people move to one town or city, they may overwhelm the social service providers and strain the resources of the host community.

Later relief efforts focus on finding longer-term solutions to homelessness and displacement. Displaced people who return to their home communities may face long-term challenges because of the destruction of homes, health care facilities, and other community buildings like schools, the loss of farmland to environmental damage and hazards like unexploded ordnance, and the displacement of their family members, neighbors, and other members of their community. Displaced people who settle in new areas often face challenges associated with learning new cultural practices, overcoming language and communication barriers, having limited occupational options, and potentially having limited access to health care. No matter where involuntary migrants settle, they are at risk of developing post-traumatic stress disorder (PTSD) and may develop chronic conditions related to illnesses or injuries sustained during their displacement.

PRISONERS

On any day an estimated 8 million to 10 million people across the globe are incarcerated, and 4 to 6 times that number spend time in jail over the course of a year.[10] In addition to housing convicted criminals, prisons and detention centers house suspects waiting for trial, juvenile offenders, and illegal immigrants. Many people entering prison already have health problems related to mental illness, drug abuse, malnutrition, and poverty. Severe overcrowding, poor ventilation, poor nutrition, unhygienic conditions, lack of access to medical care, abuse by guards, and prisoner-on-prisoner violence, including beatings and sexual assault, facilitate the spread of disease within prisons. Contracting potentially life-threatening infections is not part of any prisoner's sentence, and it is considered unjust to not provide incarcerated people with medical care, protection from infectious diseases, adequate nutrition, and safe conditions. Prisoners are entitled to all fundamental human rights, and need to be protected from abuse, starvation, medical neglect, forced medical experimentation, and other civil rights violations.

Tuberculosis has become a major health crisis in prisons, especially in the former Soviet Union, Brazil, and India. TB spreads easily in crowded prison blocks, and late diagnosis and inadequate treatment mean that prisoners with TB may have a contagious form of the disease for lengthy periods of time. Furthermore, because multiple strains of TB circulate in every population, each prisoner may become infected with several TB strains. This has contributed to the emergence of multidrug-resistant TB (MDR-TB), which is not cured by the standard antibiotics used to treat TB. The prevalence of TB in prisons has been reported to be up to 100 times higher than in civilian populations (Figure 5-1), and prison-acquired TB accounts for more than 25% of all TB cases in some countries.[11] An increase in TB in prisons will also increase the amount of TB in the general population, because once persons infected with TB are released from prison, they may

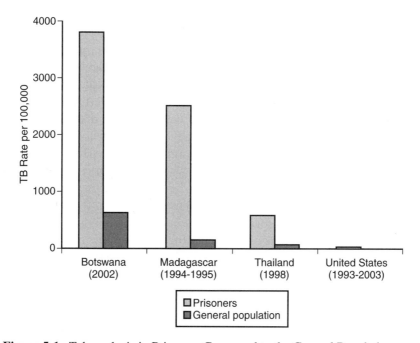

Figure 5-1. Tuberculosis in Prisoners Compared to the General Population.

Data Sources: CDC. Rapid assessment of tuberculosis in a large prison system—Botswana, 2002. *MMWR Morb Mortal Wkly Rep* 2003;52:250–252. Rasolofo-Razanamparany V, Ménard D, Ratsitorahina M, Aurégan G, Gicquel B, Chanteau S. Transmission of tuberculosis in the prison of Antananarivo (Madagascar). *Res Microbiology* 2000;151:785–795. Sretrirutchai S, Silapapojakul K, Palittapongarnpim P, Phongdara A, Vuddhakul V. Tuberculosis in Thai prisons: magnitude, transmission and drug susceptibility. *Int J of Tuberc Lung Dis* 2002;6:208–214. MacNeil JR, Lobato MN, Moore M. An unanswered health disparity: tuberculosis among correctional inmates, 1993 through 2003. *Am J Public Health* 2005;95:1800–1805.

spread TB to their family and friends. To prevent further increases in the prevalence of TB in prisons, it is important for every case of TB in prisoners to be detected early and treated consistently with no interruptions in antibiotic therapy.

PERSONS WITH MENTAL ILLNESS

Mental illnesses include anxiety disorders, mood disorders, impulse-control disorders, substance abuse, and schizophrenia and other delusional disorders (Table 5-2). Developmental disorders (like mental retardation), autism spectrum disorders, neurological disorders (like epilepsy, a seizure disorder), and dementia (often associated with Alzheimer's disease or other neurological diseases) also have mental health components. People with chronic physical ailments are vulnerable to mental illness, and people with mental health conditions often develop other health issues because of their mental illness.

Some mental health disorders cause only occasional interference with normal activities, but others are severe and cause extreme disability. For example, people with schizophrenia may have distorted perceptions of reality (including hallucinations and delusions) that cause them to behave strangely and isolate themselves from others. People with severe depression may not have the energy to get out of bed, eat, go to work, meet with friends, or conduct other normal daily activities.

A survey of mental health in 14 diverse countries found that between 1% and 5% of the populations of most countries had serious mental illnesses, and 9% to 17% of those surveyed reported having at least one episode of a mental illness in the twelve months before the survey.[12] Worldwide, an estimated 450 million people have a psychiatric disorder, including 121 million with depression, 70 million with alcohol dependence, 37 million with dementia, and 24 million with schizophrenia.[13] The World Health Organization estimates that 5 of the 10 leading causes of disability worldwide in 15- to 44-year-olds are psychiatric conditions: unipolar depression, alcohol use disorders, self-inflicted injuries, schizophrenia, and bipolar disorder (formerly called manic depression). Mental and behavioral disorders account for at least 12% of the global burden of disease, and cause as many days of lost work as physical illnesses. Nearly 1 million people commit suicide each year, and 10 million to 20 million make a suicide attempt.

In many societies, people with mental illness are treated badly.[14] They may be imprisoned or involuntarily detained in hospitals for long periods

Table 5-2. Types of Mental Illnesses.

Type of Disorder	Examples
Disorders usually first diagnosed in infancy, childhood, or adolescence	• Mental retardation • Learning, motor skills, and communication disorders • Pervasive developmental disorders like autism and Asperger's • Attention-deficit and disruptive behavior disorders like attention-deficit hyperactivity disorder (ADHD), conduct disorder, and oppositional-defiant disorder • Tic disorders like Tourette's
Cognitive Disorders	• Dementia (due to Parkinson's disease, Alzheimer's, or other causes)
Substance Abuse and Dependence Disorders	• Alcohol abuse • Drug abuse with amphetamines, caffeine, cannabis, cocaine, hallucinogens, inhalants, nicotine, opioids, phencyclidines, sedatives, hypnotics, or anxiolytics
Schizophrenia and other psychotic disorders	• Schizophrenia • Delusional disorder
Mood Disorders	• Major depressive disorder • Bipolar disorder
Anxiety Disorders	• Panic disorder • Phobias • Obsessive-compulsive disorder (OCD) • Posttraumatic stress disorder
Impulse-Control Disorders	• Anorexia nervosa • Bulimia nervosa • Pathological gambling

Source: American Psychiatric Association, DSM-IV (Diagnostic and Statistical Manual of Mental Disorders, 4th edition).

of time without any legal recourse, or they may be denied access to hospitalization when it is needed. Some people with mental illness are subjected to forced labor and some are physically or sexually abused. And because of poverty and discrimination, many people with mental illness do not have access to the health care that could improve both their mental and physical health.

Many mental illnesses are treatable. Medications can relieve symptoms and prevent relapse, therapy can help patients understand and change their thoughts and behaviors, and social rehabilitation that focuses on practical skills can help people with mental illnesses return to normal living activities. Unfortunately, mental health therapies are extremely underused (Figure 5-2). Many people do not know that help is available and do not seek treatment. For others, fear of the stigma of being diagnosed with a mental illness prevents them from seeking treatment. And some people who would like mental health assistance do not have access to a mental health specialist. In most African and Asian countries, there are more than 100,000 people for every psychiatrist.[15] And since risk factors for mental illness include living in poverty, experiencing a conflict or disaster, and having a major physical disease, the populations that have the greatest need for mental health services often have the least access to them.

The actions for improving mental health care recommended by the World Health Organization include educating the public about mental illness, providing mental health treatment as part of primary health care, and involving communities and families in caring for people with mental illnesses. When a support system is in place and public sectors like the education and justice systems are prepared to work with persons with mental disorders, an

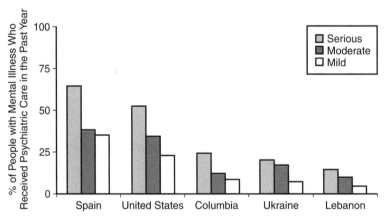

Figure 5-2. Proportion of People with Mental Illness Who Received Medical Treatment for Their Mental Health Condition in the Past Year.

Data Source: The WHO World Mental Health Survey Consortium. Prevalence, severity, and unmet need for treatment of mental disorders in the World Health Organization World Mental Health Surveys. *JAMA* 2004;291:2581–2590.

environment can be created in which most people with mental illnesses can participate in the economy, be included in social events, and be protected from discrimination and violence.[16]

Measuring the Burden of Disease

The **DALY** (disability-adjusted life year) is a way of estimating the burden of disease in a population by assigning weights to the average amount of years lost to disability and death due to various causes.[17] Chronic conditions— including mental health disorders—that limit productivity for lengthy periods of time and diseases that kill children, who would have had decades of productive life remaining had they survived, are given extra weight. The main criticism of DALYs is the difficulty in assigning weights to the burden caused by various illnesses and impairments. It will never be possible to assign an accurate rank order to the decrease in quality of life caused by blindness, loss of a limb, depression, a brain tumor, or asthma, because the experience of illness and disability varies based on the individual, the level of community support, living conditions, and other individual factors. However, the DALY is the best currently available tool for estimating the global burden of disease and disability, and it highlights the burden of mental health disorders.

While neuropsychiatric conditions are only estimated to account for 2.0% of deaths each year, they contribute at least 13.5% of DALYs.[18] (If self-inflicted injuries are included with neuropsychiatric conditions, then the adjusted estimates are 3.6% of deaths and 14.9% of DALYs, respectively.) Figure 5-3 shows the burden of disease by WHO region using the DALY as the measurement of disease burden. (You may want to compare this data for DALYs to the data for deaths presented in Figure 2-6.)

PERSONS WITH PHYSICAL IMPAIRMENTS

Impairment of anatomy (structure) or physiology (function) can affect any part of the body and may lead to activity limitations and participation restrictions. Common impairments include anatomical differences or physiological dysfunction in the skeletal, muscular, or nervous systems, intellectual or cognitive impairments, and sensory impairments that affect vision, hearing, and speech. Some impairments are present at birth and others are the result of infection (such as paralysis from polio or deafness from

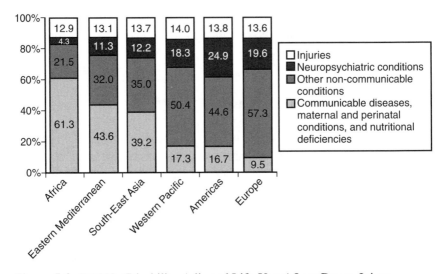

Figure 5-3. DALYs (Disability-Adjusted Life-Years) Lost Due to Injury, Non-communicable Disease (Including Neuropsychiatric Conditions), and Communicable Disease by WHO Region.

The small percentage of DALYs attributable to neuropsychiatric conditions in Africa is not because few Africans have mental health disorders but because so many Africans suffer disability and premature death due to infectious diseases and other conditions.

Data Source: WHO, Global Burden of Disease database, 2006 update.

measles), malnutrition (such as blindness caused by vitamin A deficiency), injury (such as those caused by traffic accidents, landmines, or burns), or age-associated degeneration.

A distinction is made between impairments and disabilities. **Disability** is both a health condition and a social context in which a person with impairment interacts with other people, institutions, and the environment (Figure 5-4).

One way of measuring disability is to ask how much "functional impairment" is caused by the physical impairment (Table 5-3). In other words, does the condition cause extreme limitation in personal activities and participation in society or relatively little limitation? Does the person with the condition require assistance from other people for the completion of daily activities or is the person independent? Can the person with the condition fully participate in social events or is the person marginalized?

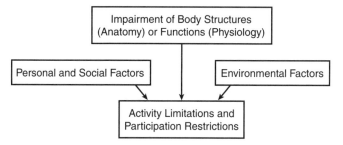

Figure 5-4. The Relationship Between Impairments and Disabilities (Activity Limitations and Participation Restrictions).

A second consideration is the environment and resources available for people with physical impairments (Table 5-4). A person who uses a wheelchair may only have minor limitations in access to buildings in the United States, but may find it impossible to navigate the unpaved pathways of rural Nigeria. A Canadian with a visual impairment may have access to books through Braille editions, electronic magnifiers, and books on tape, but a similarly impaired person in Sri Lanka may not have access to any of these tools. Poverty also limits access to resources, and disabled people and their families are more likely to be poor than people without disabilities. Disabilities are expensive because there are direct costs related to treatment, the disabled person may be unable to work, and caregivers may have to limit their paid employment and home productivity or hire others to provide care. Disabled people may also have fewer opportunities to escape poverty because they are often denied access to education, employment, and public services.

Another way to measure disability is to look at the duration of the impairment. Is the condition permanent or short-term? A person with a severe spinal cord injury will probably have life-long paralysis, but a broken bone will heal. Here, too, there are significant differences between high-income and low-income populations. Some conditions that are considered permanent disabilities in low-income regions are preventable or treatable in other parts of the world. Cataracts are the most common cause of blindness in older adults, but can be surgically corrected. Arthritis (swelling of the joints) may not be able to be cured, but the pain of arthritis can be managed with medications. Infections like onchocerciasis (river blindness) and trachoma that can cause blindness can be prevented or treated early so that they do not progress to an advanced stage.

Table 5-3. Domains of Activity and Participation.

Domain	Activities
Learning and applying knowledge	Watching, listening, learning to read, learning to write, learning to calculate, solving problems
General tasks and demands	Undertaking a single task, undertaking multiple tasks
Communication	Receiving spoken messages, receiving non-verbal messages, speaking, producing non-verbal messages, conversation
Mobility	Lifting and carrying objects, fine hand use (picking up, grasping), walking, moving around using equipment (wheelchair, skates, etc.), using transportation (car, bus, train, plane, etc.), driving (riding bicycle and motorcycle, driving car, etc.)
Self care	Washing oneself (bathing, drying, washing hands, etc.), caring for body parts (brushing teeth, shaving, grooming, etc.), toileting, dressing, eating, drinking, looking after one's health
Domestic life	Acquisition of goods and services (shopping, etc.), preparation of meals (cooking, etc.), doing housework (cleaning house, washing dishes, laundry, ironing, etc.), assisting others
Interpersonal interactions and relationships	Basic interpersonal interactions, complex interpersonal interactions, relating with strangers, formal relationships, informal social relationships, family relationships, intimate relationships
Major life areas	Informal education, school education, higher education, remunerative employment, basic economic transactions, economic self-sufficiency
Community, social, and civic life	Community life, recreation and leisure, religion and spirituality, human rights, political life and citizenship

Source: International Classification of Functioning, Disability, and Health (ICF).[19]

Early intervention is especially important for children with special needs. Babies with cleft lip or cleft palate, which is when the upper lip or the roof of the mouth is split in two, may require surgery to be able to suck properly and receive adequate nutrition. Children born with cerebral palsy, spina bifida, or other anatomical birth defects can develop their motor skills

Table 5-4. Environmental Characteristics That Relate to Activities and Participation.

Environment	Environmental Characteristics
Products and technology	For personal consumption (food, medicines), for personal use in daily living, for personal indoor and outdoor mobility and transportation, products for communication; design, construction, and building materials of buildings for public use and buildings for private use
Natural environment and human-made changes to environment	Climate, light, sound
Support and relationships	Immediate family, friends, acquaintances, peers, colleagues, neighbors, community members, people in positions of authority, personal care providers and personal assistants, health professionals
Attitudes	Individual attitudes of immediate family members, friends, personal care providers and personal assistants, health professionals; societal attitudes; social norms, practices, and ideologies
Services, systems, and policies	Housing, communication, transportation, legal, social, health, education and training, labor and employment

Source: International Classification of Functioning, Disability, and Health (ICF).

to the fullest potential only if they have physical therapy and the use of braces, crutches, and walkers at an early age. Language and communication skills are learned best in the early years (until about age 7), so children who are deaf or hearing impaired do best when they develop communication skills as early as possible. Children with other sensory impairments, such as blindness or visual impairments, or with developmental disorders also benefit from early therapy that focuses on skills such as mobility, orientation (the ability to locate oneself in space), and communication. Unfortunately many parents do not have the resources or ability to have their children start therapy at an early age and do not know what therapy to provide at home for their children. And they may not be able to demand access to education for their disabled children, even when the children are capable and intelligent.

Older children and adults of all ages who have physical impairments can benefit from access to appropriate physical therapy, occupational therapy, speech therapy, and other types of rehabilitation. For example, people who have had a stroke can re-learn language and self-care skills, especially if they receive therapy within days after the stroke. Access to assistive medical devices, such as prosthetics for people with a missing arm or leg, orthotics and braces for people with certain types of musculoskeletal disorders, hearing aids, and glasses, is also crucial. Most importantly, people with physical impairments benefit from being included to the fullest extent possible in the activities of their families, schools, workplaces, and communities.

Landmines

Although the number of landmine injuries each year is relatively small when compared to the number of injuries caused by road traffic accidents, burns, and other unintentional causes, landmines are worthy of special attention because they are an intentional and persistent environmental hazard. Landmines and other unexploded ordinance buried during wartime remain hazards to workers, children, and communities long after the conflict is over—which means, among many other problems, that lots of potential farm land is unable to be used because of the risk of encountering a mine while clearing a field. Most people injured by landmines are civilians. Men are often at greatest risk because they spend more time outside and are involved in farming and other occupations with a high likelihood of mine contact. Children are also at risk because they may not know how to recognize mines and may pick them up and even play with them. Landmines are a problem in many countries throughout the world (Figure 5-5).

Landmine Monitor, an international voluntary organization that advocates for and monitors compliance with anti-mine agreements such as the "Mine Ban Treaty" (more formally called the Convention on the Prohibition of the Use, Stockpiling, Production, and Transfer of Anti-Personnel Mines and on Their Destruction), conducts annual country surveys of landmine incidents. They estimate that there are 15,000 to 20,000 new landmine casualties each year and that there may be as many as 500,000 landmine survivors, many of whom have an amputated leg or other severe damage to limbs or other body parts.[21] Although it costs only $3 to $10 to purchase and plant a mine, it costs $300 to $1000 to safely remove one.[22]

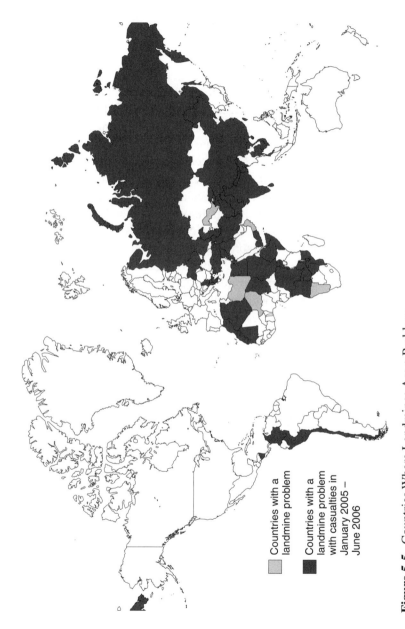

Figure 5-5. Countries Where Landmines Are a Problem.

Data Source: International Campaign to Ban Landmines, Landmine Monitor Report 2006: Toward a Mine-Free World, 2006.

More than 100 of the landmine casualties reported in 2005 were professional de-miners.

OLDER PERSONS

Many older people contribute to families and communities by taking care
of their grandchildren, providing training and guidance for younger employees, connecting younger generations to their cultural heritage, and
sharing wisdom gained from decades of life experience. However, most aging
people will eventually develop chronic health conditions that limit mobility and function. Some of the most common chronic conditions that affect
older people worldwide include cardiovascular disease, hypertension, stroke,
diabetes, cancer, chronic obstructive pulmonary disease (COPD), musculoskeletal conditions such as arthritis and osteoporosis, mental health conditions such as dementia and depression, and vision and hearing impairments.[22] The causes of death for older adults (Figure 5-6) and the mortality
rates from common non-communicable conditions (Figure 5-7) are relatively
similar for older adults in most parts of the world.

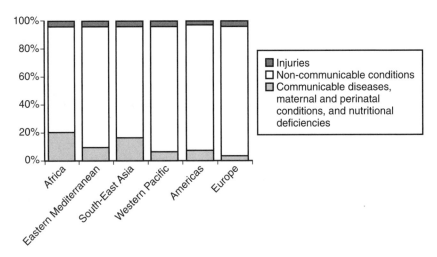

Figure 5-6. Percent of Deaths in Adults Ages 60 and Older Due to Injury,
Non-communicable Disease, and Communicable Disease by WHO Region
(2005 Estimates).

Data Source: WHO, Global Burden of Disease database, 2006 update.

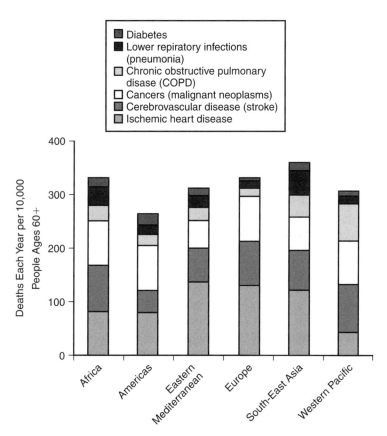

Figure 5-7. Mortality Rates per 10,000 for Several Common Causes of Death in Adults Ages 60 and Older, 2005 Estimates.

Data Source: WHO, Global Burden of Disease database, 2006 update

The health of older people is a function of a lifetime of behaviors such as tobacco and alcohol use, physical activity, healthy eating, oral health, and adherence to prescribed medical regimens.[23] Personal characteristics like biology and genetics and psychological factors also play a role. In all cases, a safe physical environment—one with clean water, clean air, and safe foods, and barrier-free housing that helps prevent falls—and a social support system are key to extending health into old age.

Arthritis, nervous system disorders like Parkinson's Disease (which causes tremors), and decreasing muscle and bone strength may result in limitations in the ability to complete normal daily functions like personal care, such as bathing and dressing, and managing a home by making meals, cleaning, and completing other tasks (Table 5-5). Mental health problems like dementia, a syndrome that leads to impaired cognitive functions, reasoning, speech, and memory, may also limit the ability of an older person to live independently and without assistance.

Declining fertility (the number of children born to each woman) and increasing life expectancy have drastically increased the percentage of the world population that is 65-years-old or older (Figure 5-8). The number of people aged 60 and over worldwide is expected to increase from 600 million in 2000 to 1.2 billion in 2025 and 2 billion in 2050.[24] Because older people are more likely than younger adults to have health problems, the increasing proportion of older adults is putting stress on health care systems. Few countries are prepared to care for a rapidly increasing number of older people with chronic illnesses and disabilities.

Staying with family is often the preference of both older people and their families. In most of the world, care of the elderly is provided by spouses,

Table 5-5. Activities of Daily Living.

Activities of Daily Living (ADLs): *Self-Care*	Instrumental Activities of Daily Living (IADLs): *Independence*
Dressing	Shopping
Eating	Housekeeping
Ambulating (mobility)	Accounting (personal finances)
Toileting	Food preparation
Hygiene	Transportation

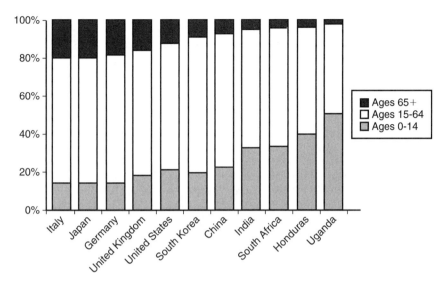

Figure 5-8. Population Distribution by Age Group, 2004.
Data Source: UNDP, Human Development Report 2006.

children, and other family members, and institutionalization of older people is uncommon. But decreasing fertility rates mean that there are fewer young people to care for the aging, and the increasing number of women who work outside the home also limits the number of people available to provide in-home care. This is creating challenges for older adults, caregivers, health care systems, and national pension systems. In Japan and much of Europe, national pension programs are on the verge of collapse because there are not enough young workers paying in to the programs to support retirees sufficiently. The age of retirement is increasing, while benefits are cut.

In developing countries where retirement accounts and pension plans are not the norm, aging is expected to become a major social issue. The migration of young rural people to cities means that adult children often live far from their aging parents and cannot provide daily care, and few families have the ability to hire additional care-givers or nursing assistants. More than two-thirds of older people live in the developing world, and this is expected to increase to 75% by 2025.[25] Concern over ability to support older persons is a growing problem in China and Russia, and will become a concern in Latin America and other parts of Asia in coming decades. All countries need to begin planning for the care of aging populations.

REFERENCES

1. FDA News, "FDA Approves BiDil Heart Failure Drug for Black Patients," P05–32, 23 June 2005.
2. United Nations Development Programme, 2004. Human Development Report.
3. Brockerhoff M, Hewett P. Inequality of child mortality among ethnic groups in sub-Saharan Africa. *Bull World Health Organ.* 2000;78:30–41.
4. Anderson WF, Chatterjee N, Ershler WB, Brawley OW. Estrogen receptor breast cancer phenotypes in the Surveillance, Epidemiology, and End Results database. *Breast Cancer Res Treat.* 2002;76:27–36.
5. World Health Organization, "International Migration, Health and Human Rights," Health and Human Rights Publication Series, Issue No. 4, December 2003.
6. UNHCR, "2005 Global Refugee Trends: Statistical overview of populations of refugees, asylum-seekers, internally displaced persons, stateless persons, and other persons of concern to UNHCR," 9 June 2006.
7. Internal Displacement Monitoring Centre, "Internal Displacement: A Global Overview of Trends and Developments in 2005," March 2006.
8. UNHCR Standing Committee Report on Nutrition, 2006 (EC/57/SC/CRP.17).
9. World Health Organization—Health Action in Crises, Annual Report 2005.
10. World Health Organization, "Tuberculosis in prisons."
11. Ibid.
12. The WHO World Mental Health Survey Consortium. Prevalence, severity, and unmet need for treatment of mental disorders in the World Health Organization World Mental Health Surveys, *JAMA,* 2004;291:2581–2590.
13. Unless otherwise noted, all statistics on mental health in this section are from the World Health Organization, World Health Report 2001: Mental Health: New Understanding, New Hope, WHO Press: Geneva, Switzerland, 2004.
14. The WHO Resource Book on Mental Health, Human Rights and Legislation, published in 2005, details poor treatment of mentally ill persons and provides a guide to creating laws that protect the human rights of all people regardless of health status.
15. A psychiatrist is a physician who is trained to provide mental health care and prescribe appropriate medications. Other mental health specialists, like psychologists, provide counseling but usually do not have the authority to prescribe drugs.
16. Helen Herrman, Shekhar Saxena, and Rob Moodie, eds. Promoting mental health: concepts, emerging evidence, practice: report of the World Health Organization, Department of Mental Health and Substance Abuse in collaboration with the Victorian Health Promotion Foundation and the University of Melbourne. Geneva: WHO, 2005.
17. The DALY was first introduced in the 1993 World Development Report.
18. World Health Organization, Global Burden of Disease database, 2006 update.
19. The International Classification of Functioning, Disability, and Health (ICF) is a series of guidelines for assessing disability. For example, the ICF has codes for indicating changes in body structure such as total absence, partial absence, additional part, aberrant dimensions, discontinuity, or deviating position. The full code is available online.
20. International Campaign to Ban Landmines, Landmine Monitor Report 2006: Toward a Mine-Free World, 2006.

21. United Nations Mine Clearance and Policy Unit, "Landmines Factsheet," September 1997.
22. World Health Organization, "Active Ageing: A Policy Framework," WHO/NMH/NPH/02.8.
23. Ibid.
24. World Health Organization, "The world is fast ageing—have we noticed?" http://www.who.int/ageing/en/.
25. Ibid.

CHAPTER 6

The Spread
of Infectious Diseases

Key Points:
- Infection transmission is related to an infectious agent's mode of transmission, reservoir, and cycle of infection.
- Not all exposures cause infection and not all infections cause disease.
- Infections may be caused by bacteria, viruses, protozoa, worms, other types of parasites, fungi, and prions.
- Antimicrobial resistance is making it harder to treat infections that were once easily cured with medication.
- A major goal of public health is to control the spread of infectious diseases.

Most North Americans and Europeans would consider cancer, heart disease, or perhaps diabetes to be their number one health concern. Few would mention infectious diseases as a top priority, unless there was a major infectious disease outbreak getting a lot of media attention. This happens occasionally when there are new fears about the emergence of a particularly bad influenza strain (like the H5N1 strain of "bird flu") or there is an outbreak linked to a food product or restaurant chain. These worries usually fade quickly. But in many parts of the world infectious diseases remain the greatest threat to health, and are responsible for a large percentage of deaths in children, the poor, and other underserved groups (Figure 6-1). This fact alone is a very good reason to care deeply about developing new methods for and increasing access to prevention and treatment. We also need to be concerned about infectious diseases because they can spread and adapt quickly, and they have the potential to affect nearly everyone. Infectious diseases are clearly associated with patterns of social interaction, and the network of human contacts is becoming more and more complex all the time as modern transportation allows travel to anywhere in the world within about 24 hours. Global health professionals must know how infectious diseases are transmitted and how they can be contained.

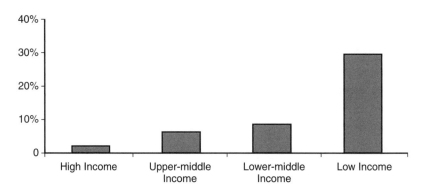

Figure 6-1. Percent of Deaths Due to Infectious and Parasitic Diseases, by Income Group, 2005 Estimates.

Data Source: WHO, Global Burden of Disease database, 2006 update.

INFECTION TRANSMISSION

An infectious agent can be transmitted to a susceptible human through several different **modes of transmission** (Table 6-1). Direct transmission, also called person-to-person transmission, occurs when a susceptible person touches an infectious person's lesions, blood, or body fluid, or is close enough to breathe in the droplets expelled when a sick person coughs, sneezes, or breathes. Direct transmission can also occur through

Table 6-1. Examples of Modes of Transmission.

Mode of Transmission	How Infection is Acquired
Direct contact	Sexual contact, contact with an infected skin lesion or contact with blood or other body fluids, injecting drug use (IDU)
Airborne	Breathing contaminated air
Vector-borne	Spread by an animal, usually by the bite of an infected insect
Food- and water-borne	Ingesting contaminated food or water
Mother-to-child (MTC)	Passed from a pregnant woman to her baby during pregnancy or delivery or through breastmilk

sexual contact or through fecal-oral contact, which is when a person who has had contact with fecal matter touches his or her mouth, eyes, nose, or another **portal of entry**.

Some infections are airborne, which means that the pathogen can become suspended in the air because it has been aerosolized or caught in dust, and people become infected by breathing the contaminated air. Influenza, SARS, and tuberculosis are airborne diseases. To prevent a contagious person from spreading an airborne infection to susceptible people, it may be necessary to treat the patient in **isolation** by limiting his or her contact with others and by protecting other people from the air breathed out by the sick person. (If the infection causes a high rate of mortality, the sick person ought to be treated in a special "positive pressure" room where the air is vented through a filter and then outside the building and is never circulated through the ventilation system into other rooms in the hospital.) Hospitals in tropical climates often do not have indoor ventilation systems and may face a challenge when trying to isolate highly infectious patients.

Vector-borne infections are spread by insect vectors like mosquitoes, sand flies, ticks, or other animals. Malaria, Lyme disease, dengue fever, and trypanosomiasis are all transmitted through insect bites, and control of these diseases can be at least partially attained through the use of insecticides or other methods of reducing the insect population. Viruses spread by arthropods—insects and arachnids (spiders, ticks, mites)—are called arboviruses (short for arthropod-borne viruses) and include yellow fever, dengue fever, and Venezuelan equine encephalitis. Many of the insect vectors become infected by biting infected mammals. Rodents are frequent carriers of diseases such as plague and typhus fever, which are both spread by ticks. Livestock may be carriers of infectious agents, such as the ones that cause African sleeping sickness and are spread by tsetse flies. In some cases, animals may directly transmit infections to humans. For example, rabies is spread through the saliva of infected mammals, some infectious agents that cause diarrhea can be passed from livestock and pets to people, and some strains of influenza that affect humans originate in bird or mammal populations.

Other infections are vehicle-borne because they are spread through inanimate objects like food, water, and fomites (other non-living objects) like doorknobs. Cholera and hepatitis A virus are both waterborne diseases, and many infections that cause diarrhea are spread through ingestion of fecally-contaminated food.

Some diseases, such as HIV, have vertical, or mother-to-child, transmission because they can be passed from a mother to her fetus during pregnancy or delivery or to her baby through breastmilk.

To control disease in a population, several other aspects of transmission must be considered. The **reservoir** is the "home" for infectious agents (Table 6-2). Some infections, like smallpox and measles, only occur in humans. (Infectious diseases that usually occur only in humans are called anthroponoses.) Some, like West Nile virus, rabies, and influenza, can infect many types of animals. (Infectious diseases that usually occur in animals and only occasionally infect humans are called zoonoses.) Other infectious agents have an environmental reservoir and live in the soil (like hookworm) or water (like cholera). Controlling an infectious disease may require controlling animal populations or altering the environment if a disease has a non-human reservoir. If the infectious agent has an animal reservoir, it may be nearly impossible to eradicate it.

The **cycle of infection** is the way an infection is spread through different species. Measles, TB, and sexually transmitted infections exist only in humans, so we can say that the cycle of infection is human—human—human. Vectorborne infections like malaria have a human—insect—human cycle. **Zoonoses**, diseases like rabies that are usually in animals and not humans, have a vertebrate—vertebrate—vertebrate cycle, which on occasion can become a vertebrate—vertebrate—human cycle. Some infectious agents have much more complex cycles and undergo life stages in several different animal hosts. An **intermediate host** is an animal that alternates with humans as the host for an infectious agent as it undergoes reproductive stages in the various host species. For example, the snail is the intermediate host for schistosomiasis.

Each host must be considered in an infection control plan. Prevention of infection can occur by decreasing susceptibility of the human host through

Table 6-2. Reservoirs for Infectious Agents.

Reservoir	Meaning
Humans	The infectious agent is an anthroponosis usually found only in humans.
Animals	The infectious agent is a zoonosis usually found only in animals.
Soil	The infectious agent can survive in dirt.
Water	The infectious agent can survive in water.

nutrition and immunization or by decreasing contact with the infectious agent through food safety practices and hygiene. Control plans must address the type of agent, mode of transmission, reservoir, cycle of infection, availability of a vaccine or drugs, and other factors.

THE DISEASE PROCESS

An **infection** occurs when an infectious agent begins to reproduce inside a person. This usually causes an immunologic response to the specific agent, which can often be detected through laboratory testing. Not all exposures to an infectious agent cause an infection. People may be more vulnerable to infections when the ability of their immune systems to fight off infection is weakened by age, malnutrition, cancer treatments and immunosuppressive drugs, or other infections. They may be protected from infection by previous infection, by immunization, or by genetics. Sometimes an infectious agent does not have genetic characteristics that allow it to easily infect people or easily make them sick. **Infectivity** is the capacity of an infectious agent to cause infection in a susceptible human (a person who does not already have immunity to the infection). Infectivity is sometimes measured by calculating the **secondary attack rate**, which is the average number of other people that one sick person infects. Measles has a high infectivity rate because it quickly spreads through a population, but leprosy has a low infectivity rate and does not easily spread to susceptible people who do not have prolonged contact with an infectious person.[1]

Pathogenicity is the capacity of an infectious agent to cause disease in an infected human. **Disease** occurs when an infected person develops symptoms or illness. Some types of viruses that cause diarrhea have a high pathogenicity rate and cause symptoms in nearly everyone who contracts the virus.[2] In contrast, hepatitis A virus has a relatively low pathogenicity rate. Most children who are infected with hepatitis A virus remain asymptomatic (do not show disease) and develop lifelong immunity to the disease following their infection.[3]

Not all infections cause disease, so it is important to keep the difference between infection and disease clear (Table 6-3). For example, nearly one-third of the world's population has been infected with TB, but only about 10% of those infected will develop active TB disease in their lifetimes.[4]

The time it takes for a disease to present or to resolve usually follows a predictable pattern called the **natural history** of the disease (Figure 6-2). During the **incubation period** when the infectious agent multiplies in the

Table 6-3. Exposure, Infection, and Disease.
Not all exposures cause infection and not all infections cause disease.

Term	Calculation
Infectivity	# infected / # of susceptible people exposed
Pathogenicity	# ill (diseased) / # infected
Virulence	# with severe illness or death / # with symptoms (disease)

host after infection, it may be possible to test for the presence of infection even if the infected person does not feel sick. Laboratory tests that detect early-stage infection can be critical for halting the spread of infection during outbreaks and for treating patients before they develop severe disease. Usually there is a subclinical stage following infection when a person may (or may not) be contagious but has no symptoms. Because infected people may unknowingly spread infection to others during this subclinical stage, it may be necessary during outbreaks to track down and **quarantine** (limit the movement of) sick individuals and all of their primary contacts and secondary contacts (people contacted by primary contacts). This was done in China during the 2003 SARS epidemic and helped to stop the spread of the epidemic.[5] For some kinds of infection, some people, called **carriers**, may harbor an infectious agent and spread it to others without ever showing symptoms. One of the most famous chronic carriers was "Typhoid Mary," a New York food services worker who was a long-term carrier of typhoid and infected hundreds of her customers.

After the onset of symptoms a person has clinical disease. Once symptoms develop, there are three possible outcomes: death, recovery with immunity,

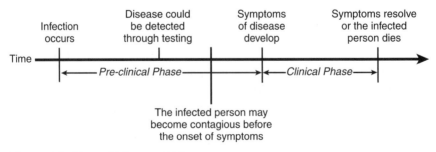

Figure 6-2. Natural History of Disease.

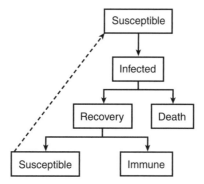

Figure 6-3. Outcomes for an Infected Individual.

or recovery without immunity (Figure 6-3). In most cases, the recovery rate is extremely high, since few infectious diseases are severe. **Virulence** is the ability of an infectious agent to cause severe disease or death in a host and is measured by the proportion of severe or fatal cases among all people who have the disease. A virulent infection will have a high **case fatality rate**. Rabies is an extremely virulent infection because no one who has been bitten by a rabid animal survives without post-bite vaccination treatment.

The body's immune system will fight off most infections even if they are left untreated. Once symptoms begin a person may seek medical care and be treated for the infection, and in some cases an infection will be fatal with or without medical intervention. Exposure to some infectious agents sparks an immune process that forms "memory" antibodies in the blood that allow the body to quickly destroy any new pathogens of the same type that may invade the body in the future. These types of infections are good candidates for vaccine development. Recovery from other infections may provide no protective immunity against future infections. These types of infections are not likely to be controlled through immunization, so prevention must focus on avoidance of exposure.

Some infections cause **acute** (short-term) disease, like influenza and the rhinoviruses that cause colds. Other infections cause **chronic** (long-term) disease, like HIV and the bacterium, *Helicobacter pylori*, that causes most stomach ulcers. Chronic infections can lead to poor nutritional status, weakness and anemia, impaired immune response, and increased susceptibility to other infections. Some chronic infections may also increase the risk of cancer. For example, hepatitis C virus increases the risk of liver cancer, schistosomiasis infection (also known as bilharzia) can cause bladder cancer, and human papillomavirus (HPV) can cause cervical cancer. Researchers expect to identify many more infectious agents that contribute to the development of cancers, which may allow for the development of more cancer vaccines, like the HPV vaccine that protects against cervical cancer.

AGENT, HOST, ENVIRONMENT

In Chapter 1, the use of person, place, and time questions in descriptive epidemiology was discussed. When the Person—Place—Time questions are applied to the study of infectious diseases, the questions that are asked are: Who are the cases? Where did the cases acquire the infection? When did the cases become infected?

Chapter 1 also discussed the use of analytic epidemiology to help investigators learn more about the conditions that cause an infection to occur and allow the infection to spread through a population. Infectious disease epidemiologists refer to an analytic epidemiology "triad"—a series of questions about the characteristics of the infectious agent, the human host, and the host's social and natural environments that facilitate the spread of the infection. The components of the Agent—Host—Environment triad are discussed below (Figure 6-4).

Agent

The infectious agent is the pathogen that causes the illness, and epidemiologists want to know what makes an agent unique. What is its type, mode of transmission, reservoir, portal of entry, cycle of infection, infectivity, virulence, pathogenicity, and natural history? An epidemiologist might also ask questions like "Does the infectious agent have a high secondary transmission rate?" and "Is the infectious agent resistant to treatment with certain drugs?"

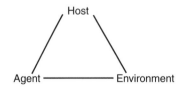

Figure 6-4. Agent—Host—Environment Triad.

There are many different types of agents that can cause infection, including bacteria, viruses, protozoa, worms, other parasites, and fungi. Different infectious agents pose different risks and require different methods of prevention and treatment.

Bacteria

Bacteria are microscopic, one-celled organisms that come in several different kinds of shapes, including rods (bacilli), spheres (cocci), and spirals (spirochetes, vibrios, and spirilla). They also can be differentiated by relative size (although all are very small) and by the amount of a substance called peptidoglycan in their cell walls. When stained with a special dye, the peptidoglycan on the surface of gram-positive bacteria will bond to the stain. Gram-negative bacteria have an outer membrane over the peptidoglycan layer so the dye will not bond.

Bacteria have been found everywhere on the planet, from the arctic tundra to hot springs deep in the ocean. They play an important role in decomposition and chemical recycling, in the fixation of nitrogen into plants, and in the production of alcohol and foods like cheese and yogurt. Millions of helpful bacteria line our digestive tract and other body parts and help make vitamins our bodies need while crowding out harmful bacteria. However, many types of bacteria can cause disease in humans (Table 6-4).

For example, *E. coli* is spread by fecal contamination of food and water, including swimming pools that are not properly maintained, and by person-to-person contact. Although many strains live in our intestines and are not harmful, some are deadly strains, like *E. coli O157:H7*, that can cause bloody diarrhea and kidney failure. Cholera is also spread through contaminated water, and because the bacteria can live in harsh environments, like ocean water and sewage, and can survive for long periods of time, cholera outbreaks have occurred in many parts of the world in recent years. Cholera infection causes severe watery diarrhea, and death can occur if rehydration and electrolyte balance cannot be maintained through fluid replacement. Typhoid, paratyphoid, shigellosis, salmonellosis, and campylobacteriosis are also diarrheal diseases spread through ingestion of fecally-contaminated food and water or the transfer of fecal matter from the hand to the mouth.

Some bacteria are spread by animals. Plague is transmitted to humans by a rodent flea. The usual symptoms of bubonic plague are swollen lymph nodes and pain, but some cases develop a more severe pneumonic plague.

Table 6-4. Examples of Infections Caused by Bacteria.[6]

Some agents could be classified under multiple features, but are only listed once.

Key Feature	Bacterial Agents
Causes diarrhea	• Campylobacteriosis (*Campylobacter jejuni*) • Cholera (*Vibrio cholerae*) • *Clostridium perfringens* • E. coli (*Escherichia coli*) • Paratyphoid fever (*Salmonella* Paratyphi) • Typhoid fever (*Salmonella* Typhi) • Salmonellosis (*Salmonella*) • Shigellosis (*Shigella dysentariae*)
Causes pneumonia	• Legionellosis (*Legionellae*)—may be spread by aerosolized water from air conditioners and humidifiers • Pneumococcal pneumonia (*Streptococcus pneumoniae*) • Psittacosis (*Chlamydia psittaci*)—spread by inhaling dried bird droppings
Can cause encephalitis or meningitis	• Leptospirosis (*Leptospira interrogans*) • Listeriosis (*Listeria monocytogenes*) • Meningococcal meningitis (*Neisseria meningitidis*)
Sexually transmitted	• Chlamydia (*Chlamydia trachomatis*) • Gonorrhea (*Neisseria gonorrhoeae*) • Syphilis (*Treponema pallidum*)
Caused by *Rickettsia*	• Typhus fever (*Rickettsia prowazekii*)—spread by fleas • Q fever (*Coxiella burnetii*) • Rocky Mountain spotted fever (*Rickettsia rickettsii*)—spread by ticks
Insect-borne	• Bartonellosis (*Bartonella bacilliformis*)—spread by sand flies (*Lutzomyia*) • Ehrlichiosis (*Ehrlichia*)—spread by ticks • Lyme disease (*Borrelia burgdorferi*)—spread by ticks (*Ixodes*)

The "Black Death" of medieval Europe was a type of plague, and it killed one-quarter to one-half of the population of affected cities.

Typhus fever is also spread by fleas that live on rats and other rodents, and causes a fever and a rash. Typhus fever is caused by a special class of infectious agents called *Rickettsia* that are cellular parasites. (Rickettsia

Table 6-4. Examples of Infections Caused by Bacteria—cont'd.
Some agents could be classified under multiple features, but are only listed once.

Key Feature	Bacterial Agents
Insect-borne—cont'd	• Plague (*Yersinia pestis*)—spread by fleas (*Xenopsylla cheopis*) • Tularemia (*Francisella tularensis*)—spread by ticks and several other insects
Spread by spores	• Anthrax (*Bacillus anthracis*) • Botulism (*Clostridium botulinum*) • Tetanus (*Clostridium tetani*)
Vaccine-preventable	• Diphtheria (*Corynebacterium diphtheriae*) • *Haemophilus influenzae* serotype b (Hib) • Pertussis/whooping cough (*Bordetella pertussis*)
Chronic seque-lae (long-term after-effects)	• Brucellosis (*Brucella abortus*, *Brucella melitensis*)—spread through ingestion of raw milk; may cause chronic relapses of disease • Buruli ulcer (*Mycobacterium ulcerans*)—causes skin lesions • Leprosy/Hansen's disease (*Mycobacterium leprae*)—causes chronic skin and nerve symptoms • *Helicobacter pylori*—causes some stomach ulcers • *Staphylococcus aureus*—can cause impetigo (skin infection), sepsis, pneumonia, toxic shock syndrome, and chronic wound infections • Group A Strep (*Streptococcus pyogenes*)—causes strep throat and impetigo (skin infection) and can cause more serious diseases like scarlet fever, toxic shock syndrome, and rheumatic fever, which can damage the heart • Trachoma (*Chlamydia trachomatis*)—can cause blindness • Tuberculosis (*Mycobacterium tuberculosis*)—chronic lung disease (can occur anywhere in body)

are sometimes classified as a distinct type of infectious agent separate from bacteria.) Typhus fever has a very high mortality rate without treatment. (Note that typhoid—a diarrheal infection—and typhus are two distinct infections.) Q fever and Rocky Mountain spotted fever are other examples of Rickettsial infections that are spread by insects.

Sexually transmitted infections (STIs) like gonorrhea and chlamydia are both often asymptomatic (causing no symptoms) but if untreated they can cause pelvic inflammatory disease (PID), which can lead to pain and to infertility in women. Syphilis, another sexually transmitted infection, can be treated in early stages when there is a chancre or rash, but if left untreated may cause weakened arterial walls and nervous system impairment.

Some bacterial infections primarily affect children. Diphtheria and pertussis, also known as whooping cough, are vaccine-preventable childhood infections. They are both spread through droplets in the air. People with whooping cough, named for the loud sound made when people with the disease inhale, may cough so hard that they break their ribs. Strep throat, an illness caused by a type of Group A *Streptococcus*, is a common childhood infection, which left untreated can lead to complications such as scarlet fever or rheumatic fever, a condition that may cause permanent damage to the valves of the heart.

Other types of bacteria can also cause chronic infections. Brucellosis can be transmitted to humans who consume dairy products that have not been pasteurized. Sometimes called undulant fever or Malta fever, brucellosis is normally a disease of cattle and goats. A person with untreated brucellosis may develop chronic fevers that last for years.

Bacteria cause illness in a variety of ways. Illness from a bacterial infection may be due to the release of endotoxins from the bacteria, which are released when the bacteria die and disintegrate. Many gastrointestinal diseases are the result of endotoxins being released from gram-negative bacteria. Some bacteria produce exotoxins, like the exotoxin produced by botulism bacilli, which can cause severe illness and death in people who eat food from cans that are contaminated with the toxin. Tetanus toxin from *Clostridium tetani* spores can cause spasms and death and is spread by "stepping on rusty nails," giving birth in unsanitary conditions, or any kind of puncture wound, but disease can be prevented with an immunization.

Some bacterial diseases are becoming less common. Leprosy, more correctly called Hansen's disease, used to be a relatively common, disfiguring disease, and people who contracted it were ostracized by their communities. Now only a few leprosy hospitals remain open. Trachoma is still the leading cause of preventable blindness in the world, but the number of new cases each year has been decreasing.[7]

Other bacterial diseases are emerging and becoming more common. *Staphylococcus aureus* causes wound infections and is developing into very difficult to treat methicillin-resistant *Staph. aureus* (MRSA). MRSA can be acquired from unsterilized hospital equipment, wrestling mats, and other everyday items. These infections can cause severe "flesh-eating" infections or even more serious systemic (internal) infections. Tuberculosis (TB) is another example of an emerging infectious disease. TB now causes more than one million deaths each year and is becoming harder to treat as multidrug-resistant TB (MDR-TB) strains become more prevalent.

Bacteria are usually susceptible to certain types of antibiotics, and will be killed when they are exposed to correct doses of the right classes of these drugs. Some bacteria, however, have developed resistance to some types of antibiotics that were once effective against them, including MRSA, MDR-TB, and some strains of sexually transmitted infections like gonorrhea.

Resistance develops because of changes in the bacterial genes. One of the main causes of the development of **antimicrobial resistance** (drug resistance in bacteria, fungi, parasites, and other microbes) seems to be the misuse of antimicrobial drugs.[8] If you have a mild bacterial infection, such as bronchitis or some ear infections, and you take antibiotics for only a few days rather than finishing the entire prescription, or you skip a couple of doses, you have killed off only the susceptible, weaker bacteria, and not the hardier bacteria (a process biologists call **selection**). The remaining bacteria may have developed resistance to the kind of drug you were taking, which makes it harder for you to fight off the infection with common antibiotics. You could also spread this hardier strain to other people, for whom the common first-line antibiotics will not work at all. Another misuse of antibiotics is taking the drugs for non-bacterial infections (like the common cold, which is caused by a virus). In this case, you are killing off helpful bacteria and allowing potentially harmful bacteria that are already in your body to proliferate. These stronger bacteria may develop drug resistance, necessitating that you take yet another antibiotic.

Viruses

Viruses are extremely tiny acellular (not cellular) parasites, which means that they are not cells themselves and can only replicate by invading the cells of a living host and taking control of the cells' nuclei. (Technically, because viruses are not cells, they are not alive.). When a virus enters the body, spikes on the outer part of the virus, called a capsid, attach to the surface of a cell. The outside of the virus is shed and the genetic material from inside the virus penetrates the cell and travels to the nucleus where it takes command. The virus directs the infected cell to make many new copies of the virus. The newly formed viruses travel to the edge of the cell and create a new capsid. When released from the cell, they travel to other cells in the body, which they infect in the same manner, or are shed to infect another person.

Influenza, colds, and many other common illnesses are viruses, as are some vaccine-preventable childhood illnesses (Table 6-5). Most children receive a series of "MMR" vaccine shots that helps them develop immunity against measles, mumps, and rubella. Measles is still a major cause of death in children in low-income countries. Mumps causes swollen salivary glands, which makes the cheeks get puffy, and can also cause brain damage and deafness. Rubella, sometimes called German measles, can harm the fetuses of pregnant women. (Appendix VII lists all currently recommended childhood immunizations. Although vaccines have been developed for many viral infections, cost limits their use in some populations.)

People who live in the tropics are also vaccinated against yellow fever, which is spread by *Aedes aegypti* mosquitoes and is named for the skin color of patients with jaundice that results when the infection makes the liver function improperly. There is also a vaccine for polio (poliomyelitis). Before the polio vaccine was available, parents lived in fear of seasonal polio outbreaks that caused paralysis in about 1% of cases and could turn an active child into an invalid overnight. Polio is slated for worldwide eradication, although the process is taking longer than expected.

Smallpox is the only disease to be eradicated by mass worldwide immunization thus far. Although no naturally transmitted infections have occurred since 1979, some of the virus is stored in laboratories and might possibly be viable (able to cause infection) if released. Smallpox lesions appear primarily on the extremities, as opposed to chickenpox, which appear primarily on the trunk. Chickenpox (varicella) is rarely fatal, but it can recur as shingles in adulthood and cause severe pain. A vaccine is now available for both chickenpox and shingles.

Most vaccines are administered before an exposure. This is the case with hepatitis B virus, which is spread through blood and body fluids and causes chronic liver disease. Because it is highly transmissible, U.S. guidelines call for vaccination of all high school athletes, people who work in health care settings or laundries, and other people who might contact body

Table 6-5. Examples of Infections Caused by Viruses.

Key Feature	Viral Agents
Vaccine-preventable	• Chickenpox (varicella) / Herpes Zoster (shingles) • Hepatitis A virus • Hepatitis B virus • HPV (human papillomavirus) • Influenza • Japanese encephalitis • Measles • Mumps • Poliomyelitis / polio • Rabies • Rotavirus • Rubella / German measles • Yellow fever
Sexually transmitted and no vaccine available	• Hepatitis C virus • Herpes simplex • HIV
Can develop into hemorrhagic fevers	• Crimean-Congo hemorrhagic fever • Dengue fever • Ebola hemorrhagic fever • Hantavirus • Lassa fever • Marburg hemorrhagic fever
Cause diarrhea	• Coronaviruses • Norovirus • Parvoviruses
Cause encephalitis (swelling of the brain) and no vaccine available	• Eastern equine encephalitis • Hendra virus • Nipah virus • St. Louis encephalitis • Venezuelan equine encephalitis (VEE) • West Nile virus • Western equine encephalitis
Others	• Chikungunya fever • Mononucleosis • Rhinovirus (colds) • Viral meningitis • Warts

fluids. (The vaccine is expensive, so people from low-income households may not be able to afford it.)

Some vaccines can prevent disease after a known exposure. Rabies is a disease of mammals spread by bites from rabid animals. The virus in their saliva spreads through nerves to the spinal cord and brain, where it multiplies rapidly over several weeks and causes dementia then death. It is 100% fatal if a post-bite series of immunizations is not received.

Many sexually transmitted infections (STIs), including HIV, herpes (HSV-2, herpes simplex virus), hepatitis C virus, and human papillomavirus are viruses. A vaccine for HPV is now available in some countries, but no vaccine has been developed for HIV, herpes, or HCV. There is no cure for these infections, and once a person is infected he or she will always have the infection. Some drugs, like interferon, can help suppress infection but will not cure it. (HIV is discussed in detail in the next chapter.)

Viral infections can never be cured by taking antibiotics. Most viral infections will go away on their own. In some cases, it might be possible to take drugs that reduce the number of virus particles present in the body and help mitigate symptoms. For example, antiviral drugs can slow the progression of HIV infection, suppress the lesions caused by herpes virus, and make influenza infections less severe. Treating viral infections inappropriately by prescribing antibiotics poses a serious threat to global health by contributing to the development of antimicrobial resistance.

Protozoa

Protozoa are generally single-celled organisms that have animal-like characteristics and live in water. *Paramecium* and *Amoeba*, which you probably looked at under a microscope in a biology class, are common protozoa (Table 6-6). Many protozoan infections cause diarrhea in infected people and are spread when people drink water that has been contaminated with feces. Amoebic dysentery causes more than 500 million cases of diarrhea each year; cryptosporidiosis (sometimes shortened to "crypto") and giardiasis are epidemic diarrheal diseases. A 1993 cryptosporidiosis outbreak in Wisconsin, USA, caused more than 100 deaths in the city of Milwaukee and made more than 400,000 people sick.[9]

Some protozoa are spread by insect bites. *Plasmodium falciparum* and other types of *Plasmodium* that cause malaria are spread to humans by the bite of infected *Anopheles* mosquitoes. (Malaria is discussed in detail in

Table 6-6. Examples of Infections Caused by Protozoa.

Disease	Agent	Type of Agent	Transmission	Where Found
African Trypanosomiasis / Sleeping Sickness	*Trypanosoma brucei*	Flagellate	Tsetse fly (*Glossina*) bite	Tropical Africa
Amoebiasis	*Entamoeba histolytica*	Amoeba	Ingesting fecally-contaminated water or food	Worldwide
Babesiosis	*Babesia*	Sporozoa	Tick (*Ixodes*) bite	Worldwide in scattered locations
Chagas Disease / American Trypanosomiasis	*Trypanosoma cruzi*	Flagellate	Kissing bug/triatomine bug (*Reduviidae*) feces infect a bug bite	The Americas
Cryptosporidiosis	*Cryptosporidium parvum*	Sporozoa	Ingesting fecally-contaminated water or food or hand-to-mouth fecal-oral spread	Worldwide
Giardiasis	*Giardia lamblia* (*Giardia intestinalis*)	Flagellate	Hand-to-mouth fecal-oral spread and sometimes ingesting fecally-contaminated water or food	Worldwide
Leishmaniasis/ Kala-azar	*Leishmania*	Flagellate	Phlebotomine sand fly bite	Worldwide in scattered locations
Malaria	*Plasmodium*	Sporozoa	Mosquito (*Anopheles*) bite	Tropical and subtropical areas
Toxoplasmosis	*Toxoplasma gondii*	Sporozoa	Contact with cat feces; mother-to-child	Worldwide
Trichomoniasis	*Trichomonas vaginalis*	Flagellate	Sexual contact	Common worldwide

Chapter 7.) African sleeping sickness (trypanosomiasis) is spread by the bite of the tsetse fly and can cause chronic fevers and headaches that lead to paralysis and death. The estimated number of cases annually in sub-Saharan Africa is between 50,000 and 70,000, although trypanosomiasis can also occur in epidemic periods in which more than half of a village may become infected in one year.[10] Without early treatment, infection with African trypanosomiasis is fatal.

Chagas disease, also called American sleeping sickness, is spread by "kissing bugs" that live in the cracks of poor-quality houses in South America and Central America. The insects emerge at night to take bloodmeals from people. The feces of the insects contain parasites that can enter the bloodstream through the wound left after the bloodmeal. Within a few days a sore may develop at the site of the bite, which is often near the eye. About one-third of people who are infected develop a chronic infection that can cause severe damage to the heart and digestive tract.[11]

Leishmaniasis is spread by female phlebotomine sandflies, which need blood from a human or other mammal in order to develop their eggs. There are several forms of leishmaniasis. The cutaneous form produces skin lesions and can lead to permanent disfigurement. The mucocutaneous form causes lesions on the mucous membranes of nose, mouth, and throat. The visceral form, also known as kala azar, causes chronic fevers, weight loss, anemia, and swelling of the spleen and liver, leading to death within a few years if left untreated.[12]

Toxoplasmosis is spread through contact with animals or their feces. Pregnant women should avoid contact with cat litter since these protozoa can cross the placental barrier and cause congenital infection in the fetus.

Some protozoan infections can be treated with drugs, but, as with bacteria, drug resistance is becoming more common. For example, nearly all malaria infections are resistant to chloroquine, formerly most common treatment for this infection. Malarial treatment drugs developed to replace chloroquine are no longer effective in many parts of the world.

Worms

Parasites are eukaryotic organisms that survive by living off of a host. (A eukaryote has a complex cell or cells that have a membrane-bound nucleus. Bacteria and viruses are not eukaryotes, but fungi, plants, and animals are.) Some parasites only minimally affect their hosts, but others can cause serious illness.

Helminths are **endoparasitic** worms that live inside the body of the host. (Protozoa are also endoparasitic. In contrast, lice and the mites that cause scabies are **ectoparasitic** animals that live outside the body.) More than one-third of the people in the world at any given time have a worm living in their body.[13] People can become hosts to roundworms, pinworms, hookworms, flatworms (which include blood, liver, lung, and intestinal flukes), tapeworms (which can be found in beef, pork, and fish), and other kinds of worms (Table 6-7).

Worms contracted from contaminated soil, water, food, or feces may take up residence in the intestine, liver, lungs, blood, or other body parts, including, sometimes, the brain. Intestinal worms increase the risk of malnutrition because nutrients from food go to the worms instead of the human host. Worms that latch onto the intestinal wall, especially hookworms, cause bleeding and increase the risk of anemia. Soil-transmitted helminths are parasitic worms that thrive in tropical climates (Figure 6-5). The most common soil-transmitted helminths (STH) are roundworm, whipworm, and hookworm. Ascariasis is the most common helminth infection in the world and occurs when a person consumes eggs from *Ascaris lumbricoides*, a common type of roundworm. The larvae hatch in the small intestine, penetrate the intestinal wall, and travel through the blood to the lungs, where they may be coughed up and swallowed, perpetuating the infection. Adult worms in the intestine may grow to 35 cm in length and eggs passed in the stool may lead to infection in others. Trichuriasis is caused by a whipworm, and may result in digestive system symptoms. Hookworm is most often contracted by walking barefoot through fecally-contaminated soil, and hookworms are a major cause of anemia in children. Trichinosis (sometimes called trichinellosis) is another worm infection that can affect the digestive tract, and is often contracted from pork and other meat products.

Although soil-transmitted helminths rarely cause serious health problems, some parasites can cause severe disability. Guinea worm disease (dracunculiasis) is an extremely painful condition. People become infected by drinking water that contains water fleas infected with guinea worm larva. A mature guinea worm may grow to up to 3 feet in length, and once the worm is mature it may crawl down the inside of an infected person's leg and emerge from a painful blister near the foot. It can take weeks for the worm to leave the body, and a person with an emerging guinea worm is usually unable to work during this time because of pain. The worm cannot simply

Table 6-7. Examples of Infections Caused by Worms.

Disease	Agent	Type of Agent	Transmission	Where Found
Ascariasis	*Ascaris lumbricoides*	Nematode: roundworm	Eating fecally-contaminated food or soil	Common worldwide
Clonorchiasis	*Clonorchis sinensis*	Trematode (flatworm): liver fluke	Eating undercooked or raw freshwater fish	Asia, especially southeast China
Dracunculiasis / Guinea worm disease	*Dracunculus medinensis*	Nematode: guinea worm	Drinking unfiltered water from a crustacean-infested source	Some parts of Africa and Asia
Echinococcosis / Hydatid cyst disease	*Echinococcus granulosus*	Trematode: tapeworm	Food or contact with infected dogs	Found in domestic dogs worldwide
Enterobiasis	*Enterobius vermicularis*	Nematode: pinworm	Hand-to-mouth fecal-oral spread	Worldwide
Fascioliasis	*Fasciola hepatica*	Trematode: liver fluke	Eating undercooked aquatic plants like watercress grown in fecally-contaminated water	Found in sheep- and cattle-raising areas
Fasciolopsiasis	*Fasciolopsis buski*	Trematode: liver fluke	Eating undercooked aquatic plants like watercress grown in fecally-contaminated water	Southeast Asia, especially in pig-raising areas
Filariasis	*Wuchereria bancrofti, Brugia malayi, Brugia timori*	Nematode: filaria	Mosquito bite	Tropical areas

Disease	Agent	Type	Transmission	Distribution
Hookworm	*Necator americanus, Ancylostoma duodenale*	Nematode: hookworm	Enters body through skin (usually bare feet)	Common in tropical and subtropical areas
Hymenlepiasis	*Hymenolepsis nana*	Trematode: tapeworm	Hand-to-mouth fecal-oral spread	Australia, the Americas, the Middle East, India
Loiasis	*Loa loa*	Nematode: filaria	Deer fly (*Chrysops*) bite	African rainforest
Onchocerciasis/ River blindness	*Onchocerca volvulus*	Nematode: filaria	Black fly (*Simulium*) bite	Some parts of Africa and the Americas
Paragonimiasis	*Paragonimus*	Trematode: lung fluke	Eating undercooked or raw freshwater crabs or crayfish	Asia (especially China), the Americas, Africa
Schistosomiasis/ Bilharzia	*Schistosoma*	Trematode: blood fluke	Contact with snail-infested water	Africa, Asia, Middle East, South America, Caribbean
Strongyloidiasis	*Strongyloides stercoralis*	Nematode	Enters body through skin	Tropical and temperate areas
Taeniasis	*Taenia solium, Taenia saginata*	Trematode: tapeworm	Eating undercooked pork, beef, or other meat	Worldwide
Trichinosis / Trichinellosis	*Trichinella spiralis*	Nematode: threadworm	Eating undercooked pork, beef, or other meat	Worldwide
Trichuriasis	*Trichuris trichiura*	Nematode: whipworm	Eating fecally-contaminated food or soil	Worldwide

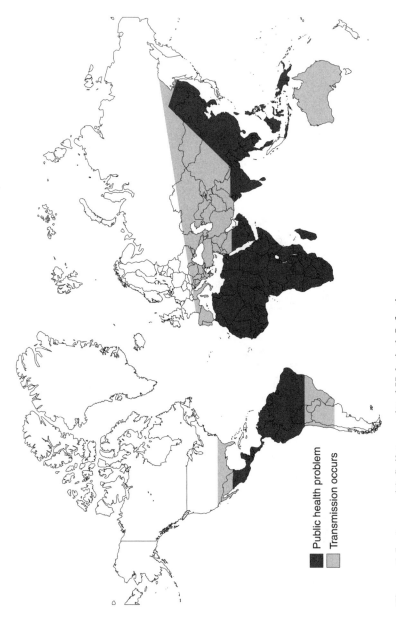

Figure 6-5. Areas with Soil-transmitted Helminth Infections.

Data Source: WHO Partners for Parasite Control, "Geographical distribution and useful facts and stats."

be pulled out of the body because if it breaks it can cause massive infection. Instead, the worm is often tied to a stick that is used to coil the guinea worm as it slowly makes its way out of the human's body. Many people with an emerging worm only feel relief from pain by putting their feet in water, but this causes the worm to release eggs and can contaminate drinking water supplies. There is no drug for dracunculiasis, but the prevalence of the disease is decreasing as use of water filters becomes more common. Found primarily in western and central Africa, the ultimate goal is to eradicate guinea worm disease.

Onchocerciasis (river blindness) is caused by a filarial (threadlike) parasite spread by the bite of infected black flies. Adult worms form nodules under the skin and release new worms (microfilariae) into surrounding tissues. If the nodules form near the eyes, the result can be blindness, if the infection is not treated with a drug called ivermectin. River blindness is found in Africa and some parts of Latin America.

Lymphatic filariasis (LF) is also caused by a filarial infection. Extreme swelling of body parts (often an arm, leg, or scrotum) is caused when worms block the flow of lymph (tissue fluid) out of body tissues. Lymphatic filariasis has sometimes been called elephantiasis because a person with LF may have a limb swell to the size of an elephant's leg and develop a coarse texture. More than 100 million people worldwide are infected with the worm that can cause LF.[14]

Schistosomiasis, sometimes called bilharzia or shortened to "schisto," is a type of flatworm that can enter the blood through the skin and may cause bladder or intestinal problems, including bladder cancer if a person has scarring from chronic infection. There are several different kinds of schistosomiasis that can be found in Africa, the Middle East, Latin America, Asia, and the Pacific. In each species, the worms infect both snails and humans and the infection cycles between these two species. Eggs released into water from the urine or feces of infected people can infect snails living in the water. After the worms undergo several developmental stages in the snails, the mature larvae are released into water and can infect humans who wade in the water while fishing, washing clothes, or bathing. An effective drug called praziquantel cures the infection, but people who are treated for schistosomiasis are immediately susceptible to new infection when they come into contact with contaminated water. Molluscicides are sometimes used to kill the snails that live in infested waters, but snails will eventually move back into the waters, and new snail habitats are created when dams and irrigation systems are built. The prevalence of schistosomiasis increased drastically when the Aswan Dam was built on the Nile River in Egypt, when dams were built on the Senegal and Volta Rivers and other locations in West Africa, and when small dams and irrigation projects have been introduced into villages in many parts of the world.[15] A similarly large increase is expected in China as a result of the Three Gorges Dam.

Fungi

Fungi come in many forms, including molds and yeasts. Fungi are important decomposers used to make bread, wine, and cheese, but some are pathogenic (disease-causing). Fungal conditions frequently occur after the normal balance of helpful microflora is disturbed by antibiotic use or immunosuppression (Table 6-8). For example, *Candida albicans* is normally found on human skin, especially around moist areas like the mouth, groin, and underarms. An imbalance of *Candida*, called candidiasis, could present as thrush (a white coating on the tongue that is common in AIDS patients), a vaginal yeast infection, or diaper rash. Other examples of fungal infections include histoplasmosis, which is spread through animal droppings, PCP pneumonia (*Pneumocystis carinii* pneumonia), which is common in AIDS patients, and dermatomycoses (fungal diseases of the skin) like ringworm and athlete's foot. Fungi thrive in moist, dark places and are especially common in the tropics.

Prions

Prions are "proteinaceous infectious particles" that appear to cause degenerative nervous system diseases and wasting diseases. Proteins are the building blocks of cells, tissues, and organs. Normal proteins are chains of amino acids that are folded into complex shapes. Mutant prion proteins lose their shape by unraveling and straightening out. A single mutant prion appears to be able to cause the normal proteins near it to also unravel. In "mad cow disease," formally called bovine spongiform encephalopathy (BSE), the brains of cows become spongy as their brain proteins unravel. The equivalent disease in humans is called Creutzfeldt-Jakob Disease (CJD). Infections are apparently transmitted by ingestion of brain and nervous tissue

Table 6-8. Examples of Infections Caused by Fungi.

Disease	Agent	Transmission	Where Found
Aspergillosis	*Aspergillus*	Airborne	Worldwide but uncommon
Candidiasis (thrush, vaginal yeast infection, diaper rash)	*Candida albicans*	Skin contact	Common worldwide
Coccidioidomycosis	*Coccidioides immitis*	Airborne	Arid and semi-arid areas of the Americas
Cryptococcosis	*Cryptococcus neoformans*	Ingesting fecally-contaminated water or food or hand-to-mouth fecal-oral spread	Worldwide
Dermatomycosis / Tinea (ringworm, Athlete's foot)	Various species	Skin contact or contact with surfaces that have been touched	Common worldwide
Histoplasmosis	*Histoplasma capsulatum*	Airborne	Worldwide in scattered locations

from infected individuals or animals. Kuru, another transmissible spongiform encephalopathy, was spread in the South Fore region of New Guinea during funeral rites that involved ingestion of the brain tissue of the deceased. (These rituals were discontinued in the 1950s.)[16] Although cooking food at sufficient temperatures will kill most bacteria and parasites, heat will not kill prions because the proteins are already denatured (unraveled).

Host

A host is a human who has contracted a particular infection or developed a particular disease. Host factors describe the personal characteristics that make a person vulnerable to infection and disease (Table 6-9). Some factors, like age and immune status, indicate level of susceptibility. For example, the

Table 6-9. Examples of Host Factors.

Unmodifiable	• Age • Sex • Birthplace • Ethnicity • Nationality
Biological	• Pregnancy (in women) • Psychological factors • Immune status • Co-morbidities (existing health problems) • Anatomical defects • Genetic makeup • Stress and fatigue • Nutritional status
Socioeconomic	• Income and wealth • Education • Occupation • Immigration status • Marital and family status
Behavioral	• Alcohol, tobacco, and drug use • Diet and exercise habits • Sexual practices and contraceptive use • Hygiene practices • Food handling practices • Religious practices • Hobbies and recreational activities • Use of health resources

risk of Alzheimer's disease increases with age and women are more likely than men to have rheumatoid arthritis. Other host characteristics, like occupation and sexual practices, indicate exposure risks.

Environment

Environmental factors include both the natural environment and the social environment (Table 6-10). The types of infections that are common in humans living in a particular area often relate to characteristics of the natural environment like temperature, rainfall, and proximity to bodies of

Table 6-10. Examples of Environmental Factors.

Natural environment	• Geography: land and water features, soil type, geology, topography • Climate and weather: temperature, rainfall, humidity, altitude, season • Proximity to animals, birds, insects, plants, and other living things • Natural disasters
Community / occupational environment	• Drinking water quantity and quality • Waste disposal and sanitation • Chemicals in the air, water, soil, and workplace • Industrial pollutants, radiation, noise, and occupational exposure to other chemical and physical agents • Population density and crowding in the household or community
Social, economic, and political environment	• Access to transportation, health services, education, and communication technology • Special environments like child-care centers, hospitals, military bases, refugee camps, prisons, and war zones • Travel to new areas

water or specific types of groundcover. The social, economic, and political environments contribute to the interaction of humans with one another and with infectious agents.

Vector

When an insect **vector** is involved in transmission, the triad can be modified to be an Agent—Host—Vector—Environment schema (Figure 6-6). The interactions of the vector with the agent, the human host, and the natural environment can all impact the spread of infection. For example, infection with the *Plasmodium* parasite that causes malaria is spread to humans by mosquito bites. For transmission to occur the environment must contain the water sites where mosquitoes breed and develop and the host must be in contact with the mosquito vector during the times of the day (dusk and dawn) when the type of mosquito that spreads malaria usually bites. The mosquito must also have acquired the parasite by biting an infected human.

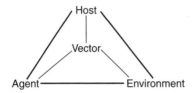

Figure 6-6. Agent—Host—Vector—Environment.

MEASURING DISEASE IN POPULATIONS

The two most common terms used to describe of describing the burden of disease in a population are incidence and prevalence. They are related concepts but have very distinct meanings. **Incidence** is the number of *new* cases of a disease occurring in a time period divided by the total number of people at risk of disease in that time period. Incidence is usually used to study infectious diseases, acute diseases (diseases that occur suddenly), and outbreaks. **Prevalence** is the number of *total* existing cases—both newly diagnosed and diagnosed before the start of the time period—divided by the total number of people at risk of disease during the specified time. Prevalence is usually used to describe the amount of chronic (long-lasting) disease in population, such as the proportion of a population with diabetes, obesity, or depression. The difference between the two terms is illustrated in Figure 6-7.

An increase in prevalence does not always mean that incidence has increased. Prevalence increases when people with a disease survive longer, diagnosis is improved so more cases are detected, or screening allows for cases to be diagnosed earlier. Cancer prevalence may increase when cases are found at an earlier, more treatable stage of the disease, which is associated with improved survival. Prevalence may decrease as the cure rates for a disease improve or if the fatality rate from the disease increases. Prevalence can also change when there is migration of sick (or healthy) people and susceptible (or immune) people in to (or out of) a community or when a population ages. The ability to understand how a population has changed over time is one reason that it is important to adjust for age when comparing health statistics. A retirement community where the average resident is 70 years old will have a very different health profile than a neighborhood near a primary school with a median age of 15 years, and it wouldn't be "fair" or accurate to compare health status in the two communities without first adjusting for the different age structures.

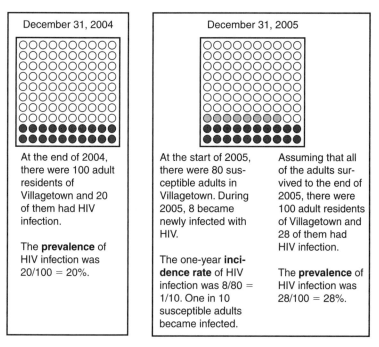

Figure 6-7. An Example of Incidence and Prevalence.

Health statistics let communities and nations know what diseases are common in their population and recognize when an unusual health situation has developed. A disease that is **endemic** is always present in a population. An **epidemic** is when a disease is occurring more often than usual. To be called an **outbreak**, there must usually be more than a few sporadic occurrences of disease. A **pandemic** is a worldwide epidemic, like influenza. Without baseline data about incidence and prevalence it is impossible to know if unusual numbers of cases are being diagnosed.

Surveillance systems track infectious disease reports to look for patterns and possible outbreaks or **clusters**, which occur when there is an unusually high incidence of disease in a particular place (spatial clustering) or time (temporal clustering). Surveillance requires continuous monitoring of diseases in a population so that changes can be detected, and control and prevention measures can be implemented. It is not necessary to track an entire population. Usually several representative clinics or communities will be selected to participate in **sentinel surveillance**, which is when data from continuous monitoring at several selected "sentinel" sites is used to alert public health officials to possible changes in community health status. If an outbreak is suspected, a more rigorous investigation involving additional sites can be conducted.

DISEASE CONTROL

A major goal of public health is to prevent the spread of infectious diseases through populations and to contain outbreaks when they do occur.

Immunizations can be used to prevent and contain epidemics of vaccine-preventable diseases.[17] Most vaccines are designed to prevent infection, and some are designed to minimize the damage caused by infection. For example, tetanus toxoid prevents damage from bacterial toxins. A vaccine is usually made from either a weakened (attenuated) living organism or an inactive killed organism that still has the same outside shell that a viable infectious agent would have. When your body responds to the contents of the vaccine, your immune system begins to create special immune cells called memory cells that remember the surface proteins they have encountered. If later on you are exposed to that same infectious agent in a live, active form, your body's immune system will be able to quickly identify the agent and kill it before it has a chance to multiply. A good vaccine will produce a strong immune response in one dose and will provide protection for several years and possibly for life. Vaccination, like a real infection, creates **active immunity** because your body has a lasting memory of the infection. (**Passive immunity** is acquired through breastmilk or immunoglobulin shots and lasts only a few months.)

When you get a vaccination you are not just protecting yourself from disease, you are protecting those around you. **Herd immunity** says that reducing the percentage of the population susceptible to an infection protects the whole population. Why? Assume each infected person has 10 contacts with others that could potentially result in infection of the person contacted. In a completely susceptible population all 10 of the people contacted might become infected—and each of those 10 people could spread the infection to many others. If 80% of the population is immune, only 2 of those 10 contacts are likely to be effective—and those 2 infected people will not be able to spread the infection to many others—so the epidemic can be stopped before it becomes a huge problem.

Environmental control and behavioral change can help reduce some infections. Reducing standing water in urban areas can reduce the breeding ground for the mosquitoes that spread dengue fever. Molluscicides can be used to reduce the snail population that spreads schistosomiasis. These kinds of infection **control** measures limit the incidence of infection in a local area. When control measures remove all risk of new infection in the area, **elimination** of the infection has been achieved.

In some cases it is possible, at least in theory, to completely eradicate an infection. **Eradication** is achieved when there is no risk of infection or disease anywhere in the world even in the absence of immunization or any other control measures. The only infectious disease eradicated (as yet) is smallpox. A massive worldwide immunization campaign that included re-vaccination in areas where any new case of smallpox occurred led to the successful eradication of the disease in 1979. (Because several laboratories kept samples of smallpox virus, the disease is not considered "extinct." Eradication is complete when an infectious agent is no longer found in nature. Extinction is complete when an agent no longer exists in nature or in the laboratory.) Polio is scheduled for eradication soon, if the global immunization plan is continued until no cases of polio exist. Dracunculiasis (guinea worm disease) is also nearing eradication. Although there is no vaccine for dracunculiasis, education programs that emphasize filtering drinking water to remove the water fleas that carry the worm larva and that teach infected people to stay out of water have contributed to a rapid decline in the number of cases reported each year. Prior to the start of the eradication program there were estimated to be more than a million new cases each year, but in 2005 there were only about 10,000 cases (Figure 6-8).

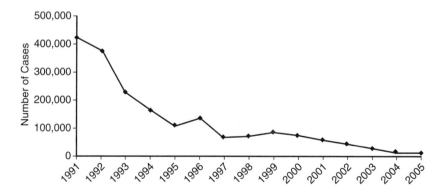

Figure 6-8. Worldwide Dracunculiasis (Guinea Worm) Incidence.

Data Sources: CDC, Guinea Worm Disease Wrap-Up, several issues from 1993 to 2006. WHO, "Dracunculiasis: Recent epidemiological data."

To be a candidate for eradication, the infectious agent must usually meet several biological criteria, such as infecting only humans and not having an animal reservoir. (If the disease also affected other animals as hosts it could be nearly impossible to track and vaccinate them all.) The infection, or the vaccine for the infection, should confer life-long or long-term immunity so that people who have had the infection are no longer susceptible to it. The disease must be highly pathogenic so that people who contract the disease have obvious symptoms and can be easily tracked and treated. And there must be an intervention, like a vaccine, that effectively interrupts the chain of transmission.

Not all infections that meet the biological criteria are appropriate candidates for eradication. For example, measles meets the biological criteria but it has such a rapid rate of transmission that it would require a massive global effort to vaccinate all susceptible people within a very short period of time. In addition to a lack of staff and structural support for a few intense weeks of immunization and several years of follow-up surveillance, many countries do not have the facilities to store the vaccine safely or the tools to deliver it. Because it takes a great deal of time, money, and organizational sophistication to achieve eradication, only diseases that are considered severe are targeted for eradication. A global eradication campaign cannot begin unless there is widespread political commitment to achieving success and a support system to ensure completion.[18]

REFERENCES

1. Heymann DL, ed., *Control of Communicable Diseases Manual*. 18th ed. Washington, DC: American Public Health Association, 2004.
2. Rooney RM, Cramer EH, Mantha S, Nichols G, Bartram JK, Farber JM, Benembarek PK. A review of foodborne disease associated with passenger ships: evidence for risk management. *Public Health Rep.* 2004;119:427–434.
3. Jacobsen KH, Koopman JS. Declining hepatitis A seroprevalence: a global review and analysis. *Epidemiol Infect.* 2004;133:1005–1022.
4. World Health Organization, 2006 Tuberculosis Facts (WHO/HTM/STB/factsheet/2006.1).
5. Ou J, Li Q, Zeng G, Dun Z, & Qin A. Efficiency of quarantine during an epidemic of severe acute respiratory syndrome—Beijing, China, 2003. *MMWR Morb Mortal Wkly Rep.* 2003;52:1037–1040.
6. Several sources were used to compile the infectious disease tables in this chapter, including: Heymann DL, ed. *Control of Communicable Diseases Manual*. 18th ed. Washington, DC: American Public Health Association, 2004.
7. Kumaresan JA, Mecaskey JW. The global elimination of blinding trachoma: progress and promise. *Am J Trop Med Hyg.* 2003;69(5 Suppl):24–28.
8. World Health Organization, "Antimicrobial resistance," Fact sheet 194, January 2002.

9. Mac Kenzie WR, Hoxie NJ, Proctor ME, et al. A massive outbreak in Milwaukee of *Cryptosporidium* infection transmitted through the public water supply. *N Engl J Med.* 1994;331:161–167.
10. World Health Organization, "African trypanosomiasis (sleeping sickness)," Fact sheet 259, August 2006.
11. UNICEF-UNDP-World Bank-WHO Special Program for Research and Training in Tropical Diseases (TDR), "Chagas Disease: Disease Information."
12. World Health Organization, "Leishmaniasis: The disease and its epidemiology."
13. WHO Partners for Parasite Control, "Geographical distribution and useful facts and stats."
14. World Health Organization. Lymphatic Filariasis: The Disease and Its Control. Technical Report 71, Geneva: WHO, 2002.
15. Steinmann P, Keiser J, Bos R, Tanner M, Utzinger J. Schistosomiasis and water resources development: systematic review, meta-analysis, and estimates of people at risk. *Lancet Infectious Diseases.* 2006;6:411–425.
16. Collinge J, Whitfield J, McKintosh E, Beck J, Mead S, Thomas DJ, Alpers MP. Kuru in the 21st century—an acquired human prion disease with very long incubation periods. *Lancet.* 2006;367:2068–2074.
17. The terms vaccination and immunization are generally used interchangeably. Technically, immunization is a more generic term.
18. Knobler S, Lederberg J, Pray LA, eds. Considerations for Viral Disease Eradication: Lessons Learned and Future Strategies. Workshop Summary: Forum on Emerging Infections, Board on Global Health, Institute of Medicine, National Academy of Sciences. Washington, DC: National Academy Press, 2002.

CHAPTER 7

HIV/AIDS, Malaria, and TB

Key Points:

- HIV (Human Immunodeficiency Virus) is a viral infection that causes the destruction of immune system cells and leads to AIDS (Acquired Immune Deficiency Syndrome).
- Malaria is a parasitic infection spread by the bites of infected mosquitoes.
- Tuberculosis is a bacterial disease that most often affects the lungs.

Three of the infectious diseases of greatest concern to people living in developing world regions are HIV/AIDS, malaria, and TB. Together these three infections account for nearly 10% of all deaths worldwide each year.[1]

HIV/AIDS

Human Immunodeficiency Virus type 1 (HIV-1) is a viral infection spread when body fluids like blood, semen, vaginal fluid, and breast milk are exchanged during sexual contact, the sharing of needles used to inject drugs, or by mother-to-child (MTC) transmission during childbirth or breastfeeding. (Transmission of HIV through blood transfusions is rare now that donated blood and blood products can be tested for HIV.) HIV is not transmitted through casual contact like shaking hands, sharing eating utensils, or using the same toilet. The virus destroys specialized white blood cells, such as $CD4^+$ T cells, that are needed by the immune system to fight infection.

(There is also an HIV-2 virus. HIV-2 accounts for only a small fraction of the HIV cases in the world, and is found primarily in West Africa. HIV-2 progresses more slowly and causes milder symptoms than HIV-1.)

Acquired Immunodeficiency Syndrome, abbreviated as AIDS, is a **syndrome** (a collection of symptoms) that occurs as a result of the destruction of immune system cells by the HIV virus. (Because AIDS is a syndrome and not an infectious agent, a person cannot "catch" AIDS from someone else. A person can become infected with HIV, and that infection can cause AIDS to develop.) The constellation of diseases, such as *Pneumocystis* *carinii* pneumonia (PCP) and Karposi's sarcoma, that occur in people with AIDS are called **opportunistic infections** (OIs) because they only occur when the body's immune system is weakened enough to give the infectious agents an opportunity to invade. The most common OIs in low-income countries include tuberculosis, bacterial pneumonia, chronic diarrhea, and fungal infections, such as *Cryptococcus.*

A person newly infected with HIV may experience flu-like symptoms for a few days or weeks but is often asymptomatic. During this stage, a person may not test positive for HIV and will still have a normal number of CD4 cells in the blood. However, the newly infected person will have a high viral load (lots of the virus in the blood) so it is possible to spread the virus (Figure 7-1).

The World Health Organization identifies four clinical stages of HIV infection and AIDS disease that follow primary infection (Table 7-1).[2] In stages 1 and 2, the person is in a latent stage, which can last from a few weeks to more than 20 years, and is asymptomatic or has only minor symptoms like skin infections and recurrent respiratory infections. Stage 3 is marked by more severe symptoms like the loss of more than 10% of body weight due to chronic diarrhea, recurrent respiratory infections, persistent fevers, TB, and mouth ulcers. The CD4 count begins to fall and the viral load in

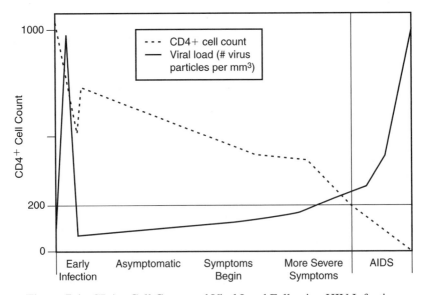

Figure 7-1. CD4+ Cell Count and Viral Load Following HIV Infection.

Table 7-1. WHO Staging System for HIV Infection and Disease: Clinical Classification.

	Primary HIV Infection	*Clinical Stage 1*	*Clinical Stage 2*	*Clinical Stage 3*	*Clinical Stage 4 (AIDS)*
Weight	Normal	Normal	Loss of less than 10% of body weight	Loss of more than 10% of body weight	HIV wasting syndrome
Activity Level	Asymptomatic	Asymptomatic, normal activity	Symptomatic, normal activity	Bed-ridden less than 50% of the day in the past month	Bed-ridden more than 50% of the day during the past month
Examples of Common Clinical Conditions	Acute retroviral syndrome: flu-like symptoms about 2-4 weeks post-exposure that resolve within a few weeks	Persistent generalized lymphadenopathy: enlarged lymph nodes in several parts of body	Minor skin problems (like fungal infections and mouth ulcers); recurrent upper respiratory infections	Chronic diarrhea and fevers for more than one month, thrush, pulmonary TB, severe bacterial infections like pneumonia and meningitis	Chronic diarrhea and fevers for more than one month, PCP, herpes simplex virus, candidiasis, atypical TB, Kaposi's sarcoma (KS), HIV encephalopathy, toxoplasmosis

Adapted from World Health Organization (WHO), Interim WHO Clinical Staging of HIV/AIDS and HIV/AIDS Case Definitions for Surveillance: African Region, WHO/HIV/2005.02.

the blood begins to rise. In stage 4, serious opportunistic infections mark the onset of AIDS and the CD4 count becomes very low (below 200 particles per mm^3 or even undetectable levels).

There is currently no HIV vaccine and no drug that can cure an HIV infection. (Antiretrovial drugs given after a known exposure, such as a nurse or doctor being stuck by a needle used on an HIV-infected patient, may lower the risk of becoming HIV infected. Drugs given after are exposure to prevent infection are called post-exposure prophylaxis, or PEP for short.) In people with an HIV infection, antiretroviral drugs (ARVs) can be used to keep the viral count low and stop the progression of symptoms. The best current treatment for HIV infection is called highly active antiretroviral therapy (HAART). HAART consists of combinations (sometimes called "cocktails") of several types of drugs, including reverse transcriptase inhibitors and protease inhibitors. The median survival time after infection with HIV if a person does not take HAART is about 10 years; after onset of clinical AIDS the expected survival without HAART is less than 2 years.[3] HAART prolongs both the duration of time between infection and the onset of clinical AIDS and the time between onset of AIDS and death, extending the lives of people with HIV infection by years or even decades.

HAART does not work for all people with HIV because some cannot tolerate the side effects, some do not adhere to the treatment regimen and skip too many doses for the drugs to be effective, and some have a drug-resistant strain of HIV. Even if the drugs do reduce the viral load, they do not cure the HIV infection or alleviate all symptoms. Once treatment is stopped the levels of HIV in the blood may quickly rise. Still, millions of people with HIV infection who would benefit from access to HAART do not have access to it because they cannot afford the treatment.

One of the alarming characteristics of HIV/AIDS is how quickly the epidemic emerged. The first cases of AIDS were identified in the United States in homosexual men in 1981.[4] By 1990 there were nearly 10 million people worldwide living with HIV, by 1995 there were 20 million people living with HIV, by 2000 more than 30 million people were living with HIV, and by 2005 there were nearly 40 million people worldwide living with HIV.[5]

More than 4 million people became newly infected with HIV in 2005 and nearly 3 million died from AIDS. HIV/AIDS occurs in every part of the world, but some regions bear a particularly heavy burden (Figure 7-2 and Table 7-2).

Sub-Saharan Africa is home to just over 10% of the world's population, but more than 60% of all people with HIV infection live in the region. More

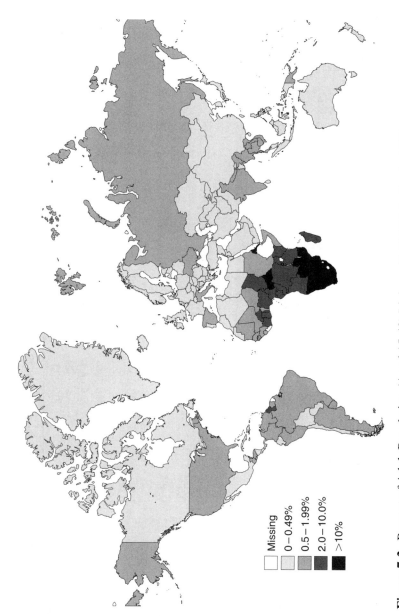

Figure 7-2. Percent of Adult Population (Aged 15-49) Living with HIV Infection in 2005.

Data Source: UNAIDS 2006 Report on the Global AIDS Epidemic.

Missing
0 – 0.49%
0.5 – 1.99%
2.0 – 10.0%
>10%

Table 7-2. HIV/AIDS Statistics, 2006.

Region	% of adults (ages 15–49) living with HIV at the end of 2006	# of adults and children living with HIV at the end of 2006	# of women (ages 15+) living with HIV at the end of 2006	% of adults living with HIV who are women	# of adults and children newly infected with HIV in 2006	# of adult and child deaths due to AIDS in 2006
Sub-Saharan Africa	5.9%	24,700,000	13,300,000	59%	2,800,000	2,100,000
Caribbean	1.2%	250,000	120,000	50%	27,000	19,000
Eastern Europe / Central Asia	0.9%	1,700,000	510,000	30%	270,000	84,000
North America	0.8%	1,400,000	350,000	26%	43,000	18,000
South and South-East Asia	0.6%	7,800,000	2,200,000	29%	860,000	590,000
Latin America	0.5%	1,700,000	510,000	31%	140,000	65,000
Oceania	0.4%	81,000	36,000	47%	7,100	4,000
Western and Central Europe	0.3%	740,000	210,000	28%	22,000	12,000
Middle East / North Africa	0.2%	460,000	200,000	48%	68,000	36,000
East Asia	0.1%	750,000	210,000	29%	100,000	43,000
TOTAL	1.0%	39,500,000	17,700,000	48%	4,300,000	2,900,000

Data Source: UNAIDS, 2006 Report on the Global AIDS Epidemic.

than 6% of African adults between 15 and 49 years old have contracted HIV, and in some southern African countries more than one-third of adults (ages 15 and older) are infected with HIV. The prevalence is especially high among young women and urban residents. About 25 million sub-Saharan Africans are infected with HIV, and nearly 2 million die each year from AIDS. AIDS has caused life expectancy to plummet in many countries (Figure 7-3) and has changed the entire social structure in some parts of Africa. Nearly all infections and deaths occur in young- and middle-aged adults (ages 15 to 49), so older adults have been forced to take on the care of their sick adult children and their young grandchildren. If the grandparents are deceased or unable to care for children, AIDS orphans (children who have lost at least one parent to AIDS) often end up homeless and living on the street. Increased access to HAART would extend the lives of millions of parents with HIV infection, but only a small proportion of Africans who would benefit from antiretroviral drugs have access to them.

Although no country in Asia or Oceania has an adult HIV prevalence rate of greater than 2%, there are more than 8 million Asians living with HIV infection. Two-thirds of HIV-infected Asians live in India and a growing number are Chinese. Both injecting drug use (IDU) and paid sex acts are facilitating the spread of HIV in the region, especially because many sex workers use drugs and many drug users have been involved in a paid sex act. Having another sexually-transmitted infection increases the likelihood of contracting HIV, so people who participate in high-risk behaviors often

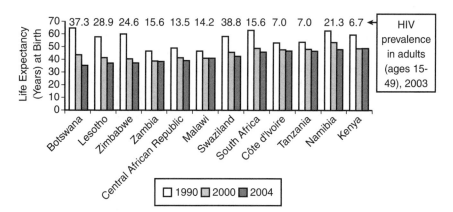

Figure 7-3. Changes in Life Expectancy at Birth Between 1990 and 2004 in Several African Countries with High HIV Prevalence Rates.

Data Source: World Bank, 2006 World Development Indicators.

have increased biological susceptibility to HIV infection. As the number of Asians with HIV infection increases, the risk of infection in people who do not participate in risky behaviors is also increasing. The Ministry of Health of Thailand estimates that one-third of new HIV infections in 2005 were in women who were infected by their husbands or long-term partners. AIDS knowledge in most Asian countries is minimal, which means that few people know that they are at risk and even fewer know how to protect themselves from HIV.

Other regions are less affected, but must maintain vigilance and continue education initiatives since the incidence (rate of new cases) increases when people stop worrying about their risk. In Eastern Europe and central Asia the prevalence of HIV infection is rapidly increasing, especially among the injecting drug users (IDUs) who now account for more than 70% of HIV cases in the region. The HIV prevalence rate in countries in the Middle East and North Africa is very low except among certain high-risk groups like IDUs. Nearly 2 million people living in South America and in the Caribbean are infected with HIV, as are an additional 2 million people living in North America and in western and central Europe.

Anyone who is exposed to blood or body fluids can contract HIV. (This is why workers are often trained to use **universal precautions**, such as wearing gloves, when caring for a sick person or cleaning up a spill or soiled laundry.) People in some population groups—such as sex workers, men who have sex with men, injecting drug users, and prisoners—are at elevated risk because they engage in high-risk behaviors that increase the likelihood of contact with blood and other body fluids. They also may have limited access to health care because of discrimination. Many people are at risk because they have not been educated about HIV and HIV prevention, or do not take preventive measures because they do not think that they are at risk.

Women have greater biological and social risk of contracting HIV than men. Anatomically, the walls of the vagina are thin and may tear during intercourse, facilitating the entrance of HIV into the bloodstream. Women are at least twice as likely as men to acquire HIV from an act of heterosexual intercourse. Socially, women marry at younger ages than men, may not have the power to demand condom use, and are more likely to be the victims of sexual violence. In sub-Saharan Africans 15- to 24-years-old, the incidence rate among women is three times higher than the incidence rate among men. In some places the majority of women with HIV infection are married and nearly all of those women contracted HIV from their husbands. Women are often hesitant to ask their husbands to use a condom, so programs that educate and encourage women to take measures to protect their health are important contributors to HIV prevention.

At the end of 2005, there were more than 2 million children under 15 years of age who were living with HIV. The vast majority (more than 90%) were infected through mother-to-child (MTC) transmission. Babies can be infected by their mothers during pregnancy, the birth process, or breastfeeding. In the absence of any drug interventions, a baby born to an HIV-infected mother has about a 15% to 30% risk of contracting HIV during delivery.[6] The likelihood of transmission is much lower if the mother takes ARVs during pregnancy, because a woman with a low viral load has a lower risk of passing the virus to her baby during delivery.[7] In high-income countries, the use of HAART has reduced the risk of mother-to-child transmission to 2% or less.[8] Even when a mother has not taken ARVs during pregnancy, the risk of mother-to-child transmission during delivery can be reduced to less than 5% if the woman is given a single dose of nevirapine at the start of labor and her baby is given a single dose of nevirapine after delivery.[9] (Zidovudine is also commonly used to prevent mother-to-child transmission.)

HIV is excreted in breastmilk, and the risk of HIV infection in babies who are breastfed for several months can be as high as 25% to 45%.[10] The risk is highest in babies whose mothers are not on ARVs. HIV-infected mothers are encouraged to use formula instead of breastmilk. However, many women living with HIV have no choice but to breastfeed their babies. Some cannot afford formula and others do not have reliable access to clean water. The risk of infant death due to diarrhea from unsafe water used to mix formula is often greater than the risk of contracting HIV through breastmilk, so women are often forced to make painful decisions about which risks they will expose their babies to.

The most important way to help control the HIV/AIDS pandemic is to emphasize prevention. One campaign uses ABC as a reminder to be *A*bstinent, to *B*e faithful if sexually active, and to consistently and correctly use a *C*ondom during every sex act. The ABC approach used in Uganda is often credited with reducing the prevalence of HIV by more than half in the 1990s. (Male circumcision has also recently been shown to significantly reduce the risk of HIV infection[11], but does not negate the need to use condoms as protection against HIV and other STIs.) The ABC approach works to prevent uninfected people from contracting HIV, and also helps keep people with HIV infection healthy. Since HIV has a lot of genetic variability, people who are infected with HIV need to protect themselves against other subtypes of the virus.

MALARIA

Malaria is a parasitic infection caused by one of four types of protozoa: *Plasmodium falciparum*, *Plasmodium malariae*, *Plasmodium ovale*, and *Plasmodium vivax*. Infection with any of the four species will cause cyclic fevers, headache, and joint pain and can in some cases cause organ failure and brain inflammation, especially in children. *P. falciparum* is generally the most serious infection, and accounts for about 90% of infections in Africa, but less than 50% of infections in South-East Asia and Latin America.[12] Some of the species (*P. vivax* and *P. ovale*) can stay dormant in the liver for years after the initial illness and can cause relapses months or even years after the initial infection.

The parasite is passed from one human to another by female *Anopheles* mosquitoes that need a bloodmeal in order to produce and lay eggs. *Anopheles* mosquitoes breed near standing water, so anyone who lives near a body of water like a pond, lake, or even a puddle could be at risk of bites. The incidence of malaria varies seasonally and generally increases during rainy seasons when the mosquito populations increase. Environmental changes related to road building, mining, logging, agriculture, and irrigation may also create breeding sites, further increasing the mosquito population.

A mosquito acquires malaria by biting an infected human. After the malaria parasites undergo a reproductive stage in the gut of the mosquito, they can be spread to humans through the saliva of the mosquito. Once in the human body, the parasites undergo a complicated life cycle (Figure 7-4). First they move to the liver and reproduce rapidly. After several days the parasites burst from the liver, enter the bloodstream, and invade red blood cells (the cells that carry oxygen throughout the body). The parasites grow and divide inside the red blood cells. Every 2 to 3 days (depending on the species) the red blood cells rupture, releasing parasites and toxins into the blood stream and causing fever, chills, and anemia. The cycle can continue for 10 to 14 days or longer if untreated.

There are 350 to 500 million acute clinical cases of malaria each year, resulting in more than 1 million deaths, mostly of children. Malaria is the leading cause of death for African children, responsible for more than 2000 deaths each day. Although anyone can contract malaria, children and pregnant women are most at risk of severe complications and death. Adults who have grown up in endemic areas usually have some degree of resistance to severe malaria, but susceptibility to disease increases during pregnancy and complications are common because pregnant women are often severely anemic,

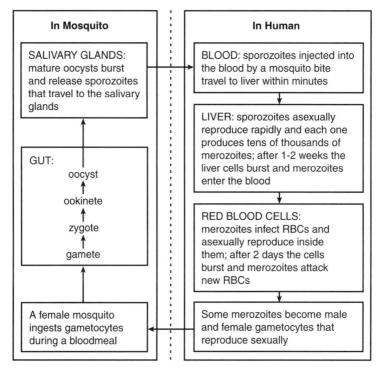

Figure 7-4. The Life Cycle of *Plasmodium*.

which means that they have too few red blood cells to carry oxygen even before additional red blood cells are destroyed by *Plasmodium*.[13,14] Babies born to mothers with malaria are at increased risk of low birthweight and other birth complications. Malaria infections in children can cause long-term impairment of health and functioning, especially for children who survive cerebral malaria or develop severe anemia. About 7% of children who survive cerebral malaria, which is characterized by coma and convulsions, have permanent neurological problems.[15,16,17]

Each bout of malaria causes, on average, about 12 days of lost productivity in terms of absence from work or school and inability to work growing food and around the home.[18] Infection is most common during the seasons when subsistence farmers grow and harvest their crops, and when malaria infection keeps family members from being in the fields at this crucial time it can result in long-term undernutrition for all members of the household. A child may have several episodes of clinical malaria every year, and children carry the risk of long-term reductions in school performance due to missed class days and continued weakness from anemia. The cost of lost productivity due to malaria extends to countries as well. A world map of the distribution of the burden of malaria (Figure 7-5) looks nearly identical to a world map of the distribution of poverty. Malaria-endemic countries also have lower rates of economic growth.[19]

The countries with the highest malaria incidence rates are in sub-Saharan Africa, where 80% of all malaria deaths occur. South-East Asia and Latin America also have relatively high incidence rates (Table 7-3). Most cases of malaria occur in the tropics where mosquitoes survive year-round and environmental control of insect populations through spraying of insecticide and land and water management is limited.

More than 40% of the world's population is at risk for malaria, but it is possible that this percentage could rise. Until the mid-twentieth century, malaria was endemic in the United States and Mediterranean, with cases reported as far north as Canada and Siberia. A massive insecticide spraying program led by WHO in the 1950s and 1960s eliminated malaria from dozens of countries, but it is possible for a re-emergence to occur, especially because of increased concern over the environmental impact of spraying insecticides and the development of insecticide-resistance in mosquitoes.

There are few anti-malarial drugs that work today. For decades the drug of choice for treating malaria was chloroquine, but in most parts of the world the common strains of malaria are chloroquine-resistant and the drug is now ineffective. Strains of malaria are also becoming resistant to other drug options such as sulfadoxone/pyrimethamine (SP or Fansidar) and mefloquine (Lariam), and artemesinin derivatives are often ineffective. The World Health Organization strongly urges the use of combination therapies that combine at least two different anti-malarials because combination drugs slow the emergence of drug resistance. Since parasites that cause malaria are very complex organisms, developing new drugs (or developing a vaccine) is a challenge.

Prevention of malaria is of increasing importance as treatment is becoming more difficult. Although travelers from non-endemic areas to places where malaria is endemic generally take prophylactic (preventive) anti-malarial drugs, these are not fully effective in preventing disease. It is not realistic or healthy to encourage prophylactic use among people living in highly endemic areas. The cost would be high, the long-term effects of drug use could be potentially harmful, and it could contribute

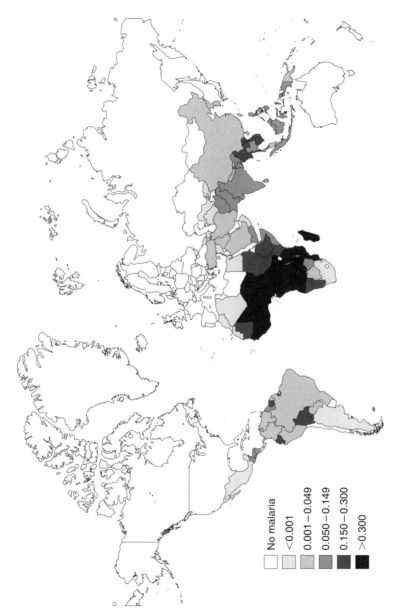

Figure 7-5. Malaria Incidence (New Clinical Cases per Person per Year) During 2004.

Data Source: World Malaria Report 2005.

No malaria
<0.001
0.001 – 0.049
0.050 – 0.149
0.150 – 0.300
>0.300

Table 7-3. Regional Malaria Burden, 2005.

Region	Africa	Asia	The Americas
% of malaria caused by P. falciparum	93%	35%	18%
% of population at risk of malaria	66%	49%	14%
Estimated % of global clinical malaria cases	59%	38%	3%
Estimated % of global malaria mortality burden	89%	10%	<1%

Data Source: World Malaria Report 2005.

to the development of drug-resistant *Plasmodium* at a time when many species are no longer susceptible to the anti-malarial drugs that are used to treat malaria.

The only guaranteed way to prevent malaria is to avoid all mosquito bites. Since the mosquitoes that spread malaria bite primarily at dawn and dusk, the use of insecticide-treated bednets (ITNs) that put a barrier between people and mosquitoes and also kill mosquitoes that are near the net is highly encouraged. Field studies of ITNs show a significant reduction in child mortality when bednets are used consistently. It is also important for malaria patients to stay under a bednet so mosquitoes cannot bite them and become carriers of malaria. Many adults who have grown up in endemic areas continue to have parasitemia (malaria parasites in the blood) even when asymptomatic, so all people who live in at-risk areas, including both children and adults, should consistently use ITNs. ITNs must generally be re-dipped in a pyrethroid insecticide once or twice a year to maintain their effectiveness.

Other barrier methods include wearing clothes that cover the arms and legs during the times of the day when mosquitoes are most likely to bite and having screens or curtains cover windows and doors of houses where it is possible to do this. Insect repellents like sprays and mosquito mats and coils are also helpful, as is reducing the number of water-filled containers near the home to minimize breeding areas. Unfortunately, most households at greatest risk for malaria have little or no money available to spend on malaria prevention.

TUBERCULOSIS (TB)

Tuberculosis (TB) is an infection caused by the bacterium *Mycobacterium tuberculosis*. TB can affect any part of the body, but usually occurs in the lungs (pulmonary TB). TB used to be called consumption because people with the disease were "consumed" by it and developed a bloody cough, persistent fever, wasting, and pale skin.

A distinction is made between having TB infection (latent TB) and having TB disease (active TB). More than one-third of the world's population has been infected with the TB bacillus, but only about 5% to 10% of infected people will develop TB disease during their lifetimes.[20] TB is spread through the air, but only people with active TB disease are contagious. A person with untreated active TB may infect 10 to 15 other people each year, especially if they have frequent and prolonged interactions.

Anyone can become infected with TB, although most infections occur in low-income nations and among people living in crowded conditions. The rates of infection are highest in Asia, Africa, and the nations that were part of the former U.S.S.R. (Figure 7-6 and Table 7-4). In 2004, there were more than 9 million new cases of TB disease, 14 million existing cases, and nearly 2 million TB deaths worldwide.

People with HIV infection are more likely to develop active TB disease than people without HIV infection, and TB is a leading cause of death in people with AIDS. Early diagnosis of TB can be critical for survival. One of the challenges of the relationship between TB and HIV, especially in sub-Saharan Africa, is that people with a lung infection may delay seeking treatment because they fear that a diagnosis of TB will likely be accompanied by a diagnosis of AIDS. Delayed diagnosis creates an unnecessarily high risk of death from TB. People with an HIV infection can be successfully treated for TB, but they must be strong enough to survive through the full course of treatment.

The standard drug regimen involves taking a combination of up to five different drugs every day for six months or longer. The first two months are the most crucial, but following through with the full course of treatment is essential so that all of the bacteria, including the hardiest organisms, are killed. The protocol for treatment that WHO recommends is called **Directly-Observed Therapy, Short-course (DOTS)**. The key part of DOTS is the "directly-observed" component. TB patients being treated under DOTS are required to have a trained observer watch them take their pills every day. This observer might be a doctor or nurse if the person is an in-patient or reports to a clinic for his or her daily treatment, a shopkeeper or other

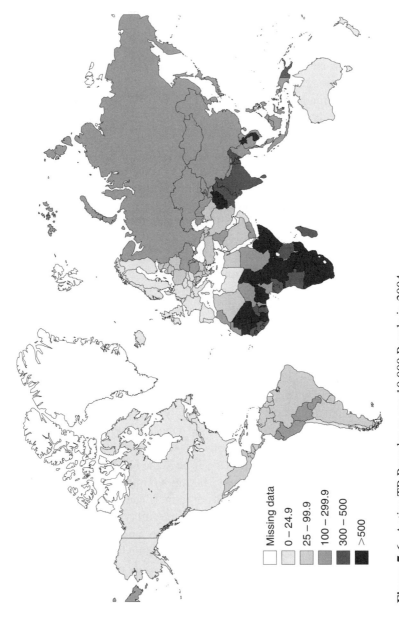

Figure 7-6. Active TB Prevalence per 10,000 People in 2004.

Data Source: Global TB Control Report 2006.

Table 7-4. Global TB Statistics, 2004.

	Incidence rate (new cases) of all forms of TB per 100,000 in 2004	Incidence rate (new cases) of smear-positive cases per 100,000 in 2004	Prevalence rate (total cases) of all forms of TB per 100,000 in 2004	TB mortality rate from all forms of TB per 100,000 in 2004	HIV prevalence rate in adult TB cases (%) in 2004
Africa	356	152	518	81	33%
South-East Asia	182	81	304	33	3.9%
Eastern Mediterranean	122	55	206	27	2.4%
Western Pacific	111	50	216	18	1.4%
Europe	50	23	65	8	4.7%
Americas	41	18	53	6	10%
TOTAL	140	62	229	27	13%

Notes: Smear-positive cases (patients with signs of active pulmonary TB based on laboratory analysis of sputum samples) are more likely than smear-negative cases to infect other people, and have higher rates of illness and death than smear-negative cases. Appendix I lists the countries in each WHO region.

Data Source: Global TB Control Report 2006.

community leader, or a family member who is supervised by another community member. If the patient misses a dose a public health worker will track the patient down and try to ensure compliance. (Some countries have public health laws stipulating that a person who is not compliant with TB treatment can be hospitalized under guard or imprisoned for the duration of their treatment, but most do not enforce these regulations.) Still, the loss to follow-up rate (the percentage of people who are diagnosed who do not complete treatment) is high in some places. WHO has set a goal of having 70% of TB cases diagnosed and 85% of diagnosed cases successfully treated under DOTS.

One of the problems that can result when patients stop taking their drugs a few months into treatment is the emergence of multidrug-resistant TB (MDR-TB). MDR-TB that does not respond to standard antibiotic therapies is a growing problem. An estimated 4% of TB cases worldwide are resistant to at least one TB drug, and in some countries more than 30% of cases are drug resistant. [21,22] Some cases of MDR-TB can be treated using DOTS (through a special protocol called DOTS Plus), but the drugs are more expensive and the course of treatment is much longer, 2 years rather than 6 months. Some cases of MDR-TB do not respond to any of the major anti-TB drugs.

A vaccine called BCG (Bacillus Calmette-Guerin) is available and used in some countries, but it provides protection for only about half of the people who receive it and the protection it provides wanes over time. The standard test for TB is the PPD test (also called the Mantoux test) in which a small amount of TB bacterial protein is injected under the skin and the reaction is monitored. A person with TB will have an immune response and develop a rash at the injection site. If a person has a positive PPD test, then a chest X-ray will be taken to look for pockets of infection. The person may also take a sputum test, in which the phlegm produced by deep coughs is analyzed for the presence of TB bacteria. Some employers and schools require employees and students to prove that they do not have TB. One of the disadvantages of BCG is that once a person has received BCG the skin test may always be positive, so more invasive tests are required to prove that a person does not have TB. Several new TB vaccines are being developed and tested, but are not yet ready for use.

COMPARISON OF HIV/AIDS, MALARIA, AND TB

Table 7-5 is a comparison chart for HIV/AIDS, malaria, and TB. Note that a different type of infectious agent is responsible for each infection and that there are distinct modes of transmission for each one. Although

Table 7-5. Comparison of HIV/AIDS, Malaria, and TB.

Disease	HIV/AIDS	Malaria	TB
Infectious agent	Virus (HIV-1)	Protozoan (several types of *Plasmodium*)	Bacterium (*Mycobacterium tuberculosis*)
Primary mode(s) of transmission	Sexual contact and injecting drug use	Mosquito bites	Airborne by droplet spread
Can it be cured?	No—drugs can suppress viral load but do not cure the infection	Yes	Yes
# deaths worldwide in 2005	2,830,000	888,000	1,411,000
% of deaths worldwide in 2005	4.9%	1.5%	2.4%
# of deaths of children under five years of age in 2005	250,000	799,000	41,000
% of under-5 child deaths in 2005	2.6%	8.3%	0.4%

Data Source: WHO, Global Burden of Disease database, 2006 update.

HIV/AIDS causes the greatest total number of deaths each year (in part because of co-infection with TB), malaria causes the greatest number of deaths in children.

REFERENCES

1. Calculated from the WHO Global Burden of Disease database, 2006 update. (See Table 7-5.)
2. World Health Organization, Interim WHO Clinical Staging of HIV/AIDS and HIV/AIDS Case Definitions for Surveillance: African Region, WHO/HIV/2005.02.
3. Jaffar S, Grant AD, Whitworth, J, Smith PG, Whittle H. The natural history of HIV-1 and HIV-2 infections in adults in Africa: a literature review. *Bull World Health Organ.* 2004;82:462–469.

4. HIV has been isolated from preserved blood and tissue samples that were collected as early as the 1950s, but the first clinical cases of AIDS were not identified until 1981 and blood tests for the virus were not developed until the mid-1980s. Zhu T, Korber BT, Nahmias AJ, Hooper E, Sharp PM, Ho DD. An African HIV-1 sequence from 1959 and implications for the origin of the epidemic. *Nature*. 1998;391:594–597.

5. Unless otherwise noted, all statistics on HIV/AIDS are from the UNAIDS 2006 Report on the Global AIDS Epidemic.

6. De Cock KM, Fowler MG, Mercier E, et al. Prevention of mother-to-child HIV transmission in resource-poor countries: translating research into policy and practice. *JAMA*. 2000;283:1175–1182.

7. Volmink J, Siegfried NL, van der Merwe L, Brocklehurst P. Antiretrovirals for reducing the risk of mother-to-child transmission of HIV infection. Art. No.: CD003510. DOI: 10.1002/14651858.CD003510.pub2. Accessed on Cochrane Database of Systematic Reviews (online), 24 January 2007.

8. Marseille E, Kahn JG, Mmiro F, et al. Cost effectiveness of a single-dose nevirapine regimen for mothers and babies to decrease vertical HIV-1 transmission in sub-Saharan Africa. *Lancet*. 1999;354:803–809.

9. McIntyre J. Strategies to prevent mother-to-child transmission of HIV. *Curr Opin Infect Dis*. 2006;19:33–38.

10. De Cock KM, Fowler MG, Mercier E, et al. Prevention of mother-to-child HIV transmission in resource-poor countries: translating research into policy and practice. *JAMA*. 2000;283:1175–1182.

11. Sawires SR, Dworkin SL, Fiamma A, Peacock D, Szekeres G, Coates TJ. Male circumcision and HIV/AIDS: challenges and opportunities. *Lancet*. 2007;369:708–713.

12. Unless otherwise noted, all statistics in this section are from the World Malaria Report 2005.

13. Mayor A, Aponte JJ, Fogg C, et al. The epidemiology of malaria in adults in a rural area of southern Mozambique. *Malar J*. 2007;6:3.

14. Roll Back Malaria Partnership, "Malaria in pregnancy." Available online at http://www.rbm.who.int/cmc_upload/0/000/015/369/RBMInfosheet_4.htm.

15. Malaria Foundation International, "Children and malaria."

16. Holding PA, Stevenson J, Peshu N, Marsh K. Cognitive sequelae of severe malaria with impaired consciousness. *Trans R Soc Trop Med Hyg*. 1999;93:529–534.

17. Murphy SC, Breman JG. Gaps in the childhood malaria burden in Africa: cerebral malaria, neurological sequelae, anemia, respiratory distress, hypoglycemia, and complications of pregnancy. *Am J Tropic Med Hyg 2001*; 64 (1 Supplement): 57–67.

18. Malaria Foundation International, "Quick Facts about Malaria."

19. Sachs J, Malaney P. The economic and social burden of malaria. *Nature*. 2002;415:680–685.

20. Unless otherwise noted, all data and statistical estimates are from the Stop TB website or the 2006 Global Tuberculosis Control Report (WHO/HTM/TB/2006.362).

21. Zignol M, Hosseini MS, Wright A, Stop TB / WHO, et al. Global incidence of multidrug-resistant tuberculosis. *J Infect Dis*. 2006;194:479–485.

22. World Health Organization, "Anti-tuberculosis drug resistance in the world report no. 3," WHO/HTM/TB/2004.343.

CHAPTER 8

Globalization and Emerging Infectious Diseases

Key Points:
- Globalization is reintroducing infectious diseases into high-income regions and introducing chronic diseases into low-income regions.
- Emerging infections, the development of antimicrobial-resistant infections, and potential acts of terrorism are creating new health threats.

THE "EPIDEMIOLOGIC TRANSITION" AND GLOBALIZATION

Less than a century ago, before the advent of antimicrobial therapy and oral contraceptives, most people died from infectious diseases and many women died in childbirth. Although the typical family had many children, the infant mortality rate was high and life expectancy even for those surviving childhood was relatively low. Modern medical technologies and improved nutrition have in some parts of the world led to a shift from high fertility, short life expectancy, and deaths from infectious diseases and undernutrition (the *pre-transition* profile) to low fertility, long life expectancy, and deaths from non-communicable diseases like heart disease, cancers, and stroke (the *post-transition* profile). This **"epidemiologic transition"** was expected to predictably follow the "demographic transition" as the economic status of a population improved.[1] According to this model, the United States, Canada, Japan, and most European countries would be considered "post-transition" whereas sub-Saharan Africa and some Asian and Latin American countries would be considered "pre-transition."

While the epidemiologic transition is a helpful model for understanding the differences in health status between more and less industrialized countries and regions, the health changes that occur with development are much less predictable than the model implies.[2] For example, in many low-income countries both pre- and post-transition populations can be found within one city. Urban professionals may have increasing rates of cancer while poor urban families continue to experience high rates of infectious disease. Furthermore, although many illnesses and deaths in low-income nations are due to infection and undernutrition and most illnesses and death in high income nations are due to non-communicable conditions like heart disease and cancers, globalization is reintroducing infectious diseases into industrialized nations and introducing new chronic diseases into developing nations. "Lifestyle diseases" related to obesity and physical inactivity are now found even in countries where the burden of infectious diseases remains high, which means that rather than experiencing a health transition, these countries are facing a dual burden of infectious and chronic diseases.

Globalization has many meanings, most of which are very specific to a particular discipline, like economics, which uses globalization to refer to the expansion and integration of economic activity and policies between nations. Globalization is seen in the increasing number of global governmental and non-governmental organizations, the proliferation of multilateral trade agreements, increases in foreign direct investment, changing production modes (such as the emergence of global supply chains), increased population mobility (including tourism, urban migration, and forced displacements), and increased cultural diffusion. The globalization of the world economy is also very evident in the items people use on a daily basis: it is likely that most of your clothes, shoes, and appliances were made in other countries, and that many of the fruits and vegetables you purchase at your local grocery store were grown in another part of the world.

Globalization is not new to the field of public health. Infectious diseases were spread across the globe when sea and land trade routes like the Silk Road and the Spice Route in the 1st century C.E. linked China, India, and the Mediterranean. Massive outbreaks occurred with the Mongol expansion to Europe in the 13th century. The infectious diseases carried by the Europeans who explored the Americas in the 15th century caused the decimation of many indigenous American populations. Infectious diseases have never stopped at national boundaries, and modern transportation allows for a new infectious disease that emerges in any part of the world to be transported by aircraft to any other part of the world within hours rather than weeks or months. The original case of SARS (Severe Acute Respiratory Syndrome), which emerged in 2003, was probably acquired in an animal market. The infection then was transmitted from person to person across parts of Asia, and within months cases were found in Canada, the United States,

South Africa, Brazil, and many European nations.[3] If a strain of highly pathogenic avian influenza develops the ability to spread easily from human to human, an even faster and more widespread dissemination of the infection across the globe is expected. Globalization means that humans are tied together and a problem in one part of the world can quickly become a global issue.[4]

EMERGING INFECTIOUS DISEASES

Even as we succeed in controlling and eradicating some diseases, other diseases previously not found in humans are emerging. **Emerging infectious diseases** occur when a new pathogen begins to affect human populations or an existing pathogen changes the kind of disease it causes. It might evolve in a way that makes it easier to transmit to a susceptible person (increased **transmissibility**) and, therefore, more common (increased incidence). It might change so that it causes a new set of symptoms or more severe symptoms (increased virulence). In some cases an infectious agent that usually affects only non-human hosts may adapt in a way that makes it infectious to humans. Sometimes an infectious agent may change in a way that allows for a different portal of entry, perhaps developing the ability to be spread through airborne transmission. Other infections, called **re-emerging infections**, were controlled at some point in the past but are becoming problematic again.[5,6]

The Institute of Medicine, one of the National Academies of the United States, issued a report on microbial threats to health in the twenty-first century. The report emphasizes that the emergence of new health threats derives from a complex interaction of genetic and biological factors, physical environmental factors, ecological factors, and social, political, and economic factors.[7] Thirteen specific risk factors have been identified: (1) microbial adaptation and change, (2) human susceptibility to infection, (3) climate and weather, (4) changing ecosystems, (5) economic development and land use, (6) human demographics and behavior, (7) technology and industry, (8) international travel and commerce, (9) breakdown of public health measures, (10) poverty and social inequality, (11) war and famine, (12) lack of political will, and (13) intent to harm.

These factors are interrelated. As the world population increases (#6), humans and domestic animals move into previously uninhabited natural environments (#5) and are exposed to new plants, animals, and microbes. Alteration of the environment (#4), such as deforestation, reforestation, dam-building, and manipulation of wetlands, creates new environmental reservoirs for infectious agents, and natural disasters (#3) like floods and droughts can alter the landscape and introduce new agents to a region. Cultural and behavioral practices (#6), including food practices, outdoor activities, and risky sexual behavior and drug use, that become trendy and spread globally may also facilitate transmission.

Both movement to urban areas and movement to rural areas can cause new diseases to emerge (#6). Urbanization facilitates the emergence of new infections as people with different infections interact with one another and creates new habitats for vectors. Dengue fever, also called breakbone fever because it causes severe joint pain, is a viral infection spread by *Aedes aeqypti* and other *Aedes* mosquitoes that thrive in urban environments where there are many small bodies of standing water, such as water that collects in old cans and discarded tires.[8] There are four serotypes of dengue, which means that there are four different strains that the body's immune system recognizes as different from one another. People who have had prior exposure to one of the strains of dengue fever may be at increased risk of developing dengue hemorrhagic fever if they contract another one of the serotypes. It will be very difficult to develop a vaccine for dengue because a vaccine would have to be effective against all four serotypes. Instead, community prevention efforts focus on eliminating the standing water that serves as breeding grounds for mosquitoes. One family that does not clean up its yard can put a whole neighborhood at risk, so all households in a community must be involved in dengue prevention projects.[9] (Dengue is common in South America, and because the mosquitoes that spread it live in the southeastern United States it is expected to cross into the U.S.)

Movement of people into rural areas, or tree-lined suburbs, also exposes people to new risks. Lyme disease is found primarily in the suburban areas of the eastern coast of the United States. It is caused by a bacterium spread by bites from infected deer ticks. The early symptoms of Lyme disease are mild, and because a bulls-eye rash (erythema migrans) at the site of a tick bite that is a sign of infection does not always occur, many people with Lyme disease are not diagnosed at an early stage.[10] Untreated Lyme disease infection can progress to arthritis-like disease and possible nervous system involvement. Hantaviruses have occurred in many parts of the world for a long time, but Hantavirus Pulmonary Syndrome (HPS) was first seen in 1993 in the isolated Four Corners region of the southwest U.S. Several young adults developed severe pneumonia after they inhaled aerosolized rat urine or feces while cleaning rural homes.[11]

Technology is also speeding up the rate of emergence. Modern transportation (#8) has made it possible for an infectious person to travel nearly anywhere in the world within hours and brings susceptible people into areas endemic for disease. This was clearly demonstrated during the SARS epidemic, which spread across the globe as visitors in Asia flew back to their home countries. Experts feared that SARS could become an annual epidemic, like influenza, but that has not (as of yet) occurred. That does not mean that the risk is over. Even recirculation of air on an airplane could spark another global outbreak if one passenger has a contagious infection.[12] The SARS epidemic was also a stark reminder of the need for responsive global public health communication systems, which have been strengthened in the years since the outbreak.[13]

Health care innovations (#7) have created new risks and risk groups. Advanced medical therapies like the immunosuppressive drugs used by people with organ transplants and the technology for keeping premature infants alive have created new populations of highly susceptible people (#2). **Nosocomial** (hospital acquired) infections may be very hardy and difficult to treat, and antimicrobial resistance is increasing (#1). Other technological advances have created new places for infectious agents to grow and new methods of dispersion.

Some infections emerge because of new distribution systems. Legionnaire's disease is a severe type of pneumonia that was first identified in 1976 following a conference of the American Legion in Philadelphia. The bacteria that cause Legionnaire's disease live in artificial water distribution systems like air cooling units, spas, and humidifiers, and infection is acquired by inhaling the aerosolized bacteria.[14] Toxin-producing *Staphylococcus aureus* causes toxic shock syndrome (TSS) and was first identified in 1980 in menstruating women using high-absorbency tampons.[15] *Escherichia coli O157:H7* is a deadly strain of bacteria that causes bloody diarrhea and kidney failure, and outbreaks of the disease have been traced to undercooked fast food burgers and contaminated swimming pools.[16]

Some infections emerge by appearing in a new location. Although relatively common in Egypt, Sudan, and Uganda for decades, West Nile Virus was found in the United States for the first time in 1999.[17] Spread by the bite of infected mosquitoes, it can affect birds and other vertebrates, including humans. Although usually asymptomatic, about 1 in 150 people, usually older people, develop serious symptoms that may involve the nervous system.[18] Five years after the first cases were identified in New York, the virus was found in birds in all 48 contiguous states.

Some newly emergent infections are still a mystery. Several types of tropical hemorrhagic fevers, like the Ebola and Marburg viruses, have emerged in central Africa, and the reservoir and modes of transmission for these infections are not entirely clear. Although rare, the infections have a high case fatality rate, which means that a large percentage of infected people die.

New infectious diseases can emerge anywhere in the world, and the distinction between a local public health problem and a global one is increasingly limited. HIV crosses borders along with truck drivers and professionals traveling for work. Bovine spongiform encephalopathy ("mad cow" disease) crosses borders when cattle or beef products are shipped to markets. Cholera, a waterborne bacterial infection that can travel in ocean waters from one nation's shores to another, appeared in South America for the first time in nearly 100 years in 1991. It was first identified in Peru but quickly spread to Ecuador and Colombia, and in less than a year it had spread throughout South America and Central America, including Mexico and several Caribbean countries.[19,20] Drug-resistant strains of bacteria are often hardier than drug-sensitive strains, so inappropriate access to drugs in one nation (infected persons taking too little of an antibiotic or healthy persons using antibiotics unnecessarily) can rapidly become a global problem. Non-communicable diseases are also being exported. As tobacco use declines in the United States, tobacco sales by American companies to Asian nations is rapidly increasing. When considering the causes of health and disease, it is increasingly necessary to think globally.

Influenza

Global health professionals are always concerned about the potential for a worldwide influenza outbreak. Influenza is the respiratory virus that causes the most deaths in the United States and other developed countries each year. About 5% to 20% of the U.S. population contracts influenza each year and more than 30,000 deaths each year are flu-related.[21] Influenza can exacerbate existing medical conditions (especially lung and heart diseases) and lead to pneumonia. ("Stomach flu" is not caused by influenza viruses.) Although the highest fatality rate from influenza is usually among the elderly and immunocompromised, anyone who contracts influenza can die from it. The most serious pandemic in the twentieth century occurred in 1918 and 1919 during World War I, and that strain killed a disproportionate number of young people, including more soldiers than those who died in combat during the war.

All infectious agents, whether newly emerging or long established in a population, are constantly adapting and changing in ways that can make them more or less transmissible, infective, pathogenic, and virulent. Influenza occurs in humans and also in birds, pigs, and other animals, and the virus constantly changes so most people and animals are susceptible to each new strain that circulates.

Influenza A virus strains differ in the kind of surface antigens they present. Surface antigens are "read" by the cells in our body's immune system and tell our bodies how to respond to the invaders. When an immune cell reads another cell that is part of the body, it recognizes that it is seeing itself. Immune cells can also recognize some of the infectious agents that the immune system has fought off before and can quickly respond to stop these infections from reoccurring. This kind of active immunity can result from either previous infection or from immunization. The two key surface antigens for Influenza A are hemagglutinin (H) and neuraminidase (N).

Influenza viruses fool the body by changing their surface antigens so that the immune system cannot recognize them. There are two processes for changing surface antigens. **Antigenic drift** occurs when small genetic mutations bring about small changes in the antigens. Antigenic drift is why infection with one version of H3N2 influenza, the most common influenza strain circulating at the start of the twenty-first century, may not confer immunity to another form of H3N2. (Antigenic drift also makes it necessary to develop a new flu vaccine every year.) **Antigenic shift** occurs when two different influenza viruses attack the same cell and the genetic material from both recombines to form a new type of influenza. Antigenic shift led to the emergence in 1997 in Southeast Asia of the H5N1 strain of avian influenza that spread rapidly through the bird population, affecting both domestic birds like ducks and chickens and wild migrating fowl. On occasion a human is infected with one of these new strains of "bird flu," and a pandemic may result if that strain develops the ability to be easily transmitted from human to human.

Influenza is a prime example of how global travel can contribute to the spread of newly modified infectious agents by allowing an infected person to fly to any part of the world and start new epicenters of infection. On the other hand, global travel and communication may also help contain a pandemic by quickly sending supplies and medical specialists to affected areas and alerting public health officials to be aware of possible flu cases.

BIOTERRORISM

Bioterrorism is the deliberate release of infectious agents that can cause illness and possibly death of people, animals, or plants. A biological weapon may be selected because it produces severe disease, has a desirable incubation period (either short so immediate disease is produced or long so that the asymptomatic contagious stage is lengthy), is highly infectious, has a low infectious dose, is environmentally stable, is inexpensive, can be produced relatively easily and rapidly, or has a simple delivery mechanism (such as through air, water, or food). While the goal of some potential bioterrorists is to kill or seriously injure people, the most common goal of bioterrorists is to cause fear, public panic, and social disruption.

Chemical and biological warfare are not new. During the Tartar siege of the city of Kaffa (now in the Ukraine) in the fourteenth century, the bodies of plague victims were launched over city walls to spark an epidemic. In 1763, during the French and Indian War, the British army sent smallpox-infected blankets to American Indians. During World War I, several European nations used biological agents against livestock of enemies. What is new is that there are now more tools available for causing and spreading infectious diseases and the scale on which such acts can occur is much larger.

In the United States, potential bioterror agents are classified into three categories (Table 8-1).[22] Category A represents high-priority agents that pose a high risk because they can be easily transmitted from one person to another or have high mortality rates. Category A agents include anthrax, smallpox, plague, botulism, tularemia, and viral hemorrhagic fevers like Ebola and Marburg virus. Naturally occurring cases of anthrax (*Bacillus anthracis*) are diagnosed every year in people who work with sheep and livestock because anthrax forms spores (dormant bacteria) that can survive in the environment for years. (Anthrax, botulism, and tetanus are all diseases caused by bacterial spores.) In the laboratory, anthrax can be made into a fine powder that can more easily cause infection in humans. Anthrax infections can affect the lungs (inhalation anthrax), skin (cutaneous anthrax), or digestive tract (gastrointestinal anthrax). Although anthrax is not passed from one person to another and it is easily cured with antibiotics if detected early, it is considered a likely agent for future attacks because it was used as a bioweapon in 2001.

Category B agents are moderately easy to spread, have a moderate illness rate, and cause few deaths. Examples of Category B agents include

Table 8-1. U.S. Classifications of Bioterrorism Agents.

Category	Agents
Category A	Anthrax (*Bacillus anthracis*), botulism (*Clostridium botulinum* toxin), plague (*Yersinia pestis*), smallpox (variola major), tularemia (*Francisella tularensis*), viral hemorrhagic fevers (like ebola, Marburg, lassa, and Machupo)
Category B	Brucellosis, epsilon toxin of *Clostridium perfringens*, food safety threats (like *Salmonella*, *Escherichia coli* O157:H7, and *Shigella*), glanders (*Burkholderia mallei*), meliodosis (*Burkholderia psudomallei*), psittacosis (*Chlamydia psittaci*), Q fever (*Coxiella burnetii*), ricin toxin, Staphylococcal enterotoxin B, typhus fever (*Rickettsia prowazekii*), viral encephalitis (like Venezuelan equine encephalitis, eastern equine encephalitis, and western equine encephalitis), water safety threats (like *Vibrio cholerae* and Cryptosporidium parvum)
Category C	Emerging infectious diseases such as Nipah virus and hantavirus

Source: CDC Emergency Preparedness & Response, "Bioterrorism Agents/ Diseases."

brucellosis, ricin (a toxin from *Ricinus communis*, which is found in castor beans), Q fever, typhus fever, and viral encephalitis infections. This category also includes food safety threats such as *Salmonella*, *Shilgella*, or *E. coli O157:H7* and water supply threats such as cholera and cryptosporidium. Category C agents are emerging infectious agents like hantavirus that are potential threats because they are unknown.

The best defense against a biological attack is early detection so that an outbreak can be contained and exposed people can receive medical treatment. Treatment will include, when possible, post-exposure prophylaxis or immunization. Defense also requires education of the public in order to prevent mass hysteria. Since the events of September 11, 2001, the United States has developed early warning systems and checklists to help households, schools, businesses, and communities prepare for natural disasters and possible terrorist attacks. For example, households are encouraged to develop an evacuation plan and to stockpile water, food, batteries, and first-aid supplies. Other nations have instituted similar programs.

REFERENCES

1. Omran AR. The epidemiologic transition: a theory of the epidemiology of population change. *Milbank Mem Fund Q.* 1971;29:509–538.
2. Caldwell JC. Population health in transition. *Bull World Health Organ.* 2001;79:159–170.
3. WHO Epidemic and Pandemic Alert and Response (EPR), "Update 95—SARS: Chronology of a serial killer," 4 July 2003.
4. Bettcher D, Lee K. Globalization and public health. *J Epidemiol Commun Health.* 2002;56:8–17.
5. Morens DM, Folkers GK, Fauci AS. The challenge of emerging and re-emerging infectious diseases. *Nature.* 2004;430:242–249.
6. Fauci AS. Infectious diseases: considerations for the 21st century. *Clin Infect Dis.* 2001;32:675–685.
7. Smolinski, MS, Hamburg MA, Lederberg J, eds. Committee on Emerging Microbial Threats to Health in the 21st Century. Institute of Medicine. *Microbial Threats to Health: Emergence, Detection, and Response.* Washington, D.C.: The National Academics Press, 2003.
8. Gubler DJ. The changing epidemiology of yellow fever and dengue, 1900 to 2003: full circle? *Comp Immunol Microbiol Infect Dis.* 2004;27:319–330.
9. Parks W, Lloyd L. Planning social mobilization and communication for dengue fever prevention and control: A step-by-step guide. PAHO/WHO, 2004. (WHO/CDC/WMC/2004.2, TDR/STR/SEB/DEN/04.1)
10. Steere AC, Coburn J, Glickstein L. The emergence of Lyme disease. *J Clin Invest.* 2004;113:1093–1101.
11. Centers for Disease Control. Hantavirus Pulmonary Syndrome—United States: updated recommendations for risk reduction. *MMWR. Recomm Rep* 2002;51 (RR-9).
12. Although rare, transmission of TB, *Neisseria meningitides*, measles, influenza, and SARS have been documented. Centers for Disease Control. Chapter 7: Air Travel, including Disinsection. In: "Conveyance and Transportation Issues" of Travelers' Health: Yellow Book, 2005–2006. Atlanta, Georgia: U.S. Department of Health and Human Services, Public Health Service, 2005.
13. Weinstein RA. Planning for epidemics—the lessons of SARS. *N Engl J Med.* 2004;350:2332–2334.
14. Centers for Disease Control, "Legionellosis: Legionnaire's Disease (LD) and Pontiac Fever," 12 October 2005.
15. Hajjeh RA, Reingold A, Weil A, Shutt K, Schuchat A, Perkins BA. Toxic Shock Syndrome in the United States: surveillance update, 1979–1996. *Emerg Infect Dis.* 1999;5:807–810.
16. Rangel JM, Sparling PH, Crowe C, Griffin PM, & Swerdlow DL. Epidemiology of *Escherichia coli* O157:H7 outbreaks, United States, 1982–2002. *Emerg Infect Dis.* 2005;11:603–609.
17. Hayes EB, Komar N, Nasci RS, Montgomery SP, O'Leary DR, & Campbell GL. Epidemiology and transmission of West Nile Virus disease. *Emerg Infect Dis.* 2005;11:1167–1173.
18. Centers for Disease Control, "West Nile Virus: What You Need to Know," 12 September 2006.

19. Update: Cholera Outbreak—Peru, Ecuador, and Colombia. *MMWR*. 40;13:225–227.

20. Update: Cholera—Western Hemisphere, 1992. *MMWR*. 11 September 1992;41(36): 667–668.

21. Centers for Disease Control, Fact Sheet: Key Facts about Influenza and the Influenza Virus, 30 August 2006.

22. The CDC's Emergency Preparedness & Response website has details about specific potential bioterrorism agents.

CHAPTER 9

Nutrition

Key Points:

- A healthy diet provides energy and nutrients from carbohydrates, proteins, fats and oils, vitamins, and minerals.
- Deficiencies in calories, protein, vitamins, or minerals can cause illness and death, especially in children.
- Undernutrition in children can cause stunting, wasting, anemia, blindness, brain damage, vulnerability to infection, and death.
- Globalization is creating new nutritional issues related to breast-feeding practices, food safety, and food security.
- The prevalence of overweight and obesity is increasing worldwide.

We all need eat on a regular basis to provide our bodies with energy and the materials needed to build and repair cells and tissue, fight infections, and stay warm. We need to consume **macronutrients** such as carbohydrates, protein, and fats and oils in relatively large quantities because they provide energy. We also need to take in small amounts of **micronutrients** like vitamins and minerals. This chapter begins with an overview of the nutrients that all people need, and then discusses the problems associated with taking in too few—or too many—calories and nutrients. Both diseases associated with undernutrition and micronutrient deficiencies and diseases associated with obesity are important contributors to global health problems.

ESSENTIAL NUTRIENTS

Carbohydrates are found in cereals like rice, maize, and wheat (the three most common staple foods in the world), in starchy roots like potatoes and yams, and in fruits and vegetables. Carbohydrates are chains of sugars (or polysaccharides, which means "many sugars"). When we need quick energy, our cells break down carbohydrates through a process called cellular respiration. Simple carbohydrates are made up of very short chains of sugars and are easily absorbed into the bloodstream. The lactose found in milk and the glucose and fructose found in fruits and honey are all simple sugars. Table sugar, or sucrose, is a disaccharide ("two sugar") composed of glucose and fructose. Complex carbohydrates, such as those found in whole grain products like whole wheat bread and oatmeal, are made up of longer chains of sugars and take longer to digest, which is why eating complex carbohydrates keeps a person from feeling hungry longer than eating simple sugars. Fiber, found in unprocessed plant-based foods, is another type of carbohydrate and is essential for healthy digestion because it provides bulk that moves food material through the intestines.

Proteins are chains of **amino acids**. Amino acids from food are broken down and reassembled in our cells to form new proteins. The keratin that makes up our hair and nails, the hemoglobin that transports the oxygen in our blood, the antibodies that help us recognize and fight infection, the actin and myosin that contract and relax our muscles, and the collagen that makes our ligaments, tendons, and skin elastic are all types of proteins. There are more than 20 different kinds of amino acids. Our bodies are unable to produce eight of these amino acids, and these **essential amino acids** must be acquired from food. Animal proteins are usually **complete proteins** that contain all of the essential amino acids. Plant proteins are usually incomplete proteins, but eating **complementary proteins** like maize (corn) with beans or hummus (chick peas/garbanzo beans and sesame seeds) with whole wheat pita bread can provide all of the amino acids in one meal. Nutritionists recommend that for most people at least 10% (but not more than 35%) of calories taken in over a day should come from high-quality proteins (Figure 9-1).

Fats and oils are both types of lipids, carbon-hydrogen chains with other chemical groups at the ends of the chains. **Fats** are lipids of animal origin like butter and lard that are solid at room temperature. **Oils** are lipids of plant origin like corn oil and olive oil that are liquids at room temperature. Lipids contain more energy per gram than any other biological molecule. **Lipids**, or fatty acids, provide long-term energy storage, insulation, protective padding around internal organs, and assistance with nutrient absorption. They are also needed for the processing of some vitamins (A, D, E, and K) and are used to make other compounds in the body. For example, polyunsaturated fats like corn oil and safflower oil are used by the body to make some types of hormones (chemical messengers). Nutritionists recommend that about 15% to 30% of calories taken in over a day should come from healthy fats and oils (Figure 9-2).

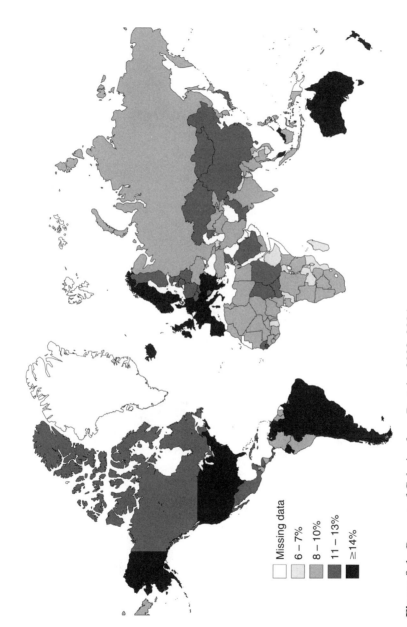

Figure 9-1. Percent of Calories from Protein, 2002–2004.

Data Source: Food and Agriculture Organization (FAO) of the United Nations, Food Security Statistics: Diet Composition—Nutrients, 30 June 2006.

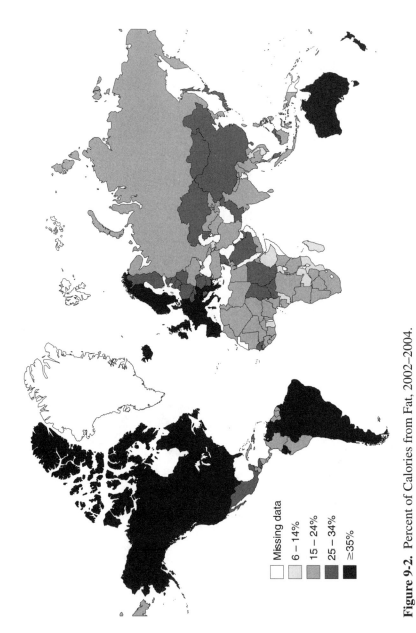

Figure 9-2. Percent of Calories from Fat, 2002–2004.

Data Source: Food and Agriculture Organization (FAO) of the United Nations, Food Security Statistics: Diet Composition—Nutrients, 30 June 2006.

But not all fatty acids are equally healthy. The relative healthiness of lipids is often related to the amount of hydrogen they contain. Unsaturated fatty acids contain at least one double bond in the carbon chain. Both monounsaturated fats like those found in olive oil, avocados, and nuts and the polyunsaturated fats in cold water fish like salmon (which contain omega-3 fatty acids) seem to be protective against heart disease. Saturated fatty acids are found in meat, butter, and other animal products and can contribute to blocked arteries. The term **saturated fatty acid** refers to the fact that the molecule is "saturated" with hydrogen, meaning that no more hydrogen can be added to it because only single bonds exist between its carbon atoms. Trans fats, liquid oils that have been transformed into solid fats by adding hydrogen to them through the use of pressure, are found in margarine and processed foods and have been shown to raise "bad" (or "lousy") LDL (low-density lipoprotein) cholesterol while depleting "good" (or "healthy") HDL (high-density lipoprotein) cholesterol. When the LDL/HDL ratio is high, the excess fat in the blood is deposited on the walls of blood vessels as plaque. When there is a lot of atherosclerosis (plaque lining the blood vessels) the risk of having a heart attack or stroke increases. The heart is a muscle, and the walls of the heart have their own blood supply to keep them healthy. A heart attack is caused when the blood vessels that bring blood to the heart's muscle tissue become blocked and the heart muscle does not get enough oxygen. A similar process can cause a stroke, if the blood vessels that become blocked lead to the brain.

Vitamins help the body use energy and act as regulators (Table 9-1). For example, vitamins C, E, and A are antioxidants that reduce free radicals, which are ions in the cells that may damage cell membranes. There are more than a dozen vitamins necessary for health, and most of them must be included in the diet. For example, folate must be ingested daily because it is not stored by the body. Folate (or folic acid) is necessary for growth and red blood cell production. Women of childbearing age need to make sure that they have an adequate intake of folate, because deficiency during the first weeks of pregnancy is associated with neural tube defects in developing fetuses. (The most common neural tube defects are anencephaly, a fatal condition in which the brain fails to develop, and spina bifida, in which the spinal cord does not develop properly.) These defects occur very early in the pregnancy, usually before a woman knows she is pregnant, so it is recommended that all women who might become pregnant take a multivitamin. Vitamin C is another vitamin that must be part of the diet. It is an antioxidant

Table 9-1. Common Vitamin Nutrients: Functions, Sources, and Problems of Deficiency.

Vitamin	Function(s)	Sources	Problems of Deficiency
Vitamin A (retinol + carotene)	Preventing infections; keeping the eyes healthy; helping children grow properly	Liver, kidney, eggs, butter; milk; orange and yellow fruits and vegetables; dark green vegetables	Increased susceptibility to infection and death, night blindness, blindness
Vitamin D	Helping the body absorb and use calcium and phosphorus to build bones and teeth	Can be made in the skin when exposed to the sun; milk, butter, cheese; fatty fish; eggs; liver	*Rickets* (if bones are still growing): bowed legs or "knock knees," chest deformities, swollen bones in wrists and ankles, muscle weakness; *osteomalacia* (if bones have finished growing): severe bone pain, broken bones, muscle weakness
Thiamine (vitamin B$_1$)	Metabolism of food	Meat, poultry, fish; liver; whole grains; legumes; seeds; milk; eggs	*Beriberi*: loss of appetite, weakness and sometimes paralysis of legs or arms, cardiac failure
Riboflavin (vitamin B$_2$)	Metabolism of food	Milk; eggs; liver, meat, fish; whole grains; green leaves; legumes	Cracked lips, sores at the corners of the mouth, rough skin
Niacin (nicotinic acid)	Metabolism of food	Liver, meat, fish; groundnuts; milk; whole grains	*Pellagra*: dark, peeling rash on skin exposed to sun; diarrhea; mental changes
Folate (folic acid)	Growth; making red blood cells	Liver and kidney; fresh vegetables; fish; beans and groundnuts	Anemia; neural tube defects in babies born to mothers who are deficient
Vitamin C (ascorbic acid)	Collagen formation and wound healing; helping with absorption of iron; antioxidant	Vegetables; fresh fruit, especially citrus; fresh potatoes; fresh milk	*Scurvy*: internal bleeding, swollen bleeding gums and tooth loss; swollen painful joints, especially knee, hip, and elbow

that helps the body absorb iron and create collagen, which is essential for maintaining healthy gums, skin, and other tissues. (Some vitamins can be produced by the body. For example, vitamin K, which is required for proper blood clotting, is made in the intestine, and vitamin D, essential for bone strength, can be made in the skin if it is exposed to sunlight.)

Minerals help in building strong bones, transmitting nerve signals, and maintaining a normal heart rate (Table 9-2). We need to include minerals like calcium, phosphorus, magnesium, sulfur, chloride, copper, selenium, and manganese in our diet. Some minerals, like zinc, promote growth and wound healing. Others, like sodium and potassium, are electrolytes that contribute to maintaining blood chemistry, blood pressure, and, in the case of potassium, a regular heartbeat. Fluoride is essential for the development of strong teeth and bones, so some communities add fluoride to drinking water to ensure that children have an adequate intake of the mineral. As with any nutrient, either a deficiency or an excess of minerals can be harmful. Some people develop problems by overdosing on vitamin and mineral supplements. Others add too much salt to their foods, and excess sodium can increase the risk of high blood pressure in some adults. Even fluoride, which has revolutionized dental health, can cause weak bones and teeth as excess fluoride (fluorosis) replaces some of the calcium in teeth, stains teeth brown, and causes teeth to become pitted or break.

And, finally, water is an essential part of the diet. Every cell in the body needs a way to take in oxygen and nutrients along with a way to get rid of carbon dioxide and waste. Blood, which is about 92% water, is the medium for transporting gases, nutrients, and wastes throughout the body, and the most common component of blood is water. Without adequate blood volume, blood pressure drops and it is difficult for the body's cells to function. A person who loses a lot of blood due to an injury or a lot of water due to excessive vomiting or diarrhea can go into hypovolemic shock, shock caused by too little blood volume. (Prevention of hypovolemic shock is one reason why paramedics usually start accident victims on IV fluids right away.) Water is also needed to regulate body temperature by sweating and to get rid of body wastes through urination and defecation. An adult loses about 2 to 3 quarts of water a day by urinating, sweating, and exhaling humidified air. More may be lost in hot climates or during intense physical activity or when a person has diarrhea. This lost water must be replaced to avoid dehydration. Severe dehydration can cause an imbalance of the acids and bases in the blood, loss of muscle tone, organ failure (especially of the kidneys), and death.

Table 9-2. Common Mineral Nutrients: Functions, Sources, and Problems of Deficiency.

Mineral	Function(s)	Sources	Problems of Deficiency
Iron	Making hemoglobin for red blood cells; helping other cells function	Heme iron from meat; non-heme iron from plants, eggs, milk, legumes, and some grains	Anemia: paleness of the tongue and mouth, tiredness, breathlessness; reduced ability to work and learn; increased risk of death for pregnant women and their babies
Iodine	Making thyroid hormones that control brain and nervous system function, the way the body uses energy, and growth	Iodine is found in soil and in plants grown in soil high in iodine; seafood; iodized salt	Goiter (enlarged thyroid gland in neck), hypothyroidism (low energy, feeling cold, dry skin, constipation); increased risk of stillbirth and sick babies, cretinism
Fluoride	Preventing tooth decay and strengthen bones	Water	Weak tooth enamel, dental caries (cavities), weak bones
Zinc	Child growth and development; wound healing; fighting infections; antioxidant	Meat, chicken, fish; whole grains and legumes	Slow growth, slow wound healing, poor appetite and impaired sense of taste and smell, apathy, skin lesions
Calcium	Making and repairing bone and teeth	Milk; small fish containing bones; beans and peas; dark green leaves	Osteoporosis; hypertension
Sodium	Cell function	Salt	Fatigue, muscle cramps
Potassium	Cell function	Fruits, especially bananas; coconuts; vegetables; legumes	Fatigue, weakness, heart arrhythmias

UNDERNUTRITION

Undernutrition is malnutrition resulting from deficiencies in the amount of food or types of nutrients eaten or from poor absorption of nutrients that have been consumed. For example, lack of protein in the diet means that the body does not have the amino acids it needs to repair itself and too little fat in the diet means that fat-soluble vitamins A, D, E, and K cannot be processed. Everyone needs a diet that includes at least some carbohydrates, proteins, fats or oils, and a variety of vitamins and minerals to stay healthy. The total amount of energy, protein, and other nutrients needed by a person varies based on age, sex, body size, activity level, climate, and pregnancy and lactation status.

Children who do not have adequate caloric intake or are nutrient deficient are at increased risk of illness and death and do not grow well. Undernourished children may have **stunting** (low height for age) and **wasting** (low weight for height). Some children develop **kwashiorkor** and have **edema** (swelling) of the arms, legs, and face, weak muscles, pale hair and skin, and an enlarged liver. Children with kwashiorkor may maintain a moderate weight and have a swollen belly. This is not because they are fat. Instead, their nutrient-deficient body is retaining fluids (causing excess weight) and the abdominal walls are so weak that the internal organs sag out. Kwashiorkor often develops in children who have been weaned early (frequently because of the birth of a younger sibling) and have a diet high in starch but low in protein. A child who has severe protein-energy malnutrition (PEM) may develop a condition called **marasmus** that is associated with very low weight, weakness, susceptibility to infections, and the eventual shutdown of body systems. Children with marasmus look skeletal, have loose and wrinkled skin, and have very little energy to move or cry. Both marasmus and kwashiorkor can have severe complications like diarrhea, dehydration, increased susceptibility to infection, hypoglycemia (low blood sugar), hypothermia (low body temperature), anemia and other nutritional deficiencies, and children with these conditions are at risk of permanent disability and death.

The statistics on childhood hunger are disturbing. Nearly 150 million children under 5 years of age are underweight (Figures 9-3 and 9-4). More than one-quarter (27%) of all under-5 children in developing countries are underweight, including nearly half (46%) the children in South Asia, a region that includes India, Bangladesh, and Pakistan.[1]

Childhood malnutrition is closely associated with poverty. Poor children are much more likely than rich children to be underweight, and poverty

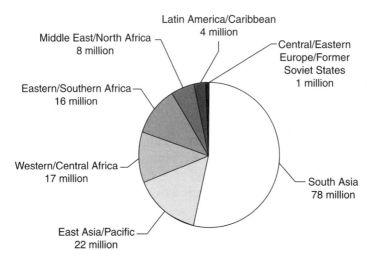

Figure 9-3. Underweight Children Under 5 Years of Age in Developing Countries.
Data Source: UNICEF, "A Report Card on Nutrition," Number 4, May 2006.

creates a cycle of malnutrition and disease that is hard to break (Figure 9-5).[2] Because poverty is greater in rural areas, rural children are nearly twice as likely as urban children to be underweight.

Undernutrition is a contributing factor in more than 50% of infectious disease-related deaths of children in their first five years of life, especially those due to diarrhea and acute respiratory infection.[3] Undernutrition also is associated with increased risk of child death due to malaria and measles.[4] Even mild and moderate undernutrition can significantly increase the risk of death.

Many babies begin life undernourished, with a low birthweight because their mothers are undernourished. Low birthweight babies have an increased risk of breathing problems and other potentially life-threatening difficulties during their first weeks of life, and some develop long-term impairments like learning disabilities, mental retardation, cerebral palsy, or blindness.

Vitamin and Mineral Deficiencies

Good nutrition requires more than just sufficient caloric intake. It also requires a balanced diet that includes all the essential micronutrients. Vitamin and mineral deficiencies are a common form of undernutrition in both children

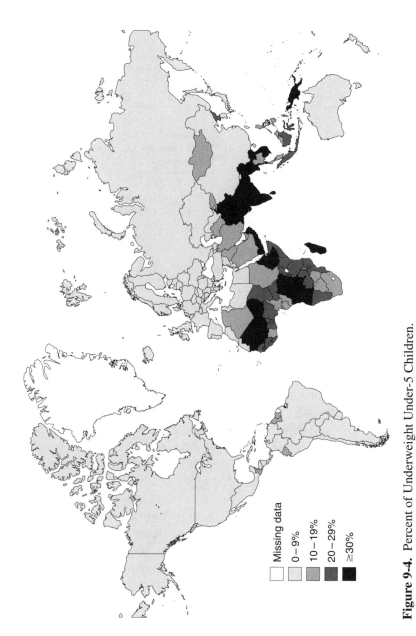

Figure 9-4. Percent of Underweight Under-5 Children.

Data Source: UNICEF, 2006 State of the World's Children Report. Table 2: Nutrition. Summary data from 1996 through 2004.

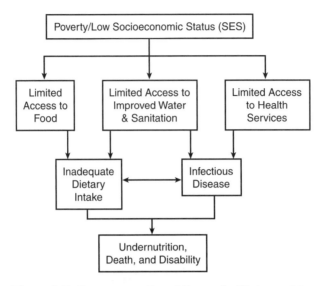

Figure 9-5. Poverty as a Causal Factor for Undernutrition.

and adults. A large percentage of the world's population is at risk of iron, iodine, vitamin A, and zinc deficiencies.

The best way to consume these micronutrients is through food. When a person's diet does not provide enough nutrients or the body is not absorbing enough of the nutrients, non-food sources may be useful. Micronutrient deficiencies can sometimes be prevented by providing **supplements** such as multivitamin pills or by enriching or fortifying food with extra micronutrients. A food is **enriched** when some of the vitamins and minerals lost during processing are added back into the food. A **fortified** food has nutrients that are not naturally present in the ingredients added to the product. Common examples of enriched and fortified foods include vitamin A fortified sugar, folic acid and iron enriched flours, and iodized salt. However, supplements and enriched and fortified foods may not provide vitamins and minerals in a form that has a high bioavailability. **Bioavailability** is the fraction of the vitamin or mineral consumed that is able to be absorbed and used by the body. Absorption can be increased by taking supplements with food. For example, the fat-soluble vitamins must be taken with fat or oil and iron absorption is boosted by vitamin C.

Most people with severe micronutrient deficiencies live in developing countries, but there are also pockets of micronutrient deficiencies in unexpected populations, like some North American teens, because of dietary habits.

Some vitamin deficiencies have relatively immediate symptoms. A person with too little niacin, which is important for metabolism, will develop pellagra and have his or her skin darken and slough off. A person with too little riboflavin (vitamin B2) will develop rough skin and cracked lips. Thiamine (vitamin B1) deficiency causes beriberi, which can damage the heart and nervous system. And too little vitamin C causes scurvy, which is characterized by bleeding gums and swollen, painful joints, and decreased immune system function.

Others vitamin and mineral deficiencies have long-term consequences. Adolescents who consume too little calcium are at risk of developing osteoporosis as they age, and porous bones can lead to hip fractures and other life-threatening injuries. Bone strength is also reliant upon sufficient vitamin D. Vitamin D deficiency in children whose bones are still growing is called rickets (or, more informally, "knock knees"). Vitamin D deficiency in adults whose bones have stopped growing is called osteomalacia and can make the bones soft and prone to breaking. Vitamin D, the "sun vitamin," can be made in the skin if it is exposed to sunlight for about 15 minutes daily, but deficiency is a problem in parts of the world where women are expected to cover themselves in public, in people who work indoors all day and avoid sun exposure, and seasonally among people who live far from the equator and have months of darkness each year.

Vitamin A Deficiency

Vitamin A is an antioxidant essential for eye health and is found primarily in yellow, orange, and dark green vegetables. Vitamin A deficiency (VAD) is the most common cause of preventable blindness in children. The World Health Organization estimates that 100 to 140 million children have VAD and 250,000 to 500,000 children with VAD go blind each year.[5] Vision problems associated with VAD usually start as dry eye (xerosis) and night blindness, then progressively worsen as the eye becomes drier and the cornea ulcerates and scars. Vitamin A also supports the body's immune system in fighting infections. VAD increases the risk of dying from diarrhea, measles, malaria, and other infections. Half of the children with blindness caused by VAD die within 12 months from undernutrition and other infections.[6]

Vitamin A is a fat-soluble vitamin, which means that it will only be absorbed by the body if it is eaten with fats or oils, so dietary prevention requires a consistent source of both vegetables and oil. In some countries, milk, sugar, or other commercial products are fortified with vitamin A, but fortified foods are not available to all households that need them. Oil-filled vitamin A capsule supplements are relatively inexpensive and would prevent hundreds of thousands of children from going blind, but distribution can be a challenge, especially since the benefits of the capsules only last for 4 to 6 months. A high-tech option is also available: *golden rice* is a genetically modified organism (GMO) that has been altered to produce the vitamin A precursor beta-carotene. Golden rice is not yet widely used, in part because of concerns by some countries about allowing GMO products to be grown, but the manufacturer grants free licenses to low-income growers and humanitarian organizations.

Iodine Deficiency Disorders

Iodine deficiency is the most common cause of brain damage in the world. The thyroid gland, located in the neck, controls body **metabolism** (the rate at which your body uses energy) and assists with growth. Thyroid hormones (chemical messengers that control metabolism) are made from the mineral iodine. If there is too little iodine in the diet, there is not enough iodine in the blood for the thyroid gland to function properly. In response, the thyroid gland will enlarge as it tries to collect more iodine from the blood and will produce a **goiter** (a swollen neck resulting from an enlarged thyroid gland). A person who cannot produce enough thyroid hormones will have a low metabolism and will feel cold, tired, and apathetic. Babies born to mothers who have hypothyroidism may be stillborn or have a type of brain damage called **cretinism**. The level of dysfunction caused by lack of iodine can range from mild to severe, but the World Health Organization estimates that iodine deficiency disorders (IDD) affect more than 740 million people (13% of the world's population) and 30% of the remainder are at risk. About 50 million people have some degree of IDD-related brain damage.[7] Most countries provide iodine in the form of iodized salt, but commercial salt may not reach the neediest households (Figure 9-6).

Iron Deficiency Anemia

Red blood cells (RBCs) carry oxygen from the lungs to the rest of the cells in the body. A molecule called hemoglobin holds the oxygen inside the RBCs, and hemoglobin is made from iron. A person with too little iron is

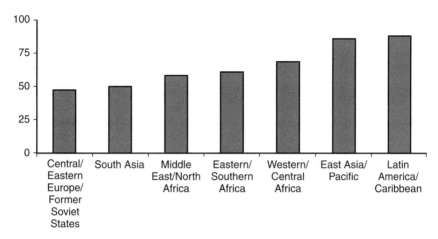

Figure 9-6. Proportion of Households in Developing Countries that Consume Iodized Salt.

Data Source: UNICEF, "A Report Card on Nutrition," Number 4, May 2006.

not able to efficiently transport oxygen. When lack of iron is caused by inadequate iron intake, this condition is called iron deficiency anemia (IDA). Symptoms of **anemia** include pale skin, fatigue, weakness, shortness of breath, headaches, an increased heart rate, and a limited ability to concentrate at work or school. Growing children, pregnant women, and women who menstruate are at high risk of IDA.[8] Children need extra iron as their body grows and their blood volume increases. Pregnant women need extra iron as their blood volume expands. Anemia increases the risk of death during delivery, and babies born to anemic women have an increased risk of illness. Anyone who loses a lot of blood due to pregnancy, menstruation, or an injury may need to replace lost iron stores.

IDA is the most common nutritional disorder in the world and affects about one-third of the world's population. More than 2 billion people are currently anemic, including the majority of pre-school children and pre-menopausal women in low-income countries.[9,10,11] Anemia can be prevented and treated through increased iron intake. Iron is found in both plant and animal sources. Heme iron is found in blood and meat from animals, birds, and fish, and about 15% to 35% is absorbed by the body. Non-heme iron is found in plants, eggs, and milk, and less than 5% is absorbed. Iron can also be added to fortified foods like pastas and flours. Control of infections that cause internal bleeding (like hookworm and schistosomiasis) or destruction of red blood cells (like malaria) is also important for preventing and treating IDA.

Zinc Deficiency

Zinc is important for immune function, growth, and development of children. Zinc is found primarily in animal sources, so people who rely solely on a plant-based diet are at risk of deficiency. Since any level of zinc deficiency can increase susceptibility to infection, it is helpful for at-risk children with diarrhea, pneumonia, and malaria to be given zinc supplements or eat food fortified with zinc.

MEASURING NUTRITIONAL STATUS

Anthropometry is the measurement of the human body. Height, weight, waist circumference, percentage of body fat, and other measurements can be useful indicators of whether a person is underweight or overweight. They can also be used to predict some health risks. For example, having a waist circumference greater than 35 inches for a woman or 40 inches for a man is associated with increased risk of heart disease. The **body mass index (BMI)** is often used to estimate body composition of adults. The BMI is calculated by taking weight in kilograms and dividing it by the square of the height in meters.

$$BMI = \frac{weight(kg)}{height(m) \times height(m)} = 703 \times \frac{weight(lb)}{height(in) \times height(in)}$$

In the United States a BMI of 18.5 to 25 is considered normal. A BMI of less than 18.5 is considered underweight. A person with a BMI greater than 25 is overweight, with a BMI greater than 30 is obese, and with a BMI greater than 35 is morbidly obese. BMI does not consider the effect of body fat, so people who are trim but have a lot of muscle mass may be incorrectly classified as overweight. BMI does not measure physical fitness levels; a person with a healthy weight may be physically unfit and have poor strength and limited cardiovascular endurance.

For children, the more accurate measures of healthy growth are weight-for-height, weight-for-age, and height-for-age. Global growth standards for children from birth through 60 months are provided by the World Health Organization. Figure 9-7 shows a sample weight-for-age chart for girls. The graph has age on the x-axis and weight on the y-axis. The graph allows a parent or health care worker to easily determine if a child is underweight (below the 15th percentile) or severely underweight (under the 3rd percentile) for his or her age.

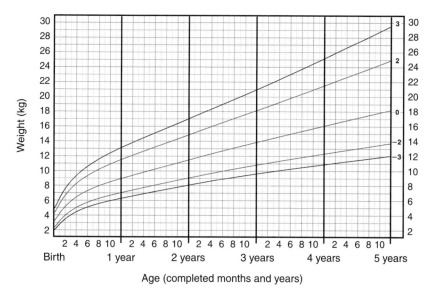

Figure 9-7. A Sample WHO Child Growth Standard Chart for Girls, Birth to 5 Years (z-scores).

Source: World Health Organization. Used with permission.

Ideally, children should be weighed often so that growth trends can emerge. A child who loses weight or fails to gain weight needs extra medical attention. Weighing of children under 5 years of age is a routine part of physical exams.

These growth charts can be used worldwide because scientific evidence shows that infants and children from geographically diverse regions experience very similar growth patterns when their health and nutritional needs are met. The most recent standards were released in 2006. Based on these standards, there are nearly 170 million underweight children under five years of age in the world and at least 20 million overweight children.[12]

One limitation of growth charts is that they require caregivers to know the birth date of the child. When this information is not available it can be difficult to determine if a child is not growing well. In emergency situations, a child's arm circumference (the mid-upper arm circumference, or MUAC) can be used to determine if the child is severely underweight.[13] Most healthy children over 12 months of age should have an arm circumference of 16 cm or greater when the measurement is taken halfway between the elbow and the shoulder. Any child at least 1 year old with a MUAC of less than 12.5 cm is severely undernourished. Children with a MUAC between 12.5 and 13.5 cm are considered moderately undernourished.

DIET		
KNOWLEDGE	**ATTITUDE**	**PRACTICE**
What is a serving size of protein? What foods are a good source of vitamin C? What are healthy sources of lipids?	What foods are essential to include in a meal? What role does food play in social events? Do you worry about your weight?	How many pieces of fruit do you eat in a week? How often do you consume meat products?

HAND-WASHING		
KNOWLEDGE	**ATTITUDE**	**PRACTICE**
How often should people wash their hands? Why should people use soap? Why should people wash their hands before eating?	Is hand washing convenient? Does it keep you healthy? Is it worth the effort? Do your friends wash their hands?	How often do you wash your hands? Do you use soap? Do you wash your hands before eating?

Figure 9-8. Example of the Kinds of Questions That Would Be Asked During KAP Surveys on Diet and Hand Washing.

Anthropometry is one way to begin to understand nutritional status, but it is also important to understand the biological, psychological, social, and behavioral factors that contribute to nutrition. Some nutritionists focus on quantifying the amount and types of nutrients in food by conducting laboratory assessments of food portions. This kind of analysis may, for example, be useful for identifying locally-available foods rich in particular nutrients that can be added to the diet to improve micronutrient status. Nutritionists may also collect data by observing food preparation and eating practices in order to understand cultural and social aspects of nutrition, which can then be incorporated by individuals and communities into plans for improving health and nutrition.

Health behaviorists often refer to a behavior triad—knowledge, attitude, and practice—that is sometimes shortened to KAP. Figure 9 8 shows the kinds of questions that might be asked during KAP surveys on diet and hand washing.

Knowledge about a subject does not always translate into changed practices unless attitudes also change. And even when both knowledge and attitude indicate a desire for changes in nutrition practice, it may not be possible to implement new practices because of resource limitations or social barriers. One example of the complex relationship between knowledge, attitude, and practice is breastfeeding.

BREASTFEEDING

Breastmilk contains all of the nutrients and water babies need, and also includes digestive enzymes and antibodies and other immune factors that protect against harmful infections and promote health. For example, "bifidus factor" encourages the multiplication of helpful bacteria called *Lactobacillus bifidus* in the baby's intestines. Colostrum, the milk produced in the first days after giving birth, is especially beneficial since it contains large quantities of an antibody called secretory immunoglobulin A (IgA).

In ideal circumstances it is recommended that an infant be exclusively breastfed for the first 6 months of life. To breastfeed exclusively means that breastmilk is the only substance the baby consumes and that no supplemental water, juice, cow or goat milk, porridge, rice water, or any other foods are fed to the baby. At six months after birth, complementary foods are introduced while breastfeeding continues for up to 2 years or more (Figure 9-9). "Complementary" means that the foods complement breastmilk, not that they replace it.

Only about one in every three children in the developing world is exclusively breastfed for the first six months of life (Figure 9-10), and this low percentage contributes to illness and death from undernutrition and diarrhea. The World Health Organization estimates that if every baby was exclusively breastfed from birth through six months, an estimated 1.5 million lives could be saved each year.[14]

Not all women are able to exclusively breastfeed. Some mothers do not produce adequate milk for their babies and have to supplement with formula at an early age. Some have HIV infection and do not want to risk passing the virus to their babies through breastmilk. Other mothers have work schedules that do not allow them to feed their baby every few hours and have

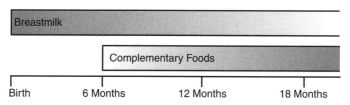

Figure 9-9. Infant Feeding Timeline.
Babies should have only breastmilk for the first 6 months of life. Complementary foods should be added as the baby is weaned.

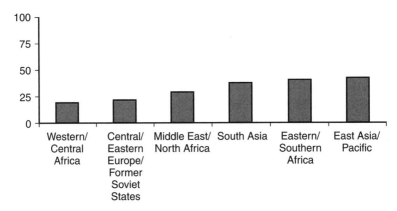

Figure 9-10. Proportion of children in developing countries who are exclusively breastfed for the first six months of life.

Data Source: UNICEF, "A Report Card on Nutrition," Number 4, May 2006.

to rely on formula. And newborns whose mothers have died in childbirth must have access to an alternate source of nutrition.

Using formula rather than breastmilk can endanger some babies because of lack of clean water, difficulties with reading and following the mixing instructions, and poor hygiene. The high cost of formula is also a burden. Mothers who have stopped breastfeeding may end up relying on cow's milk, tea, rice water, or other breastmilk substitutes that do not have the nutrients of breastmilk or infant formula.

Much of the concern about the use of formula grows out of the marketing strategies used by Nestlé and other infant formula companies in the 1970s in developing countries. Hospital maternity wards were sponsored by formula companies, and new mothers would be sent home with formula samples and no breastfeeding education. Worse, some companies hired "milk nurses" to go into communities in nurses uniforms to advertise formula, implying that formula was better than breastmilk. New mothers who do not breastfeed quickly lose the ability to produce milk and must then rely on breastmilk alternates, so providing a limited amount of free formula may create a dependency on the product.

In 1981 the World Health Assembly approved the International Code of Marketing of Breast-milk Substitutes.[15] It recognizes that "when mothers do not breastfeed, or only do so partially, there is a legitimate market for infant formula." But it stresses that breastmilk is the best option, and says that new mothers who are given information about the use of infant formula must be informed about the "social and financial implications of its use, the health hazards of inappropriate foods or feeding methods, and, in particular, the health hazards of unnecessary or improper use of infant formula and other breast-milk substitutes." The Code stipulates that marketing personnel (even if they are health care professionals) should not directly contact pregnant women or new mothers, health facilities should not promote formula use, and samples of formula should not be distributed at hospitals or by retailers. Nestlé and other formula producers have adopted the International Code of Marketing of Breast-milk Substitutes and no longer directly market to pregnant women or new mothers in developing countries.

Mothers need to be provided with the information to make an informed choice about whether to breastfeed and how long to breastfeed. Attitudes toward breastfeeding also need to be addressed since in many cultures breastfeeding is discouraged. Employers rarely have a private room available for mothers who would like to use a breast pump. Women are not always free to breastfeed in public areas, even the "public" areas of their own homes. And the mothers of new mothers may have chosen bottle feeding and may discourage their daughters from choosing breastfeeding. It is particularly important to promote breastfeeding as an option for new mothers in places where breastfeeding is not the cultural norm. The phrase "breast is best" is often heard, but it needs to be accompanied by conditions that support breastfeeding.

GLOBALIZATION AND FOOD SAFETY

Globalization of food products is seen in changing dietary habits, the increasing variety of foods on grocery store shelves, the growing number of international restaurant chains, and global marketing of food products. Cross-border trade in foods has created a new set of concerns about food safety as products from one part of the world are shipped to the far corners of the earth. Globalization is also having an impact on social and cultural practices around the world. This is evident in changed breastfeeding practices and attitudes, and also in altered perceptions of physical beauty.

Large outbreaks of foodborne illness can be caused by a variety of agents. An outbreak of *Escherichia coli* O157:H7 in 1996 made more than 6000 Japanese schoolchildren sick and was most likely spread by radish sprouts. Other *E. coli* outbreaks from across the globe have been linked to consumption of lettuce, untreated water, undercooked ground beef, and other foods. *Salmonella* outbreaks have been spread by eggs and chicken. Outbreaks of *Listeria monocytogenes*, which can be spread through cheese and processed meats, have caused miscarriages and stillbirths in pregnant women and caused septicemia in infants and immunocompromised people.

As food consumers, we want to know that our food is free from microbiological contamination and also free from contamination with toxins and harmful chemical additives. We want to be assured that our food has been prepared and stored properly, that it has not exceeded its shelf life or gone rancid, and that it was produced using safe and tested processes. We want to know that our salmon fillet does not contain high levels of mercury and that our beef is not from cattle infected with bovine spongiform encephalopathy ("mad cow" disease). It may be particularly challenging to know if imported foods are safe, and internationally-traded food now accounts for a large portion of many people's diets. (For example, the United States Department of Agriculture reports that more than half of the fish and shellfish consumed in the United States is imported, as is more than one-third of all fresh fruits.[16]) As the food industry becomes increasingly global, it will become more difficult for governments and consumers to have confidence that the food supply is safe.

New foodborne diseases can emerge as pathogens from one place are inadvertently introduced into new geographic areas through trade and by travelers who carry microorganisms from one region to others.[17] Produce that is contaminated with fecal matter or coated with pesticide and fertilizer residue can be grown in one place, injected or sprayed with preservatives or coated with wax, then shipped overnight to other countries across the globe. While the contaminated food products in many outbreaks of foodborne illness are from domestic sources, outbreaks caused by imported products are becoming more common. For example, an outbreak of hepatitis A virus in Pittsburgh, Pennsylvania, in 2003 caused several deaths and hundreds of illnesses, and its cause was fecally-contaminated green onions that had been imported from Mexico.[18] (Hepatitis A virus usually causes no symptoms in children who become infected, but infections can be serious in adults. One infection confers life-long immunity, so in countries like Mexico where nearly everyone is exposed in early childhood there are few susceptible adults and few cases of clinical disease. In countries like the United States, where a high percentage of adults are susceptible to the infection, outbreaks may cause many people to become severely ill.) Outbreaks are also associated with changes in lifestyle, such as eating out more frequently, and changes in food processing, such as butchers mixing the meat from several animals into one batch of ground meat.

There are other concerns associated with the importation of food. Labeling requirements for chemical additives and preservatives that are used to improve or maintain flavor, color, texture, or consistency of food products may not be standardized across markets. Fortification of foods with vitamins and minerals may not reach the standards of the purchaser's country. And although it currently appears that foods made from genetically modified organisms (GMO) are safe, there are no global standards for testing and labeling these foods. The international food network continues to expand and it is imperative that additional regulations be agreed upon. Both exporting and importing countries need to increase their oversight and testing of transported foods.

OVERNUTRITION

Overnutrition is a form of malnutrition caused by excessive intake of calories and nutrients. The average person needs a minimum of about 1800 kilocalories each day. A person who takes in more calories than the body uses will gain extra weight and eventually develop overweight and obesity (Figure 9-11). Obesity is already a widespread in developed countries, and there are growing numbers of obese people in developing countries. Obesity is associated with many diseases, including type 2 diabetes, hypertension (high blood pressure), gallstones and other digestive disorders, asthma, back pain, arthritis of the back and hip, and an increased risk of heart disease and strokes. Obesity is also associated with an increased risk for many types of cancers.

Overnutrition is becoming a problem in nearly every region of the world (Figure 9-12).[19,20] Some island nations in the west Pacific now have the highest prevalence of obesity in the world. Nearly all Latin American and Caribbean countries have high or moderate obesity prevalence. More than one-third of the adult populations of some oil-exporting Middle Eastern countries are obese. Even in regions like Asia and sub-Saharan Africa, where undernutrition is still a serious problem, there are pockets of obesity, especially in high-income urban areas. Urbanization contributes to obesity by lowering the amount of energy expended in labor because of mechanization and by increasing sedentary activities like watching television. Urbanization also initiates dietary changes such as increases in the amount of calories consumed during meals, total fat consumption, the number of meals eaten outside the home, and the amount of fast food consumed.[21]

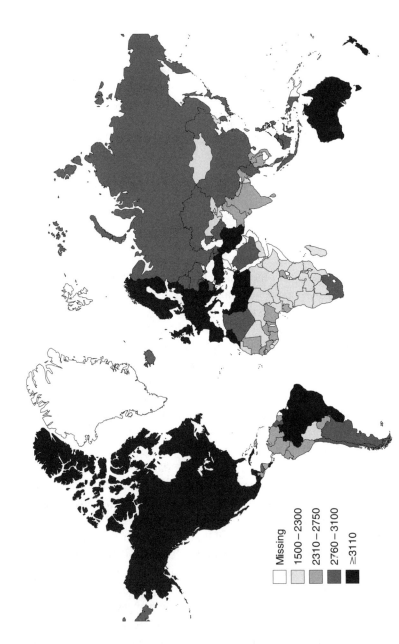

Figure 9-11. Average Energy Consumption (Kilocalories per Person per Day), 2002–2004.

Data Source: Food and Agriculture Organization (FAO) of the United Nations, Food Security Statistics: Food Consumption—Dietary Energy, Protein and Fat, 30 June 2006.

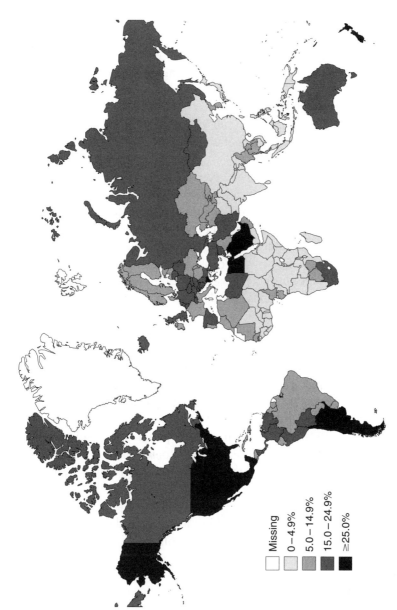

Figure 9-12. Prevalence of Obesity (BMI ≥ 30) in Adults Ages 15 and Older, 2005.

Data Source: WHO Global InfoBase

Missing
0 – 4.9%
5.0 – 14.9%
15.0 – 24.9%
≥25.0%

Genes influence metabolic rate, body shape (where a person carries excess weight), and the efficiency of the body at storing extra calories, but genetic change does not explain why obesity has become so much more prevalent in the past decade. It takes generations for genetic adaptation to occur, but it takes only a short time to change dietary and exercise habits. Although the Pima Indians of Arizona may have a strong genetic tendency toward developing diabetes, changes in diet and exercise habits explain the rapid increase in obesity and diabetes prevalence. More than half of Pima adults who live in Arizona have diabetes (and 95% of diabetics are overweight), while the rates for obesity and diabetes remain low for Pima Indians who live in Mexico.[22]

The **nutrition transition** describes a population shift from a stage in which undernutrition and nutrient deficiencies are prevalent to an intermediate stage in which undernutrition and obesity are both problems in the population to a stage in which overweight and obesity are the dominant nutritional disorders. Pre-transition populations are concerned about having too little food and may focus on eating energy-dense foods that have a lot of calories even if they are low in nutrients. Post-transition populations consume a greater variety of nutritious foods, but also eat more refined foods, foods of animal origin, and fats.[23]

Some anthropologists use the term *New World Syndrome* to refer to the "diseases of affluence" (such as obesity, diabetes, heart disease, and hypertension) that generally occur after a population replaces its traditional diet with other foods. Junk foods are often cheaper than more nutritious foods. (It often costs less to buy a cheeseburger at an American fast-food restaurant than it does to buy an apple at a grocery store.) And imported foods are often seen as more desirable than traditional foods, in part due to clever marketing by transnational food companies. Nearly every country in the world now has a McDonald's and a Pizza Hut, and Coca-Cola and Pepsi products are found worldwide. The "Coca-colonization" of food markets is creating changes in consumer behaviors and desires.

Beauty is a function of culture. Think about how the ideal woman's body has been portrayed in art. When the painters of the European Renaissance wanted to show beautiful, powerful women, they portrayed women with rolls of fat and rounded curves. In some cultures today, larger women are still seen as having ideal body shapes and excess weight is associated with perceived fertility. When resources are scarce, having excess weight is often a sign of wealth since it shows that the household has more than enough calories and does not have to expend so many of them in physical labor. On the other hand, the women who model on the fashion runways in Paris and Milan are usually bone thin and the ideal Hollywood woman is extremely skinny. In industrialized societies, being underweight is often an indication of wealth since richer households have more time and money to prepare healthy foods and exercise whereas working-class households rely on cheap fast foods and work long hours at sedentary jobs.

Globalization is bringing people together through the shared experience of food. It also is influencing attitudes toward food and body image. Although eating disorders like anorexia nervosa and bulimia nervosa are still relatively rare in non-Western cultures, there are reports from many countries of cases being identified.[24] (Anorexia nervosa is a condition in which a person has a distorted body image and feels fat even when emaciated. A person with anorexia nervosa follows a very restricted diet, exercises excessively, and may use laxatives and other methods of losing weight. Bulimia nervosa is when a person engages in frequent binge-purge cycles, eating thousands of calories at one sitting then inducing vomiting and using laxatives to get rid of the calories ingested.) More importantly, dissatisfaction with body shape is becoming more common, especially as the idealized bodies of Western movie stars and the touched-up bodies of magazine cover models are broadcast to larger audiences. For example, recent studies of ideal body size in Pacific Island nations like Fiji, Tonga, and Samoa, which have some of the highest prevalence of obesity in the world, have found growing dissatisfaction with body size, a trend toward thin bodies being seen as ideal, and the beginnings of unhealthy weight loss behaviors like purging.[25,26,27,28]

IS THERE ENOUGH FOOD IN THE WORLD?

Food security occurs when a household at all times has access to enough safe and nutritious food to be able to stay active and healthy. A food-secure household can grow or purchase an adequate quantity, quality, and variety of food during the entire year, even when it is not a growing season. Even in wealthy countries there are households that do not meet this definition of food security. The USDA estimates that 11.9% of U.S. households, including 17.6% of households with children, were food insecure for at least part of 2004.[29]

Still, the short answer to the question "Is there enough food in the world to feed everyone?" is "Yes!" Hunger and famine (which is when a large proportion of a population is hungry for an extended period of time and the result is mass migration and death) are problems of economics (poverty), politics (power), and distribution more than they are simply natural disasters. Amartya Sen, a Nobel Prize–winning economist from India, noted:

> "There is nothing inevitable about famines. Famines are typically precipitated by the loss of entitlements of one or more occupation groups, and the process can be halted by generating replacement incomes for potential victims. . . . There is nothing inescapable about endemic undernourishment either. Persistent deprivation can also be eradicated through positive public action."[30]

In other words, although drought and other natural disasters may create conditions where hunger and famine can occur, it is governmental inaction or inadequate action that determines whether a situation will spiral into famine.

Food distribution systems need to be strengthened so that those who fail to produce enough food for their families have access to surplus food, whether it is provided by domestic or foreign producers. Trade policies can also help alleviate hunger by making it attractive for growers to sell their food locally rather than shipping it out of the country for a higher profit.

Although most countries currently produce more than enough food for their residents, not all countries have the capacity to produce enough food to feed their residents. For example, Japan, Singapore, and several of the countries on the Arabian Peninsula do not have enough arable (farmable) land to produce sufficient crops for their current populations. In some cases the problem is simply population density. In others an arid climate, steeply sloped terrain, poor soil, land degradation (caused by salinization, soil erosion by water and wind, drought, overgrazing, desertification, or poor irrigation practices), water shortages, and irrigation problems contribute to low per capita food production.

The best way to ensure that everyone is food secure is to increase food production while also increasing environmental protection. This means developing new agricultural techniques or choosing to use time-tested techniques such as crop rotation that cause as little damage to the environment as possible and also increase yields. Food stores can be maximized when as little food as possible is wasted, eaten by animals, or allowed to spoil during storage. As the world population increases and available croplands shrink, crop yields will have to increase to meet demand.

REFERENCES

1. UNICEF, 2006 State of the World's Children Report.
2. Ibid.
3. Rice AL, Sacco L, Hyder A, Black RE. Malnutrition as an underlying cause of childhood deaths associated with infectious diseases in developing countries. *Bull World Health Organ.* 2000;78:1207–1221.
4. Caulfield LE, de Onis M, Blössner M, Black RE. Undernutrition as an underlying cause of child deaths associated with diarrhea, pneumonia, malaria, and measles. *Am J Clin Nut.* 2004;80:193–198.
5. World Health Organization, "Micronutrient deficiencies: Vitamin A deficiency." UNESCO, FRESH Tools for Effective School Health, "Vitamin A deficiency (VAD)," 1st edition, 2004.
6. World Health Organization, "Vitamin A deficiency." WHO, "Micronutrient deficiencies: Vitamin A deficiency."
7. World Health Organization, "Iodine deficiency disorders."
8. Anemia can have several causes, including nutritional deficiencies (such as iron, vitamin B12, and folic acid), blood loss, and inadequate production or excessive destruction of red blood cells, but iron deficiency is the most common cause. Anemia can be made worse by worm infections (which can cause small amounts of blood loss), malaria, and other infectious diseases.
9. World Health Organization, "Iron deficiency anemia."
10. World Health Organization, "Micronutrient deficiencies: Iron deficiency anemia."
11. UNESCO, FRESH Tools for Effective School Health, "Iron Deficiency Anaemia." 1st edition, 2004.
12. World Health Organization press release on "What is the double burden of malnutrition?"
13. King FS, Burgess A. *Nutrition for Developing Countries.* 2nd ed. New York: Oxford University Press, 1993.
14. UNICEF, "Key action to tackle the main causes of under-five mortality."
15. World Health Organization, "International Code of Marketing of Breast-milk Substitutes." 2001.
16. Jerardo A. Import share of U.S. food consumption stable at 11 percent, Electronic Outlook Report from the Economic Research Service, USDA FAU-79-01, July 2003.
17. World Health Organization, "Emerging Foodborne Diseases," Fact sheet 124, January 2002.
18. Hepatitis A Outbreak Associated with Green Onions at a Restaurant—Monaca, Pennsylvania, 2003. *MMWR.* 2003;52:1155–1157.
19. Popkin BM, Doak CM. The obesity epidemic is a worldwide phenomenon. *Nutr Rev.* 1998;56:106–114.
20. Kosti RI, Panagiotakos DB. The epidemic of obesity in children and adolescents in the world. *Centr Eur J Public Health.* 2006;14:151–159.
21. Caballero B. Symposium: Obesity in developing countries: Biological and ecological factors. *J Nutr.* 2001;131:S866–S870.
22. National Institute of Diabetes and Digestive and Kidney Diseases (NIDDK), "The Pima Indians: Pathfinders for Health: Obesity Associated with High Rates of Diabetes

in the Pima Indians." Betheseda, Maryland: United States Department of Agriculture, Economic Research Service, 2002.

23. Chopra M, Galbraith S, Darnton-Hill I. A global response to a global problem: the epidemic of overnutrition. *Bull World Health Organ*. 2002;80:952–958.

24. Makino N, Tsuboi K, Dennerstein L. Prevalence of eating disorders: a comparison of Western and non-Western countries. *Med Gen Med*. 2004;6:49.

25. Becker AE, Gliman SE, Burwell RA. Changes in prevalence of overweight and in body image among Fijian women between 1989 and 1998. *Obes Res*. 2005;13:110–117.

26. Becker AE. Television, disordered eating, and young women in Fiji: negotiating body image and identity during rapid social change. *Cult Med Psychiatry*. 2004;28:533–559.

27. Brewis AA, McGarvey ST, Jones J, Swinburn BA. Perceptions of body size in Pacific Islanders. *Int J Obes*. 1998;22:185–189.

28. Craig P, Halavatau V, Comino E, Caterson I. Perception of body size in the Tongan community: differences from and similarities to an Australian sample. *Int J of Obes*. 1999;23:1288–1294.

29. Nord M, Andrews M, Carlson S. *Household Food Security in the United States, 2005*. Washington, D.C.: United States Department of Agriculture, Economic Research Service (Economic Research Report, Number 29). 2005.

30. From "Public Action to Remedy Hunger," a lecture given in London on August 2, 1990, as part of the Arturo Tanaco Memorial Lecture series.

CHAPTER 10

Environmental Health

Key Points:

- Environmental health investigates the impact of the physical environment on human health. Environmental health scientists work in housing, water resources, waste management, air quality management, occupational health, and other fields.
- Access to an adequate supply of safe drinking water and to sanitation facilities for disposal of human waste are essential for preventing diarrheal diseases.
- Access to a source of energy for cooking is essential for every household, but the use of solid fuels causes indoor air pollution and increases the risk of respiratory disease.

This chapter focuses on the health of individuals and households. (The next chapter focuses on the health of communities and larger population groups.) The first part of the chapter is an overview of the variety of issues—from food safety to noise pollution to animal control—that are addressed by the field of environmental health and are relevant to all people no matter where they live. The remainder of the chapter focuses on three of the environmental issues that are most important to the health of all individuals and communities: water, sanitation, and indoor air quality.

HISTORY OF ENVIRONMENTAL HEALTH

Humans have long recognized the environment's role in disease etiology. Hippocrates (460–388 BCE) listed environmental, dietary, behavioral, and constitutional conditions and wrote that "from these things we must proceed to investigate everything else." (Hippocrates also recognized early epidemics and wrote thorough descriptions of clinical diseases, including tetanus, typhus fever, and tuberculosis.) Long before we had the technology to see microbes through microscopes, ancient people knew that some illnesses were environmental and worked to dispose of human waste, to protect water sources, and to bury the corpses of diseased animals.

211

In the early 1800s, the prevailing theory was that epidemics arose through "spontaneous generation" from a "miasma atmosphere," which was related to environmental conditions and poor sanitation. For example, during the cholera outbreak in England discussed in the section on causality in Chapter 1, investigators found a higher infection rate in places of low altitude, especially places near marshes with an abundance of foul smelling gases, and the **miasma** theory of disease blamed the spread of cholera on contact with those foul gases. This was a sensible observation, since the people who lived in the gassy, marshy areas were the same people who used the bacterium-infected water that was the true cause of the outbreak. A more modern take on this non-mechanistic approach to preventing illness is practiced by health professionals who look for a general social, behavioral, or environmental cause of illness, rather than a very specific cause, and who focus on hygiene and avoidance of environmental carcinogens as preventive measures.

By the mid-twentieth century, most medical scientists focused their efforts on identifying specific infectious agents and genes, and tended to minimize their focus on the effect of the social and natural environments on disease spread. But even with the emphasis on immunology and genetics, one of the biggest public health breakthroughs in the twentieth century was a series of studies from 1951 through 1963 that confirmed that cigarette smoking was a major cause of lung cancer, emphysema, and cardiovascular disease. Later studies indicated that exposure to secondhand smoke was an additional risk factor for lung disease.

Today, most scientists, health professionals, and health consumers recognize both environmental risk factors and biological risk factors, such as infections, genetics, and immune system disorders, as contributors to disease. Even if an infectious agent causes a disease, social and environmental factors may contribute to the likelihood of being exposed to the infection or developing disease once infected. And many diseases and disabilities, such as hearing loss, are the results of environmental exposures rather than microbial infections or genetic disorders.

WHAT IS ENVIRONMENTAL HEALTH?

Environmental health scientists assess the impact of people on their environment and the impact of the environment on human health. They specialize in areas like air quality, food protection, radiation protection, solid waste management, hazardous waste management, water quality, noise control, environmental control of recreational areas, housing quality, and vector control. A major goal of environmental health is to understand the conditions that contribute to disease so that diseases can be prevented. For example, environmental health scientists may start with questions like "What are the health effects of smog (or contaminated water, acid rain, the thinning of the ozone layer, or the spraying of pesticides on crops)?" and then use the answers they find to promote changes in environmental health laws that regulate air quality, water quality, and the disposal of waste.

Environmental health looks at all aspects of the physical environment— where we live and work and the materials these buildings are constructed from, what we eat and where our food comes from, the source and quality of our drinking water, the quality of the air we breathe, and the length and route of our commutes. A great deal of environmental research focuses on identifying environmental risk factors for cancer and for chronic diseases like asthma and arthritis. Based upon this research, we know that exposure to ultraviolet light from the sun and tanning beds contributes to the development of skin cancer and that air pollutants, including secondhand tobacco smoke, contribute to the development of lung cancer.

The physical environment also impacts health behavior. A recent study of global cancer mortality estimated that 35% of cancer deaths were due to just nine lifestyle and environmental factors—overweight and obesity, low fruit and vegetable intake, physical inactivity, smoking, alcohol use, unsafe sex, urban air pollution, indoor smoke from household use of solid fuels, and contaminated injections in healthcare settings.[1] Some of these factors, like air pollution and indoor smoke, are clearly environmental. Others are related both to the environment and to social, behavioral, and economic factors. Fruit and vegetable intake is easier for people who live where they can grow their own produce and harder for people who live in cities where produce is expensive and may not be fresh. A person who lives in an unsafe neighborhood may feel threatened when outdoors and may not have the space to be active indoors, so physical activity is curtailed.

Some environmental health researchers focus on issues related to geography, geology, and climate. Health risks are often tied to type of climate, whether the location is desert, tropical, artic, or something less extreme. Types of vegetation and animals that are native to particular climates, weather patterns and temperature, altitude, geologic formations (like volcanoes and earthquake fault lines), soil types, and other factors can influence risk for both communicable and non-communicable diseases. For example, older people who live at high altitudes and have had long-term exposure to UV light, wind, and dust are at risk of developing a pterygium, a triangular growth that starts on the white part of the eye but may eventually cover the pupil and cause blindness. And malaria is a risk only for people who live in a climate that can support the lifecycle of the mosquitoes that spread the malaria parasites.

Most environmental health experts focus on aspects of health related to the home, workplace, or community. Occupational and industrial health specialists spend their time assessing and mitigating workplace hazards, which may mean measuring noise levels in a factory and issuing appropriate ear protection or making sure that people who spend their days in front of a computer have ergonomically-designed chairs and are taking steps to minimize repetitive motion injuries. Other occupational and industrial health specialists focus on potential hazards in the home environment, such as lead paint, radon, and mold; they might also assess community risks, such as garbage dumps and runoff into waterways.

THE HOME ENVIRONMENT

Environmental health is also concerned with the health and safety of the home environment. Most buildings contain potential hazards. Construction materials may be harmful, such as paint that contains lead (which can cause mental impairment in children who ingest paint chips) or insulation that contains asbestos (which can increase risk of a certain type of lung cancer). Electrical wiring installed incorrectly may lead to the risk of electrocution. Windows without screens may let insects in. Poorly insulated and sealed walls and ceilings may not protect residents from cold and precipitation. Some residences may have high levels of radon, the second most common cause of lung cancer after tobacco, or may be infested with cockroaches, termites, or rats. There may also be hazardous chemicals stored in kitchens, bathrooms, garages, and sheds. These substances, such as cleaning agents, lawn fertilizers, and motor oil, may create new dangers when they are stored or disposed of improperly.

All of these conditions may be potentially hazardous, but in some ways it is a luxury to be able to worry about these household characteristics. For many people in the world, the most important household considerations are shelter, water, sanitation, and fuel for cooking. A shelter is a dwelling that provides at least some protection from the sun, rain, wind, and other elements. At the outskirts of large cities in low-income parts of the world, large shantytowns built from cardboard may spring up overnight to accommodate rural-to-urban migrants. These may eventually be replaced with shacks built from blocks or bricks with a tin or asbestos roof, or replaced with more permanent houses constructed from cement, but once a minimal sort of protection is built the focus of the new resident is on finding a source of safe water for drinking and washing, a place away from the home that can be used to dispose of human waste, and a source of fuel for cooking.

WATER

Everyone needs access to an adequate supply of clean water. In addition to water for drinking and cooking, we also need water for hygiene (hand-washing and bathing) and cleaning (washing clothes, cleaning cooking pots, and cleaning homes). One of the most important household benefits of getting access to an improved water source is that it saves a lot of time. Women and children, who are usually sent to fetch water when water sources are distant, may spend several hours a day walking to a water source, waiting for their turn to fill a container, and walking home. The time saved could be used for other activities, which may be social, educational, or health-oriented (such as cooking nutritious food, sleeping, or cleaning). Increased access to water is also associated with improved health. With more water available for hygiene, the incidence of diarrheal diseases decreases.

Consider five key aspects of water access: quality, quantity, proximity, reliability, and cost.

Quality: Water must be clean enough to safely drink. It needs to be free of bacteria, viruses, and parasites that can cause infection, and must also be free of harmful chemicals and sediments. The water should not appear cloudy, dirty, or strangely colored, so that it does not cause problems with cooking (such as giving food a strange flavor, color, or texture) or washing. Ideally, the source should be protected, which means that people should not wash clothes or bathe near where drinking water is collected, sewage and garbage should be kept away from the water, and there shouldn't be snails that can transmit schistosomiasis in the water or on the bank or algae on the

Table 10-1. Examples of Improved and Unimproved Drinking Water Sources.

Improved Drinking Water Sources	Unimproved Drinking Water Sources
Piped water into dwelling, plot, or yard	Surface water (river, dam, lake, pond, stream, canal, irrigation channels)
Public tap or standpipe	Cart with a small tank / drum
Tube well or borehole	Unprotected dug well
Protected dug well	Unprotected spring
Protected spring	Some bottled water and water from tanker trucks
Rainwater collection	

Information Source: UNICEF/WHO Joint Monitoring Programme for Water Supply and Sanitation, MDG Assessment Report 2006: "Meeting the MDG Drinking Water and Sanitation Target: The Urban and Rural Challenge of the Decade."

surface of the water. Table 10-1 lists examples of improved and unimproved drinking water sources.

Quantity: There must be enough water so that people can stay hydrated and clean. The average minimum amount of water needed by one person each day is about 15 to 20 liters: about 1 to 3 liters for drinking, 2 to 3 liters for food preparation and cleanup, 6 to 7 liters for personal cleanliness, and 4 to 6 liters for laundry.[2] The United Nations recommends a minimum of 50 liters per person per day.

Proximity: The water source must be close enough to the home so that distance does not prevent people from accessing the water they need. Ideally a source should be within 1 kilometer (about 0.6 miles) of the user's dwelling. This is especially necessary in areas of conflict. Some people have a water connection in the house; many people use a public community source such as a standpost (standpipe), borehole, or protected (lined) dug well. In some places it is possible to collect rainwater for drinking and domestic use, or to use a protected spring.

Reliability: The water source must be available and functioning all the time, or the household must have access to adequate water storage and water treatment methods such as filtering, boiling, and using chemicals like chlorine. One way to ensure that water systems can be maintained is to use **appropriate technology** that is simple enough that broken equipment, like water pumps, can be repaired by local residents cheaply and quickly.

Cost: Water must be affordable enough that people have access to at least the minimum amount of water necessary for healthy living. Households that use a community water system may be asked to pay a small fee for use so that the system can be maintained. These fees also promote water conservation if they are tied to the amount of water collected by a household. In most cases, community fees are minimal and recognized as essential for keeping a system running. When public water supplies are not available, exorbitant prices may be charged for bottled water.

Access to water is a requirement for life, so it is a huge concern for many people. About 20% of the world's population would be in the "No access" category of Table 10-2.

Access to water is a significant concern in Africa and the Middle East and parts of Asia and Latin America (Figure 10-1).

The lack of access to water is a particular concern in rural parts of the world (Figure 10-2). In most of North America and Europe, both urban and rural households have access to tap water. In many other world regions, however, less than 90% of the urban population and less than 40% of the rural population has access to an improved water source. Water scarcity is becoming a major issue in many parts of the world, especially the desert countries of the Middle East and North Africa where internal freshwater resources are extremely limited (Figure 10-3). Nations with less than 200 cubic meters of freshwater resources per person face ongoing challenges (Table 10-3).

As the demand for water increases, everyone needs to be concerned about the availability of fresh water. Only 2.5% of the world's water is freshwater (rather than saltwater) and two-thirds of that freshwater is in glaciers. Our main sources of freshwater are rainwater, surface water (such as water from streams and rivers), and ground water (which is accessed by drilling wells). Surface water can become contaminated by agricultural runoff, human waste, and other pollutants. Groundwater can become depleted and cause rivers, wetlands, and lakes that depend on the groundwater to dry out. About 70% of freshwater used every year is put toward agricultural uses such as irrigation and livestock production,[3] and there are increasing demands for agricultural, industrial, and domestic water use as the world population grows.

Some people predict that wars may be fought over water access issues. Scarcity of water is an obvious issue, but another set of challenges concern ownership of water. When a government privatizes water by selling the water rights or water system of a municipality, it is not just the people who are

Table 10-2. Water Service Level (Quantity, Proximity, and Quality) and Health Effects.

Service Level	Quantity (Per Person Per Day)	Proximity	Drinking Needs Met?	Hygiene Needs Met?	Level of Health Concern
No access	May be less than 5 liters	More than 1000 meters or 30 minutes round trip	Neither quantity nor quality assured	No since only available at source	Very high
Basic access	About 20 liters	Between 100 and 1000 meters or 5 to 30 minutes round trip	Quantity assured but quality not assured	Yes for hand-washing and food hygiene; No for laundry and bathing	High
Intermediate access	About 50 liters	Water delivered through one tap that is within 100 meters or 5 minutes round trip	Quantity and quality usually assured	Yes	Low
Optimal access	About 100 liters	Continuous supply through multiple taps	Quantity and quality assured	Yes	Very low

Information Source: Howard G, Bartram J. Domestic water quantity, service level and health. WHO, 2003 (WHO/SDE/WSH/03.02).

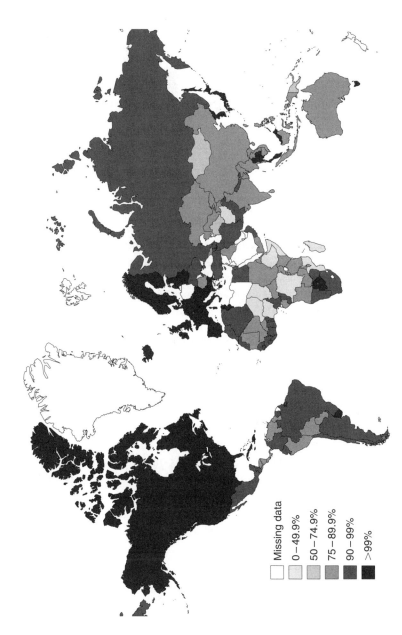

Figure 10-1. Percent of the Total Population with Access to an Improved Water Source in 2004.

Data Source: UNICEF/WHO Joint Monitoring Programme for Water Supply and Sanitation, MDG Assessment Report 2006: "Meeting the MDG Drinking Water and Sanitation Target: The Urban and Rural Challenge of the Decade."

Missing data
0 – 49.9%
50 – 74.9%
75 – 89.9%
90 – 99%
>99%

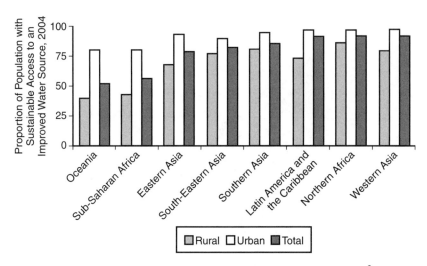

Figure 10-2. Sustainable Access to an Improved Water Source, 2004.[3]

Note: Western Asia includes Saudi Arabia, Iraq, Turkey, and other Middle Eastern countries. Southern Asia includes Iran, Afghanistan, Pakistan, India, Sri Lanka, and Bangladesh. Eastern Asia includes China, Mongolia, and Korea. South-Eastern Asia includes Myanmar, Thailand, Laos, Vietnam, Malaysia, Singapore, and the Philippines. Oceania includes the small island nations of the Pacific.

Data Source: The Millennium Development Goals Report 2006, Statistical Annex.

connected to the municipal water system that are affected. Neighborhoods that are not supplied by the municipality and have built their own systems using their own financial resources and labor may be forced to shut down their systems. People who live in the rural areas outside of the municipality may be cut off from the lakes and other water sources that have provided their families with water for hundreds of years. Wells within a certain distance of a river whose water has been sold may be forcibly capped off so that they can no longer be used as a water source.

Water privatization was a major source of contention in several South American countries in the 1990s. For example, massive protests occurred in 2000 in Cochabamba, Bolivia's third largest city, after a foreign-owned corporation took over the water system and raised water fees to what was equivalent, in some cases, to nearly half of a household's income. (Bolivia had been forced to privatize some of its national resources as a condition

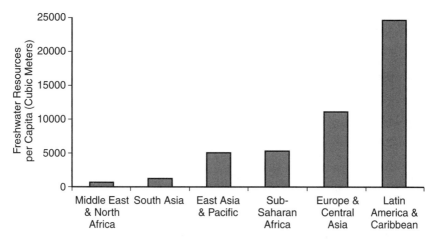

Figure 10-3. Internal Freshwater Resources per Person by World Region, 2004.

Note: Internal freshwater resources in this case are defined as "internal renewable resources, which include flows of rivers and groundwater from rainfall in the country, but do not include river flows from other countries."

Data Source: The World Bank. 2006 Little Green Data Book. Washington, D.C.: International Bank for Reconstruction and Development / The World Bank, 2006.

of a loan from the World Bank and IMF, but the company relinquished its rights to the water system after the riots.) Countries in other regions of the world are now experimenting with water privatization, notably Asian countries like China and Malaysia.

Water privatization raises important questions about whether water is a commodity that can be bought and sold to the highest bidder and denied to people who do not have the resources to purchase it. In response to the increased push for water privatization by governments, many people are calling for access to adequate water to be recognized as a human right, arguing that since access to sufficient, safe, physically accessible, and affordable water is a human need (not merely a human want), then fresh water is an entitlement and should not be treated like a commercial product.[4] Water activists also point out that the process of installing safe water systems needs to be accelerated because if water is a human right, then lack of access to water is an injustice. (Chapter 13 has more information about health and human rights.)

Table 10-3. Countries and Territories With Less Than 200 Cubic Meters of Freshwater Resources Per Person, 2004.

Country / territory	Region / type	Freshwater resources per capita (cubic meters)
Kuwait	Middle East	0
Bahrain	Middle East	6
West Bank / Gaza	Middle East	13
Egypt	North Africa	25
United Arab Emirates	Middle East	35
Bahamas	Small Island Nation	63
Qatar	Middle East	66
Maldives	Small Island Nation	93
Saudi Arabia	Middle East	100
Libya	North Africa	105
Israel	Middle East	110
Jordan	Middle East	125
Malta	Small Island Nation	126
Mauritania	North Africa	134
Singapore	Small Island Nation	141

Data Source: The World Bank. 2006 Little Green Data Book. Washington, D.C.: The World Bank, 2006.

SANITATION

Sanitation is the disposal of human excreta. There are several types of sanitation facilities that can be used for safe waste disposal (Table 10-4). One of the simplest sanitation systems is a simple pit latrine, which is basically an outhouse that covers a hole in the ground. In many communities, ownership of a latrine is a sign of prestige. A latrine also provides safety, cleanliness, comfort, privacy, and protection from dangers at night and from snakes. A slightly more advanced ventilation-improved latrine vents fumes away from the outhouse and keeps flies away. Pour-flush systems require some water for washing away the waste. Septic tanks and sewer connections are more advanced sanitation technologies. Advanced sanitation techniques are common in North America and Europe, but rare in many other regions (Figure 10-4).

Table 10-4. Examples of Improved and Unimproved Sanitation Facilities.

Improved Sanitation Facilities	Unimproved Sanitation Facilities
Flush or pour-flush to a piped sewer system, septic tank, or pit latrine	Flush or pour-flush to the street, yard or plot, open sewer, ditch, drainage way, or other location
Ventilated improved pit (VIP) latrine	Bucket or bag
Pit latrine with slab	Pit latrine without slab or open pit
Composting toilet	Bush, field, or street

Information Source: UNICEF/WHO Joint Monitoring Programme for Water Supply and Sanitation, MDG Assessment Report 2006: "Meeting the MDG Drinking Water and Sanitation Target: The Urban and Rural Challenge of the Decade."

About half of the people who live in developing countries do not have access to even the most basic sanitation systems, such as pit latrines (Figure 10-5).[5] Rural households may be able to set aside a defecation site away from the dwelling. Urban residents without access to a latrine often have no choice but to defecate on the street or into a bag that is thrown at the side of the street (sometimes called a "flying toilet"). A desire for privacy means that many people, especially women, wait until dark to defecate, even though it is often dangerous for them to be out at night.

People who do not have an improved sanitation system are at increased risk of infectious diseases that are spread through fecal-oral contact. The factors that contribute to fecal-oral diseases have sometimes been described using the "six Fs": feces, fields, fluid, fingers, food, and flies. When *feces* are not properly disposed of, they can contaminate *fields* (soil) and *fluids* (bodies of water). The fecal matter can then get onto hands, especially the hands of young children who frequently touch the ground, and *fingers* transport the fecal matter to *food* if hands are not washed before preparing it or to the mouth if hands are not washed before eating. *Flies* can also spread feces to food and water, and thrive where fecal matter is in the open. The risk of fecal-oral disease increases when there is not enough *fluid* (water) to wash hands often.

Diarrhea is a common outcome of fecal-oral infections, whether they are caused by bacteria, viruses, or protozoa. The presence of feces near homes also significantly increases the risk of helminth (worm) infections. Helminth infections can be treated through the periodic distribution of de-worming medicines to school-age children and other at-risk population groups, but

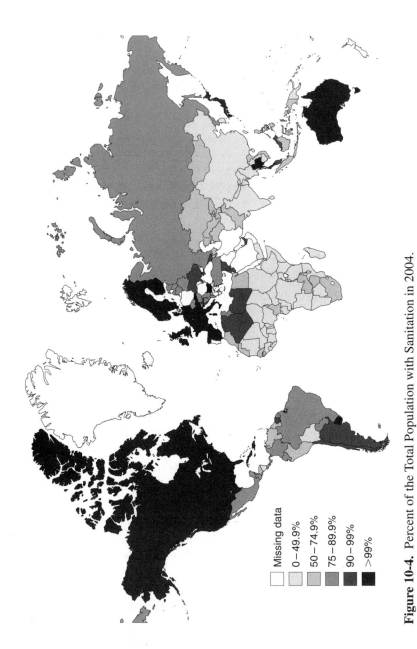

Figure 10-4. Percent of the Total Population with Sanitation in 2004.

Data Source: UNICEF/WHO Joint Monitoring Programme for Water Supply and Sanitation, MDG Assessment Report 2006: "Meeting the MDG Drinking Water and Sanitation Target: The Urban and Rural Challenge of the Decade."

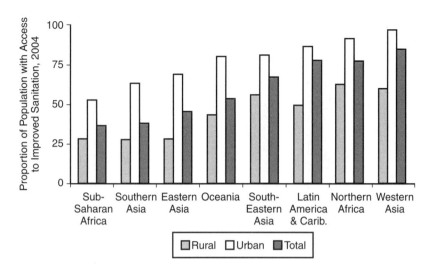

Figure 10-5. Access to Improved Sanitation, 2004.

Data Source: The Millennium Development Goals Report 2006, Statistical Annex.

improved sanitation is a necessity for preventing new worm infections. The best programs for reducing diarrhea and parasitism combine improved water supplies, excreta disposal, and hygiene promotions that focus on frequently washing hands with soap.

FUEL AND INDOOR AIR QUALITY

More than 25% of the world's people do not have electricity in their homes. Of those 1.5 billion people, 83% live in rural areas and 17% in urban areas (Figure 10-6).[7]

Energy is necessary for cooking and boiling water and for providing a source of light at night. Households without electricity rely on solid fuels (like wood, coal, dung, and crop waste) for their energy needs. These may be supplemented by the use of candles and kerosene lamps for light. Solid fuels are usually burned in open fires or in simple stoves that release most of the smoke from burning into the home. As a result, indoor air pollution levels are high and may cause respiratory problems, especially for women and young children who spend several hours a day near the fire while cooking.

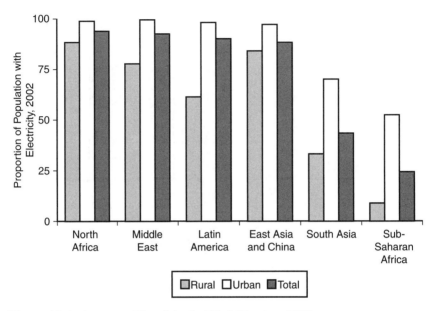

Figure 10-6. Access to Electricity by World Region, 2002.

Data Source: IEA (International Energy Agency), "World Energy Outlook 2004."

The pollutants in smoke from burning solid fuels include carbon monoxide, sulfur oxides, nitrogen oxides, aldehydes, and polyaromatic compounds.[7] These chemicals can cause lung disease by triggering inflammation, damaging the cells that line the respiratory tract, and impairing immune response. The smoke also contains particulate matter, small particles that can get deep into the lungs. The World Health Organization estimates that indoor air pollution is responsible for 1.6 million deaths every year because it increases risk of pneumonia and other respiratory infections in children, and increases risk of chronic bronchitis and of lung cancer in adults.[8]

Use of solid fuels has other health effects. Children are at risk of burns from falling into open fires or knocking over pots of boiling water. Women and children often spend hours each week collecting sticks and brush to use as fuel, and they are susceptible to injuries related to carrying heavy loads through uneven and uncleared terrain. As sources of biomass close to the home are used up, they must travel further distances to find fuel. There are also environmental consequences: burning of solid fuels contributes to outdoor air pollution, and the demand for wood and charcoal contributes to deforestation.

People without electricity can reduce their exposure to indoor air pollution in at least three ways.[9] One is to use improved cooking devices such as those that have flues to divert pollutants out of the home and those that use alternative energy sources (like solar panels). A second is to increase ventilation or move the kitchen to the outside of the home. (Obviously, relocating the kitchen does not help minimize the cook's exposure if ventilation systems are not built into the outside cooking area.) A third is to change behaviors, like keeping children away from smoke and using pot lids to conserve heat.

Access to electricity has additional health benefits. Refrigeration allows for safer food storage. The use of a radio or television allows for health and safety messages such as advertisements for immunization campaigns, information about hand-washing and other disease prevention techniques, and alerts about potential natural disasters such as oncoming hurricanes to be distributed via mass communication.

CONCLUSION

Contaminated water, poor sanitation, and inadequate water and waste management are associated with an increased risk of diarrheal diseases and other infections spread through the fecal-oral route, by contact with human or animal waste, or by poor hygiene. Air pollution is associated with acute respiratory infections (ARIs), chronic respiratory diseases, and some types of cardiovascular disease and cancer. Substandard housing can contribute to the development of these diseases. Increasing access to healthy housing, clean water supplies, sanitation, and clean air will improve health.

REFERENCES

1. Danaei G, Vander Hoorn S, Lopez AD, Murray CJ, Ezzati M, and the Comparative Risk Assessment collaborating group (Cancers). Causes of cancer in the world: comparative risk assessment of nine behavioral and environmental risk factors. *Lancet.* 2005;366: 1784–1793.
2. Hesperian Foundation and United Nations Development Programme, "Water for Life: Community Water Security," Berkeley, CA: The Hesperian Foundation, 2005.
3. The World Bank. 2006 Little Green Data Book. Washington, D.C.: The World Bank, 2006.
4. World Health Organization. "The Right to Water." Geneva, Switzerland: Health and Human Rights Publication Series, Issue No. 3, 2003.

5. United Nations, The Millennium Development Goals Report 2006, page 18, New York, NY: United Nations, 2006.
6. International Energy Agency, World Energy Outlook 2004. Paris, France: IEA, 2004.
7. Zhang J, Smith KR. Indoor air pollution: a global health concern. *Br Med Bull* 2003;68:209–225.
8. World Health Organization, "Energy and Health brochure." Geneva, Switzerland: World Health Organization, 2005.
9. Interventions adapted from Table 24.4 of Nigel Bruce, Eva Rehfuess, Sumi Mehta, Guy Hutton, and Kirk Smith, Chapter 42: "Indoor Air Pollution," page 800. In: Jamison DT, Breman JG, Measham AR, et al, eds. Disease Control Priorities in Developing Countries, 2nd ed. Washington, DC: Oxford University Press, 2006.

CHAPTER **11**

Health Effects
of Environmental Change

Key Points:
- Local environmental changes like dam buildings, deforestation, and urbanization can create new disease risks.
- Occupational and industrial hazards can lead to work-related injuries and exposure to harmful chemicals.
- Communities must work together to create healthy living and working environments.
- Global environmental changes (such as those related to climate change) create new disease risks.

Environmental change occurs whenever humans alter the natural world. We impact the environment by building permanent structures, terracing slopes for agricultural use, converting forests to fields, paving streets, installing telephone and electric lines, building dams, and extracting fossil fuels to make oil and other petroleum products. Infrastructural development contributes to greater health and safety for humans, but also creates a new set of health concerns. These changes affect the health of workers and residents in the immediate environment, but they also have implications for neighboring communities, nations, and the entire globe. This chapter examines some of the ways that environmental change affects individuals, communities, and larger populations. The first section focuses on health effects related to local environmental change, urbanization, and industry, and the chapter concludes with a look at the health effects of global environmental changes.

HEALTH IMPACTS OF LOCAL ENVIRONMENTAL CHANGE

The daily activities we conduct as humans require us to interact with the environment. We need to farm in order to eat. We need to use fresh water for drinking and bathing. We need fuel to cook and heat our homes. We need

229

to get rid of waste. We also use the environment for exercise and recreation. Changes to the local environment may contribute to better health, may create health hazards, or may solve one health problem but create another.

Many of the environmental changes we implement are beneficial for our health and have minimal impact on the environment. Digging pits for latrines reduces the incidence of diarrhea and also keeps feces from contaminating water supplies. Vector control, such as spraying insecticide to reduce the mosquito population and reduce the incidence of malaria, can be minimally damaging to the environment if applied correctly. The use of new machines and tools can help with injury prevention and may reduce impact on the land.

A recent WHO study that estimated the impact of the environment on health concluded that about 24% of the global disease burden could be attributed to environmental factors (Table 11-1).[1] Many of the environmental risk factors considered, such as water, sanitation, indoor and outdoor air pollution, noise, housing risks, chemicals, the recreational environment, water resources management, land use and the built environment, radiation, and occupational exposures, could be modified to reduce—and, in some cases, perhaps even eliminate—the risk of disease. For example, water resources management could significantly reduce the incidence of malaria, reduction of indoor air pollution could reduce the incidence of lower respiratory infections, and improving housing infrastructure could reduce the incidence of Chagas disease.

On the other hand, some activities permanently damage the environment or make extensive use of non-renewable natural resources, and these activities may create long-term environmental health risks. We are involved in mineral extraction and processing, refining of mineral ores, power generation (from fossil fuels, nuclear reactions, hydroelectric power, and other sources), and other industrial and manufacturing activities, and we alter the landscape by building dams and bridges, paving thousands of miles of roads between cities and thousands of acres of ground within cities, and creating dump sites for solid waste.

In his best-selling book *Collapse: How Societies Choose to Fail or Succeed*,[2] Jared Diamond presents many examples of societies that died out or languished because they refused to change their cultural habits of environmental interaction. For example, the Rapanui, a group of Polynesians who settled on Easter Island in the ninth century C.E., were obsessed with building large stone figures called *moai* that they transported using ramps built from trees. They ended up clear-cutting the island, which contributed to animal and plant extinctions, starvation, and social chaos. Diamond identifies eight key processes for human damage to the environment: (1) deforestation

Table 11-1. Percent of Disease Attributable to Environmental Risk Factors.

Disease	% of Cases Attributable to the Environment	Primary Environmental Risk Factor (>25% of cases attributable to the risk factor)
Intestinal nematode infections	100%	Water, sanitation, and hygiene
Trachoma	100%	Water, sanitation, and hygiene
Schistosomiasis	100%	Water, sanitation, and hygiene
Japanese encephalitis	95%	Water resources management
Dengue	95%	Housing risks
Diarrheal diseases	94%	Water, sanitation, and hygiene
Drowning	72%	Recreational environment
Unintentional poisonings	71%	Chemicals
Lymphatic filariasis	66%	Water, sanitation, and hygiene
Chagas disease	56%	Housing risks
Malnutrition	50%	Water, sanitation, and hygiene
Lower respiratory infections	42%	Indoor air pollution
Malaria	42%	Water resources management
Road traffic accidents	40%	Land use and built environment

Data Source: Prüss-Üstün A, Corvalán C. Preventing disease through healthy environments: toward an estimate of the environmental burden of disease. Geneva: WHO, 2006.

and habitat destruction, (2) soil problems such as erosion, salinization, and soil fertility losses, (3) water management problems, (4) over-hunting, (5) over-fishing, (6) the effects of introduced species on native species, (7) human population growth, and (8) increased per capita impact of people. Whenever humans change the environment there are potential health repercussions, including the risk of increased disease incidence and prevalence (Table 11-2).

Table 11-2. Health Effects of Local Environmental Change.

Environmental Change	Possible Pathways	Examples of Increased Disease Incidence or Prevalence
Dams, canals, irrigation	Increased snail habitat and human contact with water	Schistosomiasis
	Increased insect breeding sites	Malaria, onchocerciasis (river blindness), Japanese encephalitis, West Nile virus, St. Louis encephalitis
	Increased moist soil	Helminth infections
Urbanization	Lack of access to clean drinking water and sanitation and poor hygiene of residents in low-quality housing areas	Cholera, cryptosporidiosis, other diarrheal diseases and infections spread by the fecal-oral route, helminth infections
	Increased trash that attracts rodents and collects water that provides *Aedes aegypti* mosquito breeding sites	Dengue fever, plague
	Crowded housing	Mental illness, war / violence, TB and respiratory infections
	Immigration of susceptible people	Communicable diseases
Deforestation	Increased insect breeding sites and contact with insect vectors and animal reservoirs	Malaria, leishmaniasis, yellow fever, onchocerciasis, zoonotic infections
Reforestation	Increased contact with tick vectors and increased outdoor exposure	Lyme disease
Agricultural intensification	Increased pesticide use and development of insecticide-resistant vectors	Poisoning, malaria
	Increased rodent population and human contact with rodents	Venezuelan equine encephalitis, Western equine encephalitis, typhus fever

This table was adapted from several sources, including: Wilson ML, "Ecology and Infectious Disease," In: Aron JL, Patz JA, eds, *Ecosystem Change and Public Health*, Baltimore, MD: The Johns Hopkins University Press, 2001; and UNEP, Global Environmental Outlook Year book 2004/2005: Emerging and Re-emerging Infectious Diseases: Links to Environmental Change.

Unhealthy environments may be present anywhere, regardless of wealth and level of industrialization (Table 11-3). For example, people who live in less-developed areas may drink water contaminated with pathogenic microbes, whereas people who live in highly industrialized areas may have drinking water that is contaminated with pesticides and other industrial and agricultural chemicals. Many diseases attributable to environmental risk factors can be prevented if potential problems are identified and appropriate actions are taken. Ideally, the potential long-term effects of environmental change should be analyzed before large-scale projects like dam building are initiated. The risks and benefits must be balanced, and the likelihood that solving one health problem will contribute to an increase in another one must be considered.

It is possible for development to occur in a way that minimizes the impact on the environment and promotes human health. For example, planned urbanization is much healthier for humans than unplanned urbanization. Urban planning can alleviate much of the environmental stress created by increased population density. Planning can also minimize the contributions of human

Table 11-3. Sample Comparison of Environmental Hazards in Less-Developed and More-Developed Areas.

Environmental Factor	Hazards in Less-Developed Areas	Hazards in More-Developed Areas
Water and sanitation	Lack of access to safe drinking water and basic sanitation; microbial contamination of drinking water	Water pollution from industrial processes and agricultural run-off
Food	Microbial contamination of food	Food additives and preservatives; risk of pathogens in processed foods
Indoor air	Indoor air pollution from burning biomass	Indoor air pollution from building materials and paints / solvents
Workplace	Risks from agriculture and trade work	Risks from industrial work
Home environment	Risks of infectious disease due to crowding and poor hygiene	Risks of asthma and allergies due to the immune system not being exposed to pathogens and dirt

activities to polluted air, deforestation, degraded soil, scarcity of freshwater, loss of biodiversity, and declining fishery yields.

URBANIZATION

Each day, thousands of people move from rural areas to cities in search of better jobs, higher incomes, more social opportunities, and greater conveniences. On average, urban residents have greater access than rural residents to water and sanitation, to a relatively reliable public transportation system, to health care providers, and to health technologies and products. Access to electricity reduces cooking time and makes it easier to safely store food. Communications systems, such as radio and television, broadcast news and entertainment shows as well as emergency warnings and health messages. Women have more opportunities to pursue additional education and to find employment outside the home. Pregnancy is safer because of greater access to antenatal care and assistance by medical professionals during delivery.

However, these benefits are not available to all urban residents. Many people who move to cities end up living in unplanned settlements (sometimes called shantytowns, slums, or squatter camps) where the quality of life is worse than rural life. Poorly constructed homes, often made from cardboard, scraps of metal and wood, or other found items, provide little comfort or privacy. Trash and human waste may collect near the home and attract rodents and insects. Living in close proximity to large numbers of people and their animals increases the risk of insect-borne and animal-borne diseases; violence is common. It may be difficult to grow or to purchase nutritious foods, and there may be little time or space for exercising. Unplanned communities often form in undesirable locations near noisy and polluted highways or industrial centers. They are often built in floodplains or other vulnerable lands, and lack of drainage systems means that floods carry feces and other waste into homes. Urban workers may also face new occupational hazards. Table 11-4 compares rural, unplanned urban, and planned urban communities.

Although a large percent of Asians and Africans still live in rural areas (Figure 11-1), the urban populations in these regions are growing rapidly. Six of the 10 largest cities in the world are now located in Asia (Table 11-5).

Urbanization affects both urban and rural residents. Rural women, for example, may bear a particularly heavy burden when their husbands leave the

Table 11-4. Comparison of Health Risks Associated with Rural Living, Unplanned Urban Living, and Planned Urban Living.

Sector	Rural	Unplanned Urban	Planned Urban
Water	Minimal access to improved sources and high risk of contamination	Minimal access to improved sources; inadequate quantity of water; risk of contamination; may be expensive	Safe clean drinking water system
Sanitation	Inadequate sanitation facilities mean that people may defecate in a field away from the house	Inadequate sanitation facilities mean that people may defecate in the street	Sewage system
Trash disposal	Solid waste is burned or buried	No collection of solid wastes, which creates a habitat for insect and rodent vectors.	Solid waste is collected and removed
Fuel	Solid fuels, which may be able to be collected locally	Solid fuels, which may be expensive	Electricity
Nutrition	May have limited options and ability to purchase food products, but can usually grow food or hunt/gather food	May have limited access to healthy foods and foods may be expensive; may not have space for a garden	Adequate access to healthy dietary choices
Health facilities	May be distant and may provide only basic care; may be expensive	May be expensive and crowded	Basic, emergency, and specialty care (including mental health and rehabilitation facilities) are available
Air quality	Indoor air pollution	Both indoor and outdoor air pollution; noise pollution	Outdoor air pollution
Chemical Hazards	Potential exposure to agrochemicals like fertilizer and pesticides	Potential exposure to industrial waste	Little exposure to industrial or agricultural hazards

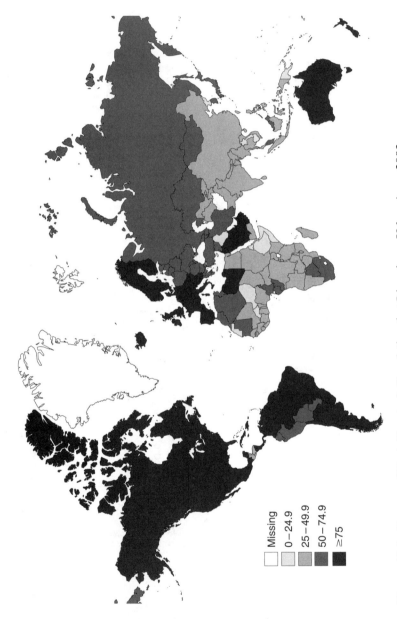

Figure 11-1. Percent of Each Country's Population that Lives in an Urban Area, 2003.

Data Source: Human Development Report 2005.

Table 11-5. 10 Largest Metropolitan Areas in the World, 2005.

Rank	Metropolitan Area	Population of Metropolitan Area
1	Tokyo, Japan	35.2 million
2	Mexico City, Mexico	19.4 million
3	New York City, USA	18.7 million
4	São Paulo, Brazil	18.3 million
5	Mumbai, India	18.2 million
6	Delhi, India	15.0 million
7	Shanghai, China	14.5 million
8	Kolkata, India	14.3 million
9	Jakarta, Indonesia	13.2 million
10	Buenos Aires, Argentina	12.6 million

Data Source: United Nations World Urbanization Prospects Report 2005.

household and go to the cities to find wage employment, leaving the women with the responsibility of completing all the household chores.

THE WORK ENVIRONMENT

Occupational health was one of the first public health specialties. In 1700, Bernardino Ramazzini published *Diseases of Workers*, a book that detailed the environmental hazards—including poisoning, respiratory diseases, problems related to prolonged postures and repetitive tasks, and even psychological stress—encountered in 52 occupations.[3] In 1747, James Lind designed an experiment that proved that sailors could prevent scurvy if they carried citrus fruit with them on long journeys. (After this discovery, sailors were sometimes called "limeys" for the limes and other citrus fruit they carried on ships.) In 1775, Percival Pott identified chimney soot as the cause of elevated rates of scrotal cancer in chimney sweeps. The coal tar in chimneys is carcinogenic and since sweeps rarely bathed or changed their trousers, they had nearly constant exposure to the carcinogen.

Every worker may face a particular mix of biological, chemical, physical, mechanical, and psychosocial challenges as part of work. Some occupations carry specific risks. Those who work with heavy machinery are at risk of crush wounds from moving parts. Those exposed to loud noises are at risk of permanent damage to their hearing. Medical workers are at risk of contracting infectious diseases from needle-sticks and by contact with body fluids. And the people who have long-term exposure to industrial chemicals are at increased risk of developing certain types of cancers. Office workers have their own set of occupational risks, including repetition injuries, such as carpal tunnel syndrome, that can develop after performing the same tasks over and over. All workers may be subject to stress that can impair mental health.

The International Labor Organization (ILO) estimates that each year more than 2 million people die as a result of occupational injuries, nearly 270 million miss at least 3 days of work due to an injury, and at least 160 million become ill.[4] It is estimated that 3.9% of all deaths are attributable to work-related accidents and illnesses, and 15% of people worldwide suffer a minor or major occupational accident or work-related disease in any given year. Workplace hazards are responsible for an estimated 37% of back pain, 16% of hearing loss, 13% of chronic obstructive pulmonary disease, 11% of asthma, 10% of injuries, 10% of lung cancers, and 2% of leukemias.[5] Fatal injuries sustained at job sites are increasing, especially in Asia and Latin America. Many of these injuries and deaths could be prevented if worksite managers and government officials enforced compliance with safety regulations.

Toxicology is the study of the harmful effects of chemicals and other environmental hazards like radiation on living things. Toxicologists study the way variations in exposure frequency (how often a person is exposed), duration (length of exposure at a given time), and dose (amount of chemical contacted) influence health. They also assess the various exposure routes (like inhalation, ingestion, and absorption through the skin) and pathways (through air, water, food, soil, or other mechanisms) related to hazardous exposures. Substances identified as carcinogens, **teratogens** (that cause birth defects), or other hazards can be regulated or banned. Hazardous exposures include radiation, chemical pollutants, toxic substances like PCBs (polychlorinated biphenyls), dioxins, asbestos, lead, mercury, cadmium, DDT, organic solvents, and pesticides. Many of these are released into the environment through industrial activities. Some of the most common toxic substances are listed in Table 11-6.

Hazardous substances cause more than 400,000 deaths each year, including 100,000 occupational deaths from asbestos and 70,000 poisoning deaths due to agricultural pesticides. Although these hazardous substances are used and produced in industrial settings in both developed and developing countries, workers in developing countries have greater risks. Many highly toxic

Table 11-6. Top 8 Hazardous Substances, U.S. Agency for Toxic Substances and Disease Registry (ATSDR), 2005.

	Substance	Uses
1	Arsenic	Used to make "pressure-treated" lumber, as a pesticide for cotton plants, and in copper and lead smelting
2	Lead	Used in production of batteries, ammunition, metal products (solder and pipes), and devices to shield X-rays; released from the burning of fossil fuels and during mining and manufacturing; used in some gasoline, paints, caulks, and ceramic products
3	Mercury	Used in thermometers, dental fillings, batteries, and some antiseptic creams and ointments
4	Vinyl chloride	Used to make polyvinyl chloride (PVC) used plastic products like pipes, wire and cable coatings, and packaging materials
5	Polychlorinated biphenyls (PCBs)	Used as coolants and lubricants in transformers, capacitors, and other electrical equipment
6	Benzene	Used to make other chemicals that form plastics, resins, nylon and synthetic fibers, rubbers, lubricants, dyes, detergents, drugs, and pesticides
7	Polycyclic aromatic hydrocarbons (PAHs)	A group of over 100 different chemicals that are formed during incomplete burning of coal, oil, gas, garbage, tobacco, charbroiled meat, and other organic substances; also found in coal tar, crude oil, creosote, roofing tar, some medicines and dyes, plastics, and pesticides
8	Cadmium	Extracted during production of metals like zinc, lead, and copper for use in batteries, pigments, metal coatings, and plastics

Data Source: U.S. Agency for Toxic Substances and Disease Registry, "Top 20 Hazardous Substances from the 2005 CERCLA Priority List of Hazardous Substances."

agents that have been banned for use in the United States and other industrialized nations are still used in low-income nations. Occupational regulations in low-income countries are rarely enforced, so workers generally have very little access to protective gear and safety training. And in low-income countries where jobs are scarce, workers may have to choose between repeated exposure to very high doses of dangerous chemicals and being unemployed.

When industrial accidents occur, they do not just affect people who work at the site of an incident. The pollutants, toxins, and other substances released into air or water as a result of an accident can affect the local community and may spread to a much larger area. The radioactivity released during the meltdown of the nuclear reactor at Chernobyl in Ukraine (then part of the U.S.S.R.) in April 1986, spread a radioactive cloud across most of Europe. One health-related outcome of the meltdown was an increase in the incidence of thyroid cancer in children in the most contaminated regions. An accident at a chemical plant in Bhopal, India, in December 1984, released liquid and vapor methyl isocyanate. At least 6000 people died when they were exposed to the fumes, some in their beds and others in the street after they staggered out of their homes to try to escape from the chemical. Hundreds of thousands of people sustained lung injuries.

Another example of widespread environmental damage that can be created by industrial processes is air pollution. Air pollution can be produced by transportation (exhaust from cars and trucks), power plants (which burn coal and oil to produce electricity), industrial processes, forest fires, and the disposal of solid waste. The substances released into the air from these processes include carbon monoxide, sulfur oxides, hydrocarbons, nitrogen oxides, and particulates, which are particles of solid or liquid substances that are small enough to remain suspended in the air for long periods of time and are easily moved by wind. Poor air quality can cause reduced visibility and unpleasant odors, interfere with plant growth and agricultural quality, and endanger health by irritating the eyes and respiratory tract, increasing the risk of asthma, and exacerbating symptoms of chronic diseases like cardiovascular diseases, chronic obstructive pulmonary disease (COPD), and anemia. Pollutants produced in one place can end up affecting air quality thousands of miles away, so international regulations are designed to regulate the amount of emissions produced in each country. For example, the Kyoto Protocol, an agreement made under the Framework Convention on Climate Change, asks countries to commit to reducing their emissions of carbon dioxide, methane, nitrous oxide, and other greenhouse gases.

COMMUNITY HEALTH ACTION

Whether they are rural or urban, households, businesses, and communities are inextricably linked. Everyone who lives and works in a community shares the same air, water, and other environmental components. This can be a problem if each individual and group pursues only its own interests at the expense of the other parties and the environment. Ideally, all parties can work together to protect their communities and to promote health. Relatively simple examples include community action to enforce transportation policies that protect pedestrians and bicyclists and voluntary groups that maintain recreational space to promote physical activity. Sometimes community health problems call for more dramatic and far-reaching solutions. Two examples, arsenic poisoning from tube wells in Bangladesh and the debate over the use of DDT for malaria control, highlight different approaches to community health action.

In Bangladesh, surface water is often contaminated with feces from humans, cattle, and water buffaloes, so an initiative begun by UNICEF in the 1970s promoted the installation of tube wells that tap ground water. Only after millions of wells had been dug did geologists determine that the wells extract water that flows through fluvial deposits that contain arsenopyrites. As a result the concentration of arsenic in water from these wells can be more than 100,000 times the recommended maximum exposure, (exceeding a concentration of 1:1000 when the World Health Organization recommends a maximum concentration of 1:100,000,000). Millions of Bangladeshis are at risk of arsenicosis, chronic arsenic poisoning from drinking contaminated water over a long period of time.[6] The most visible symptom is a change in skin color (hyperpigmentation) and the formation of hard skin patches (keratosis). Arsenicosis can cause skin cancer and cancers of the lung, kidney, and bladder, liver damage, gangrene, and peripheral vascular disease.

An initial solution is to promote the use of a low cost filter system that can remove arsenic from drinking water, but since even a very low cost filter is more expensive than many Bangladeshi families can afford, other steps are needed. Besides, filters produce toxic waste so they are at best only a temporary solution. The amount of arsenic in each well varies widely, so workers are testing wells and then painting green handles on safe pumps and red handles on contaminated pumps. Another solution is to collect rain water during the rainy season or dig deeper wells that bypass the geologic formations that contain arsenic. There is no one approach that will work for all communities, so local communities must be involved in making decisions about what will work best for their geologic, social, and economic situation.

Many communities struggle against malaria. In the middle part of the twentieth century, DDT (dichloro-diphenyl-tricholoethane) was sprayed in large quantities over cities and crops to control malarial mosquitoes in the United States and other countries. DDT does not easily degrade, so it persists in the environment and builds up in the food chain, killing birds and fish. The United States banned DDT in 1972 (in large part because of the uproar caused by Rachel Carson's book *Silent Spring*, which had been published in 1962), and many other countries, both developed and developing, also enacted DDT bans. The DDT ban led to a drastic increase in the incidence of malaria in many countries.

In recent years, many communities have begun using DDT in homes. The environmental persistence that makes DDT an environmental hazard when it is sprayed outdoors makes it appealing for in-home insecticide use. DDT sticks to the walls so that pesticides only need to be used once or twice a year. Spraying a tiny amount of DDT on the walls of houses twice a year kills mosquitoes that land on the walls but seems to be harmless to humans and animals. DDT is also cheaper and more effective than other pesticides.

In 2001, a global treaty sponsored by the United Nations Environment Program (UNEP) and many private environmental organizations banned eleven other persistent organic pollutants, but made a special exemption for public health use of DDT. Its use is now limited, but not banned. DDT is not a cure-all. It only protects people from bites while indoors, and some mosquitoes are resistant to the effects of DDT. Still, the World Health Organization now endorses the use of indoor residual spraying for vector control in areas that have endemic or epidemic malaria transmission[7] and DDT could contribute, if used correctly, to preventing millions of malaria deaths. Although still controversial, the re-implementation of minimal use of DDT for home protection may end up being an example of how people with different views on the risks and benefits of an intervention can find a middle ground that is acceptable to most parties involved.

GLOBAL ENVIRONMENTAL CHANGE

The immediate effects of most human activity are local, but some cause global problems by polluting the air and water. The distinction between local and global environmental change is not always clear. For example, the air pollution created by millions of commuters driving to work each day does not just damage their airspace, but contributes to the destruction of the ozone layer, increasing everyone's risk of developing asthma and skin cancer.

Some environmental changes, especially those related to climate change, are by definition global (Figure 11-2). While cycles of climate change have occurred throughout history, there is growing concern about the pace of

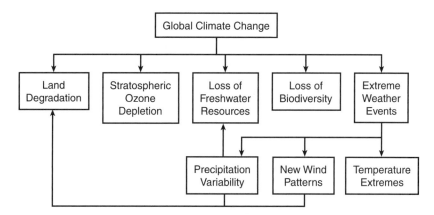

Figure 11-2. Examples of the Signs of Global Environmental Change.

global warming. The Intergovernmental Panel on Climate Change (IPCC) recently released a consensus document that expresses certainty that global warming is occurring and will continue to occur for centuries to come—and that the observed changes are very likely due to human activity.[8]

The IPCC predicts that climate change will mean more frequent hot days and nights and fewer cold days and nights, an increasing frequency of warm spells and heat waves, an increase in the frequency of heavy precipitation events in some areas and an increase in droughts in others, an increase in tropical cyclone (hurricane) activity, and an increase in the incidence of extreme high sea levels. In addition to temperature extremes and variable weather cycles, there may be continued ozone depletion and increased UV radiation. Global warming can also lead to acid precipitation (acid rain), loss of biodiversity, deforestation and desertification, and resource depletion (such as the loss of potable water supplies). These changes can have direct effects on human health (Table 11-7).

Climate change will affect every individual, community, and nation, creating a cycle of events with tremendous significance for human societies, especially because of the increasing human population and the greater per capita impact of people on the environment due to industrialization. Heat waves have killed hundreds of people, especially the elderly and those with respiratory diseases, in the United States, Europe, India, and other regions of the world. Each year, floods cause the deaths of thousands of people and animals, destroy homes and crops, and damage infrastructure, including hospitals, roads, and sewage systems. The

Table 11-7. Health Effects of Global Environmental Change.

Environmental Change	Possible Pathways	Examples of Increased Disease Incidence or Prevalence
Ozone depletion	Increased exposure to ultraviolet radiation	Skin cancer, cataracts
Temperature extremes	Heat waves	Heat stroke and death
	Increased geographic range for insect vectors	Malaria and other vector-borne diseases
	Destruction of agricultural products	Malnutrition
Decreased precipitation	Increased drought	Malnutrition
	Increased air pollution, including spores, pollen, smoke, and dust	Asthma, allergies, other respiratory illnesses, and meningitis caused by *Neisseria meningitides*
Elevated precipitation and increased frequency of floods and hurricanes	Flooding and rising sea level	Drowning; cholera and other diarrheal diseases caused by contaminated water supplies
	Increased pools of standing water for mosquito breeding	Rift Valley fever, dengue fever
	Increased rodent population	Hantavirus pulmonary syndrome
	Destruction of agricultural products	Malnutrition

This table was adapted from several sources, including: Wilson ML. Ecology and Infectious Disease. In: Aron JL, Patz JA, eds. *Ecosystem Change and Public Health*. Baltimore: The Johns Hopkins University Press, 2001; and UNEP, Global Environmental Outlook Year Book 2004/2005: Emerging and Re-emerging Infectious Diseases: Links to Environmental Change.

poor bear the highest burden, since most of the deaths from extreme weather occur in low-income areas.

The globalization of the world economy increases our ability to influence the way people in other parts of the world relate to their environment. The movement of waste products, including hazardous materials, across national boundaries is one example of how the prospect of immediate financial gain can influence a nation to take on a long-term environmental risk. But global markets can also increase the use of sustainable practices. The growing demand for organic foods and other organic products has created an incentive for farmers to avoid the use of chemicals on their crops. Our choices about where to live, work, travel, and what to purchase have an effect on our health and the health of others around the world.

Regardless of arguments about whether global warming is currently occurring and possible future directions of climate change, we do know that humans alter the environment. It makes sense to take steps to limit our contribution as humans to global warming and other climate changes. We can, for example, work to find alternative energy sources. We know that air pollution is created when we burn biomass fuels and fossil fuels, that hydropower requires the building of massive dams which flood large swaths of land, and that nuclear power remains dangerous because of the risk of a meltdown. Alternative energy sources that are able to harness solar, wind, or wave power or other sources of energy, may be able to produce energy that creates less pollution and less environmental damage. Although it may not be possible to prevent weather extremes, it is possible to prepare for them by not building in especially vulnerable locations, using appropriate building styles and materials, and instituting early warning systems. Other actions need to be proposed and enacted. All of us have a stake in creating and sustaining a healthy global environment.

REFERENCES

1. Prüss-Üstün A, Corvalán C. Preventing disease through healthy environments: toward an estimate of the environmental burden of disease. Geneva: World Health Organization, 2006.
2. Diamond J. *Collapse: How Societies Choose to Fail or Succeed.* New York: Viking, 2005.
3. The first edition of *De Morbis Artificum Diatriba* was published in 1700. A second edition was published in 1713.
4. Unless otherwise noted, the occupational health statistics in this section are from the ILO (International Labour Organization), "World Day for Safety and Health at Work 2005: A Background Paper." Geneva, Switzerland: ILO, 2005.
5. World Health Organization. World Health Report 2002: Reducing Risks, Promoting Healthy Life. Geneva, Switzerland: World Health Organization, 2002.
6. Smith AH, Lingas EO, Rahman M. Contamination of drinking-water by arsenic in Bangladesh: a public health emergency. *Bull World Health Organ* 2000;79:1093–1103.
7. World Health Organization, "WHO gives indoor use of DDT a clean bill of health for controlling malaria," 15 September 2006.
8. Intergovernmental Panel on Climate Change. Climate Change 2007: The Physical Science Basis. Summary for Policymakers. Switzerland: Intergovernmental Panel on Climate Change, February 2007.

CHAPTER 12

Global Health Payers and Players

Key Points:
- In most low-income countries individuals must pay out-of-pocket for personal health care. In most high-income countries everyone has access to government-funded health services.
- Public health programs in low-income countries are often funded through bilateral and multilateral aid, private foundations, and loans from the World Bank and IMF.
- Health programs are often implemented by national governments, United Nations agencies, international development and cooperation agencies, and non-governmental organizations (NGOs).
- NGOs may focus on relief, development, advocacy, logistics, or a combination of these areas.

WHO PAYS FOR HEALTH?

Payment for health can be divided into two categories, money spent on personal health and money spent on public health. Examples of personal health costs might include purchasing chloroquine to treat a case of malaria and paying for a midwife to help deliver a baby. Examples of public health costs might include mass polio vaccination days, using molluscicides to kill the snails in a schistosomiasis-infected lake, and developing and testing a new antibiotic.

Paying for Personal Health

Expenses related to medical care of individuals are paid by a combination of government funds, health insurance, and private funds of the individual or family. Some countries have a health system that is primarily privately-funded and others sponsor a publicly-funded health care system (Figure 12-1).

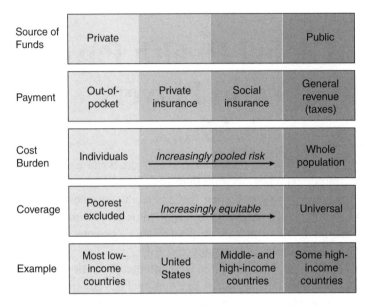

Figure 12-1. Public and Private Approaches to Health Care Funding, Risk Burden, and Coverage.

Source: Model from the World Health Report 1999, Figure 3.5.

In countries with a publicly-funded health care system, everyone receives the same level of coverage regardless of how much money they have paid in to the system. Funds are raised through general taxation or through social security systems (sometimes called "sickness funds") in which premiums are determined based on a percentage of the person's income. Individuals may be required to pay a small fee at the time of service or may choose to supplement the coverage provided by the national health plan with private insurance that pays for services not covered by the national health plan, but most people are adequately covered by the national health system.

Most high-income countries have a government-sponsored health care system. Canada's Medicare program and Italy's health system are funded from general government revenues collected through taxation. In Japan, France, and Germany, everyone pays into a government-run social security system that is separate from general taxes. The services covered vary for different plans. Some systems cover dental care and eye care and others do not. Some pay for all the expenses of hospitalization while others require the patient to pay for a percent of the cost of a hospital stay. The ownership of the health infrastructure also differs between countries. For example, the United Kingdom's National Health Service (NHS) owns some hospitals and employs some medical personnel, but in Canada and Japan most health providers are in private practice even though the government pays for the services provided. Common complaints about publicly-funded health care include long waiting times for access to specialists and advanced procedures, inefficiency because the health consumer does not pay directly for services and may over-use the system's resources, and shortages of health care providers.[1]

The United States is one of the few developed countries that does not have a universal health care system with adequate coverage for its entire population. The United States relies primarily on private health insurance, although the government sponsors Medicare for the elderly and disabled and Medicaid for the country's poorest citizens, and provides health care to injured veterans through the Veterans Administration (VA) hospital system and to indigenous Americans through the Indian Health Service (IHS).

Health insurance systems and government-sponsored systems are funded based on pooled risk. Pooled risk assumes that if many low-risk people and a few high-risk people all pay in to the insurance system over many years, then there will be a pot of money that can be used to pay for major illnesses when they occur. Only a few people will suffer a catastrophic injury or develop a very serious chronic condition, but everyone is at risk. The risk is small, but real and worrisome, so many people are willing to pay additional taxes or purchase insurance that protects them against the possibility of incurring an overwhelming amount of debt due to a serious illness.

Some countries have a social insurance system that employers and employees are required to pay into. Other countries rely primarily on private insurance systems, in which insurance is purchased by individuals or provided by employers, and health care is provided by private practitioners at private clinics and hospitals. The services provided by health insurance companies vary greatly. Some low-cost insurance plans only cover conditions serious enough to require hospitalization. Higher-cost insurance plans may cover clinic visits, preventive care, and medications in addition to paying for hospitalizations and surgeries. Private insurance companies may charge higher premiums to people with pre-existing conditions, older people, and people who are in high-risk groups, and insurance companies have the option of denying coverage to people who have applied to be insured.

Some of the features of the various models for health financing are summarized in Table 12-1. People who do not participate in a health insurance program may have to pay out-of-pocket for all health care expenses.

Table 12-1. Examples of Health Financing Models.

Model	Coverage	Financing	Ownership of Health Sector Inputs
National Health Service	Compulsory universal coverage	Taxes (general revenue)	Public
Social Insurance	Compulsory universal participation in "sickness funds"	Employers and individuals must pay in to the system	Public and private
Private Insurance	Voluntary	Employers or individuals may purchase private insurance	Private

Countries vary both by the type of health financing system they use and by the amount of money that is spent on health care. High-income countries spend more on health care per person and more on health care as a percent of GDP than low-income countries, and a greater proportion of the spending on health is covered by the government (Table 12-2).

The countries with the least total spending on health generally require the greatest contribution from individuals through out-of-pocket payments, as

Table 12-2. Health Expenditures by Country Income Level, 2001.

Country Income Level	Health Expenditure Per Capita (US$) in One Year	Health Expenditure as a % of GDP	Public Sector Expenditures Are a % of Total Health Expenditures
Low income countries	23	4.4	26.3
Middle income countries	118	6.0	51.1
High income countries	2841	10.8	62.1

Data Source: World Development Report 2004.

shown in Figure 12-2. People who live in low-income countries must often pay for the majority of their health care themselves through out-of-pocket spending. (This is not always true, because even within one region there may be many different levels of wealth and different approaches to health spending. For example, although most sub-Saharan African countries require large out-of-pocket expenditures, such as Guinea and Nigeria, not all do, such as Botswana. Botswana has an average income nearly ten times higher than that of Guinea and Nigeria.)

Spending on out-of-pocket health expenses as a percentage of income is much higher in low-income countries than higher-income countries. Since people in low-income countries generally have very little income, this means that they usually have only a very limited ability to purchase health care. An illness can quickly bankrupt a family, and that the poorest people might not have access to any health care since they cannot pay for it. The amount of money spent on health care by people in low-income countries is dwarfed by the amount spent in higher-income areas (Figure 12-3).

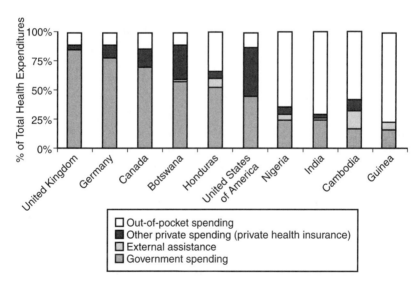

Figure 12-2. Examples of Distribution of Total Spending on Health by the Government and by Private Sources (Out-of-pocket Spending and Private Insurance) in 2003.

Data Source: World Health Report 2006.

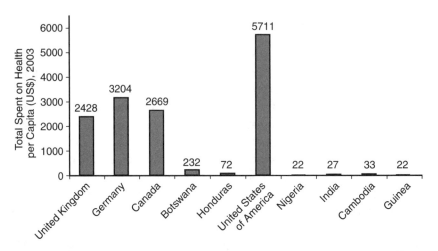

Figure 12-3. Total Expenditure on Health per Capita in U.S. dollars in 2003.
Data Source: World Health Report 2006.

Paying for Public Health

Since individuals do not typically pay for public health programs (other than through taxation), the money that is spent on major global health initiatives usually comes from different sources than the money spent on individual health care.

Bilateral aid is money given directly from one country to another. Although some aid is given simply to fight poverty, bilateral aid is often tied to the political and economic interests of the donor country. For example, an aid agreement may require that the recipient country purchase certain goods and services from companies based in the donor country. These kinds of bilateral aid agreements sometimes pay more attention to the business interests of donor nations than to the needs of the recipient country. **Multilateral aid** is money pooled from many donors. The World Bank, International Monetary Fund, and other United Nations agencies are the largest multilateral development funding institutions. The five donor nations that provide the greatest amount of "ODA" (official development assistance) are the United States, Japan, Germany, France, and the United Kingdom. As a percentage of their GNI (gross national income) the largest donors are Norway, Sweden, Luxembourg, the Netherlands, and Denmark.[2]

Private funding sources are making an increasingly significant contribution to spending on public health. Some private foundations, such as the Bill

& Melinda Gates Foundation and the Carter Center, work directly on global health projects. The Gates Foundation supports efforts to prevent and to treat diseases that cause widespread illness and death in developing countries, represent the greatest inequities in health between developed and developing countries, and receive inadequate attention and funding. Some of the priority diseases and conditions targeted by the Gates Foundation include acute diarrheal illnesses, acute lower respiratory infections like pneumonia, HIV/AIDS (with a focus on vaccine development), poor nutrition, reproductive and maternal health, tuberculosis (especially the development of new drugs and diagnostic tools), and vaccine-preventable childhood illnesses. The Gates Foundation also supports efforts to eradicate less common diseases through partnerships with organizations. For example, a partnership with The Carter Center, established by former U.S. President Jimmy Carter, is working to eradicate Guinea worm disease. Other foundations, such as the Ford, Carnegie, Kellogg, MacArthur, and Rockefeller Foundations, provide funding for projects that are implemented by other organizations. Non-governmental organizations working on health-related projects in low-income regions raise funds from individuals, private donors, and some governmental sources. A variety of public-private partnerships—like the Global Alliance for Vaccines and Immunizations (GAVI), the Global Fund to Fight AIDS, Malaria, and Tuberculosis (GFATM), and the Global Alliance for Improved Nutrition (GAIN)—are also working to set and accomplish goals for selected health issues. The role of each of these types of organizations in implementing global public health initiatives is discussed later in this chapter.

International Funding and Debt Relief

The two international agencies most involved in offering grants (money that does not have to be repaid) and loans (money that needs to be repaid and usually requires payment of interest on the money that has been loaned) are the World Bank and the International Monetary Fund.

The World Bank Group consists of five institutions: the International Bank for Reconstruction and Development (IBRD), the International Development Association (IDA), the International Finance Corporation (IFC), the Multilateral Investment Guarantee Agency (MIGA), and the International Centre for Settlement of Investment Disputes (ICSID). When people use the term "World Bank" they are usually referring specifically to the IBRD and the

IDA. The IBRD focuses on middle-income nations and the IDA focuses on the poorest countries. Both institutions provide low-interest loans, interest-free credit, and grants to developing countries for education, health, infra-structure, communications, and many other purposes. The World Bank functions as a cooperative that is run by representatives of member countries, who are usually member countries' ministers of finance.

Unlike the World Bank, the International Monetary Fund (IMF) does not lend money for specific projects. The goal of IMF loans is to allow countries to rebuild their monetary reserves, stabilize their currencies, continue paying for imports, and create conditions for economic growth and high employment rates. Loans are typically extended to member countries that have a "balance of payment" need—that is, countries that cannot afford to make their required payments on international loans.

As a condition of getting a loan, the IMF frequently requires recipient countries to adhere to a Structural Adjustment Program (SAP) that might require tax increases, reduced government spending, currency devaluation, elimination of price controls and subsidies, and increased production of exports. SAPs are often designed to encourage capitalism through privatization of government-owned utilities and industries and deregulation of markets. The SAP rules put farmers and other workers in low-income countries at a competitive disadvantage, because richer nations do not have the same restrictions on subsidies. SAPs have been criticized for creating even tougher economic situations for poor households. The short-term consequences of implementing SAPs often include falling incomes, decreased social expenditures, rising food prices, and an increased burden on women who must shift from formal wage labor to informal, low-paid work as the unemployment rate rises.

Because loans must be repaid with interest, lending nations make a profit by lending money to poor countries, assuming that the principal is repaid with interest. A major criticism of the international loan system is that payments on debt divert money away from education, health, clean water, and other essential human services. This often means that the rich benefit the most from loans (because the loans can be used to support the companies owned by the wealthy and have sometimes gone directly into the bank accounts of dishonest leaders) and the poor suffer the most because of the debt.

Many low-income nations spend more on repaying debt each year than they do on primary education and health care combined.[3] Some countries even have debt that exceeds the total national income in a year (Figure 12-4). The amount that must be repaid grows larger if debt payments are not made, creating a level of debt that could burden the country and stifle economic

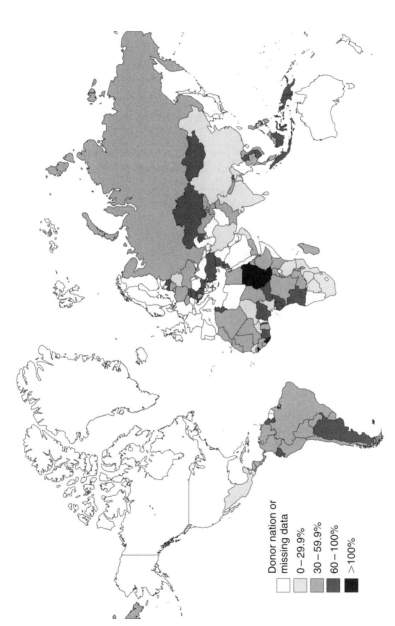

Figure 12-4. Debt as a Percent of Gross National Income (GNI), 2004.

Data Source: Human Development Report 2007.

growth for decades. Unlike individuals and companies that can file for bankruptcy protection, poor countries are not given legal protection from debt.

Lending nations have agreed to forgive some of the debts of the most burdened poor countries. The World Bank's Enhanced Heavily Indebted Poor Countries (HIPC) Initiative has committed to forgiving $17 billion in debt, and the leaders of the G8 nations (eight large industrialized countries—Canada, France, Germany, Italy, Japan, Russia, the United Kingdom, and the United States) pledged in 2005 to cancel debts in the most indebted nations. But the cancellation only applies to loans from the IMF, World Bank, and African Development Fund, and not to other bilateral and multilateral donors or private lenders. Furthermore, because interest rates may increase over time, the amount that must be paid each year may not decrease significantly even if the principal and interest from some loans are forgiven. Countries that have crushing debt burdens are unable to put resources toward improving their health and educational systems, and this contributes, in turn, to perpetuating a cycle of poverty and poor health.

WHO IMPLEMENTS HEALTH PROGRAMS?

The majority of health services are implemented by, or with the approval and assistance of, national ministries of health and their provincial and district health offices. Health services, health supplies, and technical assistance may also be provided by United Nations Agencies (such as WHO, UNICEF, and other specialized programs), other governments through their international development or international cooperation agencies, non-governmental organizations (NGOs), businesses and public-private partnerships, and individuals. Sometimes the coordination between groups is poor and the groups end up "competing" and duplicating their efforts in an area. Sometimes the various players work together to promote health or agree to focus on different aspects of health, such as when one organization working in a community specializes in water and sanitation and another focuses only on child vaccination.

National and Local Governments

National governments provide the bulk of health services and payment for health care systems. They decide, at least in part, who gets to use the health care system, the choice (if any) that people have about where to seek care, the kinds of services that are covered by social security or health insurance, the level of training required for health care practitioners, and the types of facilities available. Even when the health care system is not nationalized, the government can still dictate, for example, what services must be covered by insurance and what educational and testing requirements must be fulfilled before people are licensed as doctors, nurses, and therapists.

The national government is also responsible for the public health system. It can set guidelines for nutrition, vaccination schedules, screening, and other preventive measures, and can regulate the production and sale of health supplies, medications, and food products. It can also form public health partnerships with other nations and agencies that allow it to share information and quickly respond to infectious disease threats that require an international response. And it can negotiate with companies, for example, to secure cheaper prices on medications and supplements.

The implementation of any public health program almost always requires the approval of national or local government officials and local leaders. For example, if a voluntary organization from Canada wants to distribute free insecticide-treated bednets (ITNs) in a village in Zambia, the leaders of the organization should first meet with local government, tribal, or church leaders to get their approval and support. The local leaders will be able to help the visiting group set up a distribution system that is culturally appropriate and will help spread the word about the free ITNs to the community. The local leaders will also be able to tell the visitors if they do not need or want ITNs, if the visitors have come at a bad time (say, during harvest time or on a day when there is a funeral), or if the presence of the visitors (who might need meals or a place to sleep) will place an undue burden on the community. Organizations that want to work on a bigger scale might need to get the approval of the national Ministry of Health and other national governmental offices. This is true for all intervention programs, and essential for any projects that might involve testing a new product or medical protocol. When a new health product is being tested, the sponsoring organization must obtain Institutional Review Board approval from the national IRB of the Ministry of Health before starting a trial, and needs to communicate frequently with a national supervisory committee during the trial.

United Nations Agencies

The United Nations (UN) was founded in 1945 by 51 member states and by 2006 had expanded to 192 member nations. The goal of the UN is to provide a forum for nations to come together to debate and discuss areas of disagreement, make and enforce trade agreements and other international regulations, and implement multilateral humanitarian actions.

The United Nations addresses human rights, economic and social development, international peace and security, international law, and humanitarian action. These functions are carried out by the specialized agencies, offices, funds, and programs of the UN (Table 12-3). The Office of the United Nations High Commissioner for Human Rights (OHCHR) coordinates human rights activities. The Economic and Social Council and its commissions work on economic, social, and sustainable development in partnership with other UN groups like the UN Environment Programme (UNEP), the Office of the UN High Commissioner for Refugees (UNHCR), the UN Drug Control Programme (UNDCP), and the Joint UN Programme on HIV/AIDS (UNAIDS). The 15-member Security Council is responsible for peace-building, mediation, and security operations. The General Assembly, which is composed of one voting representative from each member state and is the main policy-setting group for the UN, and other governing bodies propose and adopt international laws. Organizations like the International Court of Justice provide legal judgments and advisory opinions. Humanitarian operations are conducted by specialized groups including the United Nations High Commissioner for Refugees (UNHCR), United Nations Development Programme (UNDP), United Nations Children's Fund (UNICEF), and the World Food Programme (WFP).

The World Health Organization (WHO) is the primary health organization of the United Nations, and conducts research on health issues of international importance, monitors disease epidemics, collects health statistics, develops standards such as child growth charts and procedures for laboratory and diagnostic work, and creates educational materials. (Other mandated functions are listed in Appendix II.) WHO also provides assistance to national governments that ask for technical assistance and coordinates the health work of other UN agencies. For example, WHO coordinated the smallpox eradication campaign in the 1960s and 1970s and is now coordinating the global polio eradication campaign. The annual World Health Report provides current health statistics and addresses key policy issues, and several divisions and regions also publish regular journals and reports.

WHO is governed by the World Health Assembly, composed of one representative from each UN Member State, which convenes every May to approve a budget, make policy decisions, and approve conventions, agreements, and regulations. The first global health treaty negotiated by WHO is the Framework Convention on Tobacco Control (FCTC), which details specific measures, such as increased taxation and comprehensive bans on advertising of tobacco products, that should be taken to reduce the demand for tobacco and the supply of tobacco.[4]

The diversity of global health issues addressed by the World Health Organization is impressive, especially given the limitations of its small budget. Common concerns expressed about the organization include criticism of the areas of focus (with some people complaining that the organization puts too much emphasis on diseases with easily measurable outcomes instead of tackling less-measurable conditions like mental illness), unease about slow reaction time because of the need to involve regional and national offices in decision-making, and the fear that WHO takes the most capable health professionals away from their home countries to work in Geneva or a regional office.

Several other United Nations agencies, funds, and programs with health-related functions are listed in Table 12-4.

National Governmental Organizations

National governments are often involved in sponsoring relief and development work internationally and cooperatively. Most governments of high-income countries sponsor medical and public health research and have an international development or cooperation agency that works with the governments and people of lower-income countries.

In the United States, the National Institutes of Health (NIH) is the federal focal point for medical research. The NIH is divided into more than twenty separate institutes, and research funded by nearly any of the divisions can be conducted internationally, provided that the research protocol meets rigorous standards for conducting ethical human subjects research. The United Kingdom's Medical Research Council (MRC), the Canadian Institutes of Health Research (CIHR), and the South African Medical Research Council (MRC) are other examples of nationally funded health research agencies. Although most research funds are spent on health issues of national concern, some money is used for international research.

The U.S. Centers for Disease Control and Prevention (CDC) is somewhat unique in the lead role it plays in responding to international public health crises. The CDC responds to international health emergencies when invited to do so by the country or countries affected, and works with the ministries of health of other nations to conduct field research, to set up monitoring and surveillance systems, and to train public health workers.[5]

Table 12-3. Selected Agencies, Funds, and Programs of the United Nations.

Principal Organs

General Assembly	Security Council	Economic and Social Council	International Court of Justice	Secretariat

Specialized Agencies

ILO (International Labor Organization)	FAO (Food and Agriculture Organization)	UNESCO (UN Educational, Scientific, and Cultural Organization)	WHO (World Health Organization)	UNIDO (UN Industrial Development Organization)
World Bank Group	IMF (International Monetary Fund)	IFAD (International Fund for Agricultural Development)	WIPO (World Intellectual Property Organization)	WTO (World Tourism Organization)
ICAO (International Civil Aviation Organization)	MO (International Maritime Organization)	ITU (International Telecommunication Union)	UPU (Universal Postal Union)	WMO (World Meteorological Organization)

Programs and Funds

UNDP (UN Development Programme)	UNFPA (UN Population Fund)	UNHCR (Office of the UN High Commissioner for Refugees)	WFP (World Food Programme)	UN-HABITAT (UN Human Settlements Programme)

UNEP (UN Environment Programme)	UNCTAD (UN Conference on Trade and Development)	UNDCP (UN Drug Control Programme)	UNICEF (UN Children's Fund)	UNRWA (UN Relief and Worlds Agency for Palestine Refugees in the Near East)
Commissions of the Economic and Social Council				
Commission on Human Rights	Commission on Sustainable Development	Commission on the Status of Women	Statistical Commission	Commission on Science and Technology for Development
ECA (Economic Commission for Africa)	ECE (Economic Commission for Europe)	ECLAC (Economic Commission for Latin America and the Caribbean)	ESCAP (Economic and Social Commission for Asia and the Pacific)	ESCWA (Economic and Social Commission for Western Asia Commission for Africa)
Commission on Narcotic Drugs	Commission on Crime Prevention and Justice	Commission on Population and Development	Commission for Social Development	PFII (Permanent Forum on Indigenous Issues)
Other UN Agencies and Related Organizations				
OHCHR (Office of the UN High Commissioner for Human Rights)	UNOPS (UN Office for Project Services)	UNAIDS (Joint UN Programme on HIV/AIDS)	WTO (World Trade Organization)	IAEA (International Atomic Energy Agency)

Table 12-4. Selected United Nations Agencies with Health Functions.

Agency, Program, or Fund	Primary Work Area
Food and Agriculture Organization (FAO)	Rural development
UNAIDS	HIV/AIDS
United Nations Development Programme (UNDP)	National development
United Nations Environment Programme (UNEP)	Environmental health
United Nations Population Fund (UNFPA)	Population and reproductive health issues
United Nations High Commissioner for Refugees (UNHCR)	Refugees
UNICEF	Children
World Food Program (WFP)	Hunger
World Health Organization (WHO)	All health issues

Most developed countries also have a governmental division dedicated to working with developing countries, and many of these agencies have a visible presence on the ground in low-income countries (Table 12-5). Several types of assistance may be offered. Monetary aid is when funds are provided for a particular project, such as the distribution of science textbooks to children attending urban primary schools, the promotion of drought-resistant crops, or the installation of boreholes for water at rural health clinics. Technical aid is when highly trained people are sent to work alongside nationals of the recipient country on a specific project. Sometimes international development assistance takes the form of military training grants and technical security assistance. The type of aid countries donate depends on the goals of the donor country. This is illustrated by describing the organizational strategies and funding priorities of agencies from three high-income countries: the United States, the United Kingdom, and Japan.

The international development agency of the United States is USAID. USAID is run by the U.S. Department of State and supervised by the Senate Foreign Relations Committee, which makes funding and assistance allocations based on political goals. The U.S. supports five different types of foreign aid: bilateral development assistance (34.7% of the 2005 budget), military assistance (23.6% of the foreign aid budget, which is in addition to military assistance paid for from the much larger defense

Table 12-5. International Development and Cooperation Agencies.

Country	Abbreviation	Agency
Australia	AusAid	Australian Agency for International Development
Austria	ADA	Austrian Development Agency
Belgium	DGDC	Belgian Development Cooperation
Canada	CIDA	Canadian International Development Agency
Denmark	DANIDA	Danish International Development Agency
Finland	FINNIDA	Department for International Development Cooperation
France	AfD	Agence française de Developpement
Germany	DED	Deutscher Entwicklungsdienst
	GTZ	Deutsche Gesellschaft für Technische Zusammenarbeit
Greece		Ministry of Foreign Affairs
Ireland	Irish Aid	Irish Development Cooperation Directorate
Italy		Ministry of Foreign Affairs—Directorate General for Development Cooperation
Japan	JICA	Japan International Cooperation Agency
Luxembourg		Lux-Development
The Netherlands		Dutch Development Cooperation
New Zealand	NZAid	New Zealand Agency for International Development
Norway	NORAD	Norwegian Agency for Development Cooperation
Portugal	IPAD	Instituto Português de Apoio ao Desenvolvimento
Spain	AECI	Agencia Española de Cooperación Internacional
Sweden	SIDA	Swedish International Development Cooperation Agency
Switzerland	SDC	Swiss Agency for Development and Cooperation
United Kingdom	DFID	Department for International Development
United States	USAID	U.S. Agency for International Development

budget), economic aid supporting U.S. political and security objectives (21.8%), humanitarian assistance (12.6%), and multilateral assistance (7.3%).[6] The three "strategic pillars" of foreign aid identified by the Bush Administration are (1) economic growth, agriculture, and trade; (2) global health; and (3) democracy, conflict prevention, and humanitarian assistance. These pillars have been refined by USAID into five "core" operational goals: (1) promoting transformational development, especially in the areas of governance, institutional capacity, and economic restructuring; (2) strengthening fragile states; (3) providing humanitarian assistance; (4) supporting U.S. geostrategical interests, particularly in countries such as Iraq, Afghanistan, Pakistan, Jordan, Egypt, and Israel; and (5) mitigating global and international ills, including HIV/AIDS.[7] The largest recipients of foreign assistance from the United States in recent years have been Iraq, Israel, and Egypt, and several South American countries receive large amounts of aid focused on anti-drug efforts. Other major recipients include countries involved in counter-terrorism activities (like Afghanistan, Pakistan, Turkey, Jordan, and Indonesia) and countries receiving HIV/AIDS funds.

In the United Kingdom, the Department for International Development (DFID) is overseen by the Secretary of State for International Development, who is a Cabinet member. The goal of DFID is to fight world poverty and the problems associated with poverty like conflict, crime, pollution, and infectious diseases, and DFID has adopted the United Nations' eight Millennium Development Goals as part of its own mission.[8] In 2004-2005, the top five recipients of bilateral aid from the United Kingdom were India, Bangladesh, Tanzania, Sudan, and Afghanistan.[9]

The agency in Japan is JICA, and its mission is to be "a bridge between the people of Japan and developing countries."[10] JICA's three pillars are (1) a field-oriented approach, (2) human security, and (3) effectiveness, efficiency, and speed. JICA distributes assistance based on: (1) reaching those in need through a people-centered approach, (2) empowering people as well as protecting them, (3) focusing on the most vulnerable people, (4) comprehensively addressing both "freedom from want" and "freedom from fear," (5) responding to people's needs by assessing and addressing threats through flexible and inter-sectorial approaches, (6) working with both governments and local communities to realize sustainable development, and (7) strengthening partnerships with various actors to achieve a higher impact from assistance.[11] The top recipients of "cooperation" in 2004 were all Asian nations—Indonesia, China, Vietnam, the Philippines, and Thailand.[12]

While each of these agencies works to alleviate poverty and improve health, the goals, methods, and targeted recipient countries vary based on the political situations and historic connections of the donor nation.

Non-Governmental Organizations (NGOs)

Non-Governmental Organizations (NGOs), sometime called **Private Voluntary Organizations (PVOs)**, are non-profit organizations that are independent of any government and get at least some of their funding from private sources. NGOs working internationally include Oxfam, CARE, Helen Keller International, Save the Children, the International Rescue Committee, Habitat for Humanity, Freedom from Hunger, Heifer Project, Rotary International, and thousands of other organizations (Tables 12-6 and 12-7).

NGOs may focus on one particular issue, like cultural awareness or environmental preservation, or address multiple issues in a particular town or region. NGOs may be involved in direct action like distributing food aid or may focus entirely on lobbying and advocacy. Some NGOs, called **Faith-Based Organizations (FBOs)**, are sponsored by religious organizations, and although they rarely require that aid recipients adhere to a particular faith or listen to an evangelistic message, they are representing a particular religious tradition. Examples of FBOs include Catholic Relief Services, Lutheran World Relief, Church World Service, World Vision, Islamic Relief, and the Aga Khan Foundation.

Some international NGOs focus primarily on **relief**—meeting the immediate needs of people who might otherwise not have access to water, food, shelter, health services, and other urgent necessities. Relief agencies include groups like Médecins Sans Frontières (MSF, or Doctors Without Borders) and the International Rescue Committee that provide emergency medical care, food, tents, and blankets after natural disasters and conflict. Other agencies focus primarily on **community development**, working with local communities to improve living conditions and build up small businesses, often through the use of microcredit programs. **Microcredit** programs give very small loans (**microloans**) to people who are unable to get a loan through a conventional bank because they do not have collateral, steady employment, or a credit history, or because they are women. The interest rates are much lower than those offered by conventional banks, and most microcredit programs also provide some form of financial education and community

Table 12-6. Major International Relief and Development Organizations Based in the United States.

Name	Total Spent on Program Expenses, 2004 or 2005	Target
World Vision	$752,209,000	Diverse
Feed the Children	$745,390,856	Children
CARE	$513,924,000	Diverse
Catholic Relief Services	$490,307,000	Diverse
United States Fund for UNICEF	$426,955,593	Children
Samaritan's Purse	$216,066,505	Diverse
Save the Children	$293,165,008	Children
Catholic Medical Mission Board	$182,640,122	Health Care
Compassion International	$173,447,349	Children
International Rescue Committee	$165,228,335	Refugees and Displaced People
Christian Children's Fund	$150,203,121	Children and Families
Mercy Corps	$146,903,110	Diverse
Project HOPE	$123,051,219	Health Care
The Rotary Foundation of Rotary International	$110,024,876	Diverse
The Carter Center	$108,744,344	Human Rights
Adventist Development and Relief Agency (ADRA)	$ 97,027,009	Diverse
Children International	$ 85,998,014	Children
PATH	$ 74,884,142	Health Technology
International Medical Corps	$ 73,225,732	Health Care
Church World Service	$ 72,149,275	Diverse

Sources: Charity Navigator (www.charitynavigator.org). Because results are based on IRS (Internal Revenue Service) forms, religious organizations exempt from filing Form 990 are not evaluated. Data for Catholic Relief Services (2003) from the Better Business Bureau Wise Giving Alliance (www.give.org).

Table 12-7. Top International Health Charities in the United Kingdom.

Name	Annual Expenditure	Target
Oxfam	£225,900,000	Diverse
British Red Cross	£154,920,000	Emergency Response
Save the Children UK	£126,783,000	Diverse
ActionAid UK	£108,756,000	Diverse
International Planned Parenthood Foundation	£ 95,854,000	Reproductive Health
Christian Aid	£ 70,995,000	Diverse
UNICEF UK	£ 61,991,000	Children
Disasters Emergency Committee	£ 53,514,785	Disaster Response
World Vision UK	£ 42,434,000	Diverse
Marie Stopes International	£ 42,176,000	Reproductive Health
CARE International UK	£ 40,210,000	Diverse
Tearfund	£ 40,114,000	Diverse
Islamic Relief	£ 36,940,156	Diverse
World Emergency Relief	£ 35,307,580	Children
CAFOD (Catholic Agency for Overseas Development)	£ 34,152,000	Diverse
Voluntary Service Overseas	£ 32,992,000	Diverse
Plan International UK	£ 30,456,000	Child Sponsorship
Sight Savers International	£ 29,981,000	Vision / Eye Health

Source: Intelligent Giving (www.intelligentgiving.com).

support. (One of the first major microcredit organizations is the Grameen Bank of Bangladesh, founded by Muhammad Yunus, the winner of the 2006 Nobel Peace Prize.) Logistics organizations like MAP International gather medical supplies and pharmaceutical donations and ship them to under-stocked clinics. **Advocacy** organizations, like Amnesty International, Human Rights Watch, and the Population Council, promote a specific cause like human rights or AIDS awareness. Many NGOs cover the spectrum of relief aid, development work, and advocacy.

One challenge for NGOs is balancing the goals of donors and the desires of recipients. Directed donations occur when a donor gives money and stipulates that it must go to a particular cause. Sometimes this works well, but other times donors may not be aware of conditions in the recipient community. A community that wants to upgrade its local health clinic by adding a solar panel to provide electricity for boiling water may instead receive a microscope that they cannot use without electricity. A school may receive a donation of textbooks written in a language not spoken by any of the students. Or a donor may send old medical equipment that cannot be maintained by the community or a water pump that cannot be locally repaired. Donors may also create tensions between the NGO, host country, and recipient community by requiring the NGO to adopt a particular stance on a political issue or to hire a certain person for its staff before the funds will be released.

Another concern is that not all "non-governmental" organizations are completely independent from governments. For example, several of the largest U.S.-based international NGOs listed in Table 12-5 receive a large proportion of their budget from the U.S. government. CARE received more than $270 million in federal funds in 2003, Church World Service received more than $30 million in 2004, and the Adventist Development and Relief Agency (ADRA) received more than $20 million in 2002.[13] Some people worry that governments may restrict where NGOs can work and what services they can provide. Others are concerned about the safety of NGO workers whose safety may be threatened if they are considered to be government agents.

Another challenge for NGOs operating internationally is deciding what aspects of budget and operations should be handled at the local level. Some NGOs hire primarily in-country staff while others prefer to hire "expats" as managers, accountants, and field staff. (Expatriates are people working in a foreign country for their home government, a business, the press corps, an NGO, or other organization.)

International NGOs must also decide how closely they will work with officials from host countries. Some humanitarian groups feel that it is important to remain publicly neutral so that they can assist victims on all sides of a conflict, while other humanitarian groups feel compelled to speak openly about injustices they have witnessed. This decision may impact the ability for the organization to send personnel and supplies to places they would like to work. Human rights activists may be denied visas, while medical or engineering teams may be welcomed graciously. Cross-cultural communication skills are a must for all people working for an NGO because they must be able to relate to both the funding agency and the host community.

NGOs also have to consider the social and political impact of their actions. Does the presence of a relief NGO exacerbate conflicts by potentially providing supplies that allow violence and instability to continue (perhaps by feeding soldiers or guerrillas) or encouraging displaced persons to congregate in one area that could be targeted for attack or facilitate the spread of infectious diseases? Does the presence of a community development NGO in a community promote a "culture of dependency," contribute to corruption, or limit the advancement of government or private-sector service providers? Does the message being spread by an advocacy NGO lead to greater suppression of marginalized populations?

International Committee of the Red Cross

The International Committee of the Red Cross (ICRC) works with national Red Cross and Red Crescent Societies and the International Federation of Red Cross and Red Crescent Societies to provide humanitarian aid to people in areas affected by war and other armed conflicts. It is unique among private organizations because it is an independent organization guided by its own set of rules and principles (humanity, impartiality, neutrality, independence, voluntary service, unity, and universality) but is officially sanctioned by the Geneva Convention and international law to provide certain humanitarian services. ICRC is funded through governmental funds, contributions from national Red Cross and Red Crescent societies, and private donations.

ICRC aids both civilian and military victims of conflicts by visiting prisoners of war, searching for missing persons, transmitting messages between separated family members, reunifying dispersed families, monitoring compliance with the international laws that pertain to armed conflict, and providing basic services to civilians such as food, water, and medical assistance. National Red Cross and Red Crescent societies are autonomous from ICRC and provide a variety of services that meet needs in their communities. Examples of local Red Cross activities include maintaining blood banks, providing first aid training, responding to house fires to offer assistance to victims, and responding to natural disasters.

International Businesses

All businesses can be involved in promoting health by making sure that their employees have adequate access to health care at a reasonable price. Although company health care plans can be expensive, lack of productivity by sick and disabled workers is also costly. Sick workers mean that companies have to pay higher health insurance rates, cover additional sick leave and death benefits, and recruit and train new staff as replacements. Companies can also implement and enforce occupational safety protocols in every country where they have facilities and can encourage international business partners to create healthy work environments for their employees. This can be thought of as a form of risk management. Both the employees and the company benefit by implementing health education programs such as information sessions about nutrition, weight control, and correct lifting technique (from the legs not the back), subsidizing the cost of drugs, and enforcing safety measures.

Business associations, professional societies, transnational corporations, and other companies can also choose to become directly involved in international health efforts. For example, Unilever and Colgate-Palmolive have donated soap to hygiene campaigns and DuPont has donated nylon cloth for use in filters for prevention of Guinea worm disease. In addition to being a form of humanitarian aid (and often a tax deduction), these are ways of developing international markets and bringing brand names to new potential customers. Furthermore, economies are weaker when a large proportion of the population is sick or caring for sick people, but populations with increased income and decreased health expenditures have more money to spend on other goods and services. By helping potential consumers stay healthy, companies are expanding their markets.

Businesses directly involved in health, such as private health providers, insurance agencies, and pharmaceutical corporations, have special moral obligations to make sure that their products reach the most vulnerable people. While they have the legal rights to protect intellectual property, they should also work to ensure that technology transfer is available during humanitarian emergencies. In many cases, governments, businesses, and NGOs work together to provide products and services to underserved populations.

REFERENCES

1. Hurst J. Challenges for health systems in member countries of the Organisation for Economic Cooperation and Development. *Bull World Health Organ* 2000; 78:751–760.
2. Organisation for Economic Cooperation and Development (OECD). *OECD Factbook 2005*. Paris, France: OECD, 2005.
3. United Nations Development Programme (UNDP). Human Development Report 2007: Human Development and Climate Change. New York, NY: UNDP, 2007.

4. Shibuya K, Ciecierski C, Guindon E, Bettcher DW, Evans DB, Murray CJL. WHO Framework Convention on Tobacco Control: development of an evidence based global public health treaty. *BMJ* 2003; 327:4–157.

5. CDC, "Protecting the Nation's Health in an Era of Globalization: CDC's Global Infectious Disease Strategy." Atlanta, GA: CDC, 2002.

6. Tarnoff C, Nowels L. "Foreign Aid: An Introductory Overview of U.S. Programs and Policy," CRS (Congressional Research Service of The Library of Congress) Report for Congress, updated 19 January 2005.

7. Bureau for Policy and Program Coordination, U.S. Agency for International Development (USAID), "U.S. Foreign Aid: Meeting the Challenges of the Twenty-First Century." Washington, DC: USAID, January 2004.

8. U.K. Department of International Development (DIFD), "About DFID: Mission Statement." http://www.dfid.gov/uk/aboutdfid/missionstatement.asp. Accessed 8 May 2007.

9. Statistical Reporting and Support Group, U.K. Department of International Development (DIFD), "Top Twenty Recipients DFID Bilateral Aid." Statistics of International Development 2001/02–2005/06. East Kilbride, UK: DFID, 2006.

10. Japan International Cooperation Agency (JICA), Mission Statement. http://www.jica.go.jp/about/miss.html. Accessed 8 May 2007.

11. Japan International Cooperation Agency (JICA), "Human Security." http://www.jica.go.jp/english/about/policy/reform/human/index.html. Accessed 8 May 2007.

12. Office of Evaluation, Planning and Coordination Department, JICA, *Annual Evaulation Report 2005: Moving Forward Together.* Tokyo, Japan: JICA, 2006.

13. Financial data from the Better Business Bureau Wise Giving Alliance.

CHAPTER 13

Global Health Priorities

Key Points:
- If health is a human right, then everyone is entitled to affordable basic health services and health products.
- The Millennium Development Goals (MDGs) and other global development initiatives are promoting programs that reduce child mortality, improve maternal health, combat HIV/AIDS, malaria, and other diseases, and address other global health problems.
- Cost-effective solutions for many global public health issues are available for implementation now.

HEALTH AND HUMAN RIGHTS

Ethics are norms of conduct for individuals and societies that help people understand duties and obligations, virtues and values, and the ideas of justice and fairness. Ethics are influenced by culture, religion, and other complex factors, and they define human responsibilities. Human rights, on the other hand, define governmental responsibilities. **Human rights** are considered universal (available to everyone) and irrevocable (something that cannot be taken away). Only truly essential needs are protected as human rights. National and international human rights laws limit state power and protect fundamental individual rights such as human dignity and human freedoms. (A non-derogable human right is one that is constant, such as the right to freedom from slavery and the right to freedom from torture. A derogable right can be temporarily suspended under special circumstances when the rights of some may need to be restricted to secure similar rights of others. For example, freedom of movement may be temporarily limited during an epidemic so that the right to health can be protected. The rules that govern when some rights may be temporarily suspended must not be discriminatory and must apply equally to all people.)

The right to health is one of many human rights (Table 13-1) recognized in the Universal Declaration of Human Rights, which was unanimously adopted by the member nations of the United Nations in 1948. Article 25 states that "everyone has the right to a standard of living adequate for the

Table 13-1. Human Rights Listed in the Universal Declaration of Human Rights.

Human Right	UDHR Article(s)
Right to equal dignity and human rights for all humans	1,2,6
Right to life, liberty, and security of person	3
Freedom from slavery and servitude	4
Freedom from torture and cruel, inhuman, or degrading treatment or punishment	5
Freedom from discrimination	7
Freedom from arbitrary arrest, detention, or exile	9
Right to a fair trial	8,10,11
Right to privacy	12
Freedom of movement	13
Right to asylum	14
Right to a nationality	15
Right to marry and found a family	16
Right to own property	17
Freedom of thought, conscience, and religion	18
Freedom of opinion and expression	19
Freedom of peaceful assembly and association	20
Right to participate in government	21
Right to social security	22
Right to work	23
Right to rest and leisure	24
Right to a standard of living adequate for the health and well-being of the individual and his/her family, including food, clothing, housing, medical care, and necessary social services, and the right to security in the event of unemployment, sickness, disability, widowhood, or old age	25
Right to education	26
Right to participate in the cultural life of a community	27

health and well-being of himself and of his family, including food, clothing, housing, and medical care and necessary social services, and the right to security in the event of unemployment, sickness, disability, widowhood, old age or other lack of livelihood in circumstances beyond his control." (The complete declaration is in Appendix IV.) If health is a human right, then it is a violation of human rights when national and international laws and practices interfere with a person's access to health care and to health care technology.

If health is a human right then it is unjust that poor people so often do not have access to even the minimum level of health care that will allow healthy and productive lives, especially since most poor people are born into poverty. Paul Farmer, a physician and anthropologist, is one of the best-known advocates for improved health care for the poor and the imprisoned. Although he works as a professor at Harvard and travels the world giving speeches and meeting with other activists, he prefers to spend his time at a clinic in rural Haiti. Farmer has written several books including *Pathologies of Power: Health, Human Rights, and the New War on the Poor*, in which he argues that health is a human right and should not be sold like a commercial product. He writes: "Healthcare can be considered a commodity to be sold, or it can be considered a basic social right. It cannot comfortably be considered both of these at the same time."[1]

The distribution of health care raises tough economic and social questions. Many medical professionals in industrialized regions devote their lives to the development and distribution of new technologies. Who should have access to new assisted reproductive technologies like *in vitro* fertilization, and who should pay for it? How should we balance the desire to conduct rigorous tests of new drugs with the desire to quickly get new products to patients who could benefit from them? Who should have first priority for receiving a donated organ? When should surgery for conditions that are not life-threatening, such as hip replacements and LASIK eye surgery, be offered? When is the cost of using a high-tech diagnostic machine like an MRI worth the expense? Is it justifiable to spend millions of dollars using advanced technology to prolong the life of a severely injured person or a very premature newborn? Paul Farmer points out that it is a luxury for doctors, policy-makers, and other professionals in high-income countries to struggle with these questions:

> The ethical dilemmas that are the primary focus of conversation in the literature or on hospital rounds are often about an

embarrassment of riches. Making choices that involve options. How long should we continue life support? What constitutes brain death? Should we perform liver transplants for people who are alcoholics? Of course these are serious problems for families facing grave decisions for their loved ones. But in Haiti and in other similar places it's about no options, about lack of access to just the basics: vaccines, clean water, food, and treatment for tuberculosis or AIDS.[2]

While people who live in high-income countries may experience limitations in timely access to health care resources (supplies, facilities, trained personnel, and other factors) and may have limited amounts of money to pay for health care, they usually have options that are not available to most people in other parts of the world.

In places where health resources are extremely scarce, health care providers must sometimes make tough decisions about how to prioritize distribution of health care. Because there are not enough workers and supplies to treat everyone, patients must be triaged according to need, urgency, and the likelihood of a good outcome. In situations like this, should the young receive priority over the old? Should people who care for dependent children and parents receive priority over single people without dependents? Should priority be given to the people with the worst diseases and injuries or to the ones who have the best odds of survival and complete recovery? Who should be seen first when there is only one clinician available: a pregnant woman experiencing labor complications, a young child with cerebral malaria, or a teenage pedestrian struck by a motorcycle? Many clinicians who work at hospitals and clinics have to make these sorts of life-and-death triage decisions every day.

The United Nations High Commissioner for Human Rights has clarified what is meant by the right to health:

> The right to health does not mean the right to be healthy, nor does it mean that poor governments must put in place expensive services for which they have no resources. But it does require governments and public authorities to put in place policies and action plans which will lead to available and accessible health care for all in the shortest possible time. To ensure that this happens is the challenge facing both the human rights community and public health professionals.[3]

The UN suggests using four basic criteria to evaluate access to health[4]:

1. *Availability*: There are an adequate number of medical and public health facilities that are functioning, staffed, and stocked with the necessary supplies.
2. *Accessibility*: Everyone has access to health care and health information and health care is economically accessible (affordable). People are not discriminated against because of sex, age, marital status, or any other characteristic and the facilities are accessible to all people regardless of physical ability.
3. *Acceptability*: Health care practices adhere to the standards of medical ethics and are respectful of cultural, gender, and life-cycle requirements. Confidentiality is always maintained and health care practitioners treat all patients with respect and dignity.
4. *Quality*: Health facilities, goods, and services are scientifically and medically appropriate and of good quality.

These set a minimum standard for access to health. They do not specify what constitutes an appropriate level of access to health personnel, medications, tests and procedures, and health technology. They merely indicate that everyone should have access to at least a minimum level of health care.

Trade Agreements, Intellectual Property Rights, and Health

A major rallying point for health activists around the world has been the limited ability of poor countries and poor individuals to buy medications that are essential for saving and prolonging human life. New drugs typically are under patent for a minimum of twenty years. While under patent, no other companies can legally produce the drug, and the lack of competition means that the manufacturer of the drug can charge a high price. Prices only drop after the patent expires, when generic versions of the drug can be produced and sold.

The need for low-cost antiretroviral drugs (ARVs) to combat HIV/AIDS in Africa has been a particular concern. When low-income and middle-income countries (such as South Africa, Thailand, Brazil, and India) have produced or stated their intention to produce their own generic drugs, the United States, on behalf of its pharmaceutical companies, has sued or threatened to sue to keep them from producing low-cost ARVs. The

United States has even stronger opposition when low-income countries without the facilities or technical skill to make their own medicines begin to import generics from other countries that are violating international patent laws.

Drug companies, represented in the United States by the trade group PhRMA, argue that if they are not guaranteed global patents they will have to cut back on the amount of money they spend on the development of new drugs. They say that a balance must be found between the goal of innovation and the goal of access to medicine.[5] They also point out that they have responsibilities to their shareholders to produce profits.[6]

Health activists argue that patent protection leads to higher prices because it eliminates competition and that pharmaceutical companies do not devote enough research to development of new drugs for diseases that primarily affect low-income countries. One example of an organized effort to expand drug access is the Médecins Sans Frontières (Doctors Without Borders) Campaign for Access to Essential Medicines. In addition to lobbying for lower prices and limits on patents, the Campaign is pushing for the development of new diagnostic tests and medicines for common infectious diseases like HIV, TB, and malaria, and what they refer to as "neglected diseases" such as Chagas disease, African sleeping sickness (trypanosomiasis), and leishmaniasis (kala azar). They are also pushing to bring certain abandoned drugs back into production.

Many of the protests have been directed at the World Trade Organization because of its role in inhibiting the ability of low- and middle-income countries to take action to procure or to produce their own cheaper drugs. World Trade Organization (WTO) agreements set the legal ground-rules for international commerce and function as contracts between member countries. Several of the WTO agreements have components that can limit access to health (Table 13-2).

Another United Nations agency, the World Intellectual Property Organization (WIPO), also works to protect intellectual property rights such as patents (for inventions), copyrights (for creative works like books, films, and images), and registered trademarks (for logos, slogans, and brand names). It is also involved in agreements about health-related property rights, such as the duration of drug ownership by the inventor.

Bilateral and multilateral trade agreements between two or more countries may also include clauses that restrict the ability of developing nations to access cheaper drugs. (These are sometimes called "TRIPS Plus" agreements because they require more protections on intellectual property than

Table 13-2. Health Aspects of International Trade Agreements.

Trade Agreement	Health Aspects
General Agreement on Trade in Services (GATS)	Treats human services such as health care, water, sanitation, and education as commodities subject to trade rules. Could also potentially affect safety regulations, handling of hazardous materials, licensing of medical practitioners, and other aspects of health.
General Agreement on Tariffs and Trade (GATT)	Allows for countries to ban certain products to protect public health, but directs more attention to protecting intellectual property rights like drug patents.
Trade-Related Aspects of Intellectual Property Rights (TRIPS)	Protects patents, copyrights, trademarks, and industrial designs across national boundaries and, therefore, limits the production of certain protected medications. Contains safeguards that are supposed to ensure access to essential medications.

TRIPS does.) For example, trade agreements might extend the duration of a patent on pharmaceutical agent and enforce rules that prohibit generic versions of the drug from being produced or imported.

PRIORITIES IN GLOBAL HEALTH

Where is the place to begin when addressing the huge demands of global public health? The Disease Control Priorities Project, a collaboration of the Fogarty International Center of the U.S. National Institutes of Health, the World Bank, the World Health Organization, and the Population Reference Bureau, developed a list of what they see as the developing world's ten most significant health problems (Table 13-3) and constructed a list of priority actions to address them. Note that in addition to the focus on infectious disease prevention and control (2, 4, 5), improved nutrition (3), and maternal and child health (1), this "top ten" list also emphasizes that every country in the world needs to begin preparing to provide health care (9, 10) to a large number of people with cancer (7), disabilities (8), and chronic conditions like heart disease, stroke, and hypertension (6).

Table 13-3. Top 10 Global Health Priorities.

1	Ensure healthier mothers and children.
2	Stop the AIDS pandemic.
3	Promote good nutrition.
4	Stem the tide of tuberculosis.
5	Control malaria.
6	Reduce the toll from cardiovascular disease.
7	Combat tobacco use.
8	Reduce fatal and disabling injuries.
9	Ensure equal access to quality health care.
10	Forge strong, integrated, effective health systems.

Source: Disease Control Priorities Project. Investing in Global Health: 'Best Buys' and Priorities for Action in Developing Countries. April 2006.

Because the top ten priorities are costly and will take time to address, the Disease Control Priorities Project also created a list of the top ten "best buys" in global health (Table 13-4). The "best buys" list is especially helpful because the solutions are very specific. It would be possible, and relatively inexpensive, to implement these steps around the world.

Global health can also be improved by the development of new scientific technologies. The Grand Challenges in Global Health initiative was launched in 2003 by the Bill & Melinda Gates Foundation and is administered with the Foundation for the National Institutes of Health, the Wellcome Trust, and the Canadian Institutes of Health Research. It focuses on creating new and improved vaccines, vector control methods, and therapies (Table 13-5).

Health is more than just access to a doctor and appropriate drugs when sick. It also means having a clean and safe environment that is free of pollutants, landmines, and violence—and having the health knowledge necessary for making good health decisions. Lists of global health priorities might reasonably include much broader goals, such as facilitating the social and economic conditions that lead to good health and promoting environmental protection programs. Other goals could include advocating for community water rights, supporting female literacy programs, promoting prevention and screening for early detection of disease, and developing detection systems for disease outbreaks.

Table 13-4. Top 10 "Best Buys" in Global Health.

	Target	Action
1	Child Health	Vaccinate children against major childhood killers, including measles, polio, tetanus, whooping cough, and diphtheria.
2	Child Health	Monitor children's health to prevent or, if necessary, treat childhood pneumonia, diarrhea, and malaria.
3	Tobacco Use	Tax tobacco products to increase consumers' costs by at least one-third to curb smoking and reduce the prevalence of cardiovascular disease, cancer, and respiratory disease.
4	HIV/AIDS	Attack the spread of HIV through a coordinated approach that includes: promoting 100 percent condom use among populations at high risk; treating other sexually transmitted infections; providing antiretroviral medications, especially for pregnant women; and offering voluntary HIV counseling and testing.
5	Maternal and Child Health	Give children and pregnant women essential nutrients, including vitamin A, iron, and iodine, to prevent maternal anemia, infant deaths, and long-term health problems.
6	Malaria	Provide insecticide-treated bednets in malaria-endemic areas to drastically reduce malaria.
7	Injury Prevention	Enforce traffic regulations and install speed bumps at dangerous intersections to reduce traffic-related injuries.
8	TB	Treat TB patients with short-course chemotherapy to cure infected people and prevent new infections.
9	Child Health	Teach mothers and train birth attendants to keep newborns warm and clean to reduce illness and death.
10	Cardiovascular Disease	Promote use of aspirin and other inexpensive drugs to treat and prevent heart attack and stroke.

Source: Disease Control Priorities Project. Investing in Global Health: 'Best Buys' and Priorities for Action in Developing Countries. April 2006.

Table 13-5. Grand Challenges in Global Health.

Improve childhood vaccines	1	Create effective single-dose vaccines
	2	Prepare vaccines that do not require refrigeration
	3	Develop needle-free vaccine delivery systems
Create new vaccines	4	Devise testing systems for new vaccines
	5	Design antigens for protective immunity
	6	Learn about immunological responses
Control insects that transmit agents of disease	7	Develop genetic strategy to control insects
	8	Develop chemical strategy to control insects
Improve nutrition to promote health	9	Create a nutrient-rich staple plant species
Improve drug treatment of infectious diseases	10	Find drugs and delivery systems to limit drug resistance
Cure latent and chronic infection	11	Create therapies that can cure latent infection
	12	Create immunological methods to cure latent infection
Measure health status accurately and economically in developing countries	13	Develop technologies to assess population health
	14	Develop versatile diagnostic tools

Source: Grand Challenges in Global Health (http://www.grandchallengesgh.org).

Millennium Development Goals

The **Millennium Development Goals (MDGs)** adopted by the United Nations in 2000, are eight major goals for reducing global poverty that could, under ideal circumstances, be accomplished by 2015 (Table 13-6). Three MDGs are directly related to health.

- Goal 4: Reduce child mortality.
- Goal 5: Improve maternal health.
- Goal 6: Combat HIV/AIDS, malaria, and other diseases.

Table 13-6. Millennium Development Goals.

1	Eradicate extreme poverty and hunger.
2	Achieve universal primary education.
3	Promote gender equality and empower women.
4	Reduce child mortality.
5	Improve maternal health.
6	Combat HIV/AIDS, malaria, and other diseases.
7	Ensure environmental sustainability.
8	Develop a global partnership for development.

The full list of MDG goals, targets, and indicators are in Appendix V, and a list of preventive and treatment interventions that could help accomplish these goals is in Appendix VI. Eighteen targets (benchmarks that indicate progress toward reaching the goals) accompany the goals. For example, a target associated with Goal 5 is to "reduce by two-thirds the mortality rate among children under five." There are also 48 specific indicators that are used to assess whether the targets are being reached. Indicators for Goal 5 include the maternal mortality ratio and the proportion of births attended by skilled health personnel. All the UN agencies are now collecting data on the indicators relevant to their work and are implementing programs that will support reaching the targets. Table 13-7 shows several health-related MDG indicators for selected countries in different parts of the world.

One of the main reasons the MDGs have been so influential is that they provide a clear strategy for evaluation. Progress on each of the 48 indicators is collected from each country on an annual basis so the status of each target can be tracked and countries can determine what progress they have made toward reaching their goals. The assessment data allows donors to conduct cost-benefit analyses that determine whether a program is being efficient (making good use of its resources) and effective (reaching the desired outcomes).

Some people are concerned that assessment puts too much emphasis on quick results and too little emphasis on creating socially, economically, and environmentally sustainable development. **Sustainability** aims to provide for current human needs without compromising the ability of future generations to meet their needs. For example, a program that depletes natural resources and promotes over-consumption is not sustainable, nor is a program that is fully dependent on outside donors and that does not involve recipients in decision-making.

Table 13-7. MDG Indicators in 2000 for Selected Countries.

Country		USA	Mexico	Thailand	Botswana	India	Sierra Leone
15% of Under-5 children underweight for age		1.4%	7.5%	17.6%	12.5%	46.7%	27.2%
Under-5 mortality rate (per 1000 live births)		9	29	31	93	96	316
1-year-olds immunized against measles		91%	95%	94%	90%	56%	53%
Maternal mortality ratio (per 100,000 live births)		14	83	44	100	540	2000
Births attended by skilled health professional		99%	85.7%	85%	98.5%	42.3%	41.7%
HIV prevalence among 15 to 49-year-olds		0.6%	0.2%	1.9%	37.5%	0.8%	2.0%
Malaria-related mortality rates (per 100,000)		0	0	7	8	3	321
Tuberculosis prevalence (per 100,000)		4	49	225	288	431	573
Tuberculosis mortality rate (per 100,000)		0	4	18	28	41	63
Population using solid fuels		<5%	76%	72%	65%	81%	92%
Sustainable access to an improved water source	Urban	100%	95%	95%	100%	95%	75%
	Rural	100%	69%	81%	90%	79%	46%
Access to improved sanitation	Urban	100%	88%	96%	88%	61%	88%
	Rural	100%	34%	96%	43%	15%	53%

Data Source: World Health Report 2004.

HOW MUCH WILL IT COST?

When we consider the cost of finding solutions to global health crises, a first question to ask is how much it would cost to do nothing. Bill and Melinda Gates have put the loss of human life and human productivity due to disease into economic terms:

> We believe health is the cornerstone of human development. When health takes hold, life improves by all measures. Conversely, poor health aggravates poverty, poverty deepens disease, and nations trapped in this spiral will not escape without the world's help. In Africa, the cost of malaria in terms of treatment and lost productivity is estimated to be $12 billion a year. The continent's gross domestic product could be $100 billion higher today if malaria had been eliminated in the 1960s. And if HIV infection rates continue at their present levels, the world will likely see 45 million new infections by 2010 and lose nearly 70 million people by 2020. That's 70 million of the most productive members of society—health workers, educators, and parents.[7]

Continued disparities in health between countries and within countries can also contribute to violence and instability.

So how much will it cost (in U.S. dollars)? Former World Bank President James Wolfensohn estimated in 2002 that "it will take on the order of an additional $40 to $60 billion a year to reach the Millennium Development Goals—roughly a doubling of current flows—to roughly 0.5 percent of GNP, still well below the 0.7 target agreed to by global leaders years ago."[8] UNICEF estimates that it will cost about $63 billion to achieve the water targets and $29 billion to achieve the sanitation targets over ten years (2005–2015).[9] Implementing the Global Plan to Stop TB, which aims to reverse the rise in TB incidence by 2015 and to cut in half the prevalence and death rates globally in all regions except Africa and Eastern Europe, would probably cost about $56 billion over ten years (2006–2015).[10] The Medicines for Malaria Venture (MMV) estimates that it will cost about $150 million to develop one new anti-malarial drug.[11] None of these estimates is so expensive that it would be impossible to raise the needed amount. As a comparison, in 2005 the United States produced chocolate and other candies worth more than $20 billion, soft drinks worth more than $40 billion, and tobacco products worth more than $40 billion.[12]

Another challenge is to find **cost-effective** solutions and to determine which interventions create the greatest good for the greatest number of people at the lowest cost. One way to calculate cost-effectiveness is to compare the cost of an intervention with the resulting increase in years of healthy life. Table 13-8 shows some of the ways that $1 million could be used to drastically improve health and survival for large numbers of people. The center column on the table shows the estimated cost to prevent one disability-adjusted life year (DALY) from being lost. A large number of DALYs averted indicates a highly cost-effective intervention.

Some of the most cost-effective interventions are hygiene promotion for the prevention of diarrheal diseases, preventive treatment of malaria in pregnant women in endemic areas, and childhood immunizations against measles, polio, and tetanus. These are cheap interventions that can be easily distributed to many people and can avert many years of life lost to premature death because they target infants and children. Some of the least cost-effective interventions are high technology solutions, such as coronary artery bypass surgery for treatment of heart disease, which costs more than $10,000 per patient.

There are, however, times when we need to think beyond cost-effectiveness. For example, vaccine programs, if successful, are extremely cost-effective, but there is a chance of failure and the up-front cost of research and development is extremely high. Some funding agencies and research organizations need to be willing to risk failure so that they can work toward achieving these important health goals. Also, sometimes the moral necessity to act outweighs concerns about sustainability and payment plans. Paul Farmer, for example, has created several very successful health programs in resource-poor areas: "The experience of my own group suggests that ambitious goals can be met even without a large springboard . . . We didn't argue that it was 'cost-effective,' nor did we promise that such efforts would be replicable. We argued that it was the right thing to do."[13]

The cycle of disease and poverty can only be broken when health technologies are made available to the poor, which might mean offering them at low or no cost. In some cases the technology that would cure or prevent disease, such as a vaccine against HIV, does not yet exist. But in many cases the technologies are available, proven to be effective, and relatively affordable. For example, hundreds of thousands of the children who died from malaria this year could have been saved if they had slept under mosquito nets that cost less than $5 each, and tens of thousands of cases of blindness caused by vitamin A deficiency could have been prevented by a few

Table 13-8. How Much Health Can $1,000,000 Buy?

Service or Intervention	Cost per DALY (US$)	Estimated number of DALYs averted per $1,000,000 spent
Reducing under-five mortality		
Improving care of children under 28 days old (including resuscitation of newborns)	10–400	2,500–100,000
Expanding immunization coverage with standard child vaccines	2–20	50,000–500,000
Adding Hib and Hepatitis B vaccines to the standard child immunization program	40–250	4,000–24,000
Switching to the use of combination drugs for malaria where there is drug resistance in sub-Saharan Africa	8–20	50,000–125,000
Preventing and treating HIV/AIDS		
Preventing mother-to-child transmission	50–200	5,000–20,000
Treating STIs to interrupt HIV transmission	10–100	10,000–100,000
Using ARV that achieves high adherence for a large % of patients	350–500	2,000–3,000
Preventing and treating non-communicable disease		
Taxing tobacco products	3–50	24,000–330,000
Treating acute heart attacks with an inexpensive set of drugs	10–25	40,000–100,000
Treating heart attack and stroke survivors with a daily combination drug	700–1000	1000–1400

Data Source: Table 1.3 from Jamison DT. Chapter 1: Investing in Health. In: Jamison DT, Breman JG, Measham AR, et al, eds. Disease Control Priorities in Developing Countries, 2nd edition. Washington, DC: Oxford University Press, 2006, p. 25.

doses of a vitamin A capsule that costs only a few cents. For households these costs may be prohibitive, but the biggest barrier to saving lives in these cases is not cost but the lack of collective will to see that the technologies are distributed to the people who need them most.

It is not impossible to address global health inequities. Bill Gates, for one, is certain that we can work together to make a significant difference:

> I am optimistic that in the next decade, people's thinking will evolve on the question of health inequity. People will finally accept that the death of a child in the developing world is just as tragic as the death of a child in the developed world. And the expanding capacities of science will give us the power to act on that conviction. When we do, we have a chance to make sure that all people, no matter what country they live in, will have the preventive care, vaccines, and treatments they need to live a healthy life. I believe we can do this—and if we do, it will be the best thing humanity has ever done.[14]

REFERENCES

1. Farmer P. Pathologies of Power: Health, Human Rights, and the New War on the Poor. Berkeley, CA: University of California Press, 2003.
2. Paul Farmer in an interview with Patricia Cohen for The New York Times, 29 March 2003. The text of interviews with Dr. Farmer are available from Partners in Health.
3. World Health Organization. "Twenty-five Questions & Answers on Health & Human Rights," Health and Human Rights Publication Series, Issue No. 1, July 2002.
4. These evaluation criteria were approved by the UN Committee on Economic, Social and Cultural Rights in May 2000. World Health Organization, "Twenty-five Questions & Answers on Health & Human Rights," Health and Human Rights Publication Series, Issue No. 1, July 2002.
5. Writing in the Financial Times on January 4, 2006, the chairman and CEO of Abbott Laboratories, Miles White, said in an article entitled "Drug Patents Are Good For Our Health": "The problem is that our global needs and global systems are in conflict. This threatens to harm one goal, innovation, in the name of another, access to medicine. Access is the goal the world cares about and one taken seriously by innovator companies (those that conduct research and development of new medicine) that have made significant contributions to this end across the developing world . . . But it must be recognized that access is inseparable from innovation: without access, innovation is meaningless; without innovation, there is nothing to have access to."
6. Miles White, CEO of Abbott Laboratories, went on to say in the Financial Times op-ed piece that: "Today, creating a single new medication costs, on average, about $1 billion.

That massive funding comes from one source alone: private investors. Without a promise of return on that investment—the 'fuel of interest'—that funding will go elsewhere, to opportunities that are less vital and less risky." One solution to this claim is to support private non-profit pharmaceutical research and development firms.

7. Gates B, Gates M. available at: http://www.gatesfoundation.com/AboutUs/Our Values/GatesLetter.htm. accessed June 27, 2006.

8. Wolfensohn JD, "A Partnership for Development and Peace." Address at the Woodrow Wilson International Center on March 6, 2002. Washington DC. Wolfensohn followed the estimate with a comment asking "Does anybody really believe that the goal of halving absolute poverty by 2015 is not worth this investment?"

9. Lenton R, Wright AM, Lewis K, and the UN Millennium Project Task Force on Water and Sanitation. "Health, dignity, and development: what will it take?" Sterling, VA: United Nations Development Programme, 2005.

10. World Health Organization, Global Tuberculosis Control: Surveillance, Planning, Financing. WHO Report. Geneva, Switzerland: WHO, 2006.

11. Medicines for Malaria Venture, "How cost effective is MMV?" http://www.mmv.org/article.php3?id_article=131. Accessed 8 May 2007.

12. US Bureau of the Census. *Statistics for Industry Groups and Industries: 2005*. Annual Survey of Manufactures. Washington, DC: US Bureau of the Census, 2006.

13. Farmer P. Pathologies of Power: Rethinking Health and Human Rights. American Journal of Public Health 1999;89:1486–1496.

14. Gates B, Address to the 2005 World Health Assembly on May 16, 2005. Geneva, Switzerland.

CHAPTER 14

Learning More about Global Public Health

Key Points:
- The WHO, CDC, and other organizations provide global health information on their websites.
- Abstracts from original research articles provide detailed information about health research.
- Epidemiological studies assess the association between exposures and health outcomes.
- Health research is supervised by ethics committees.

If you want to learn more about global public health, an essential first step is to understand research documents. This chapter provides an introduction to the available resources and a guide to reading and understanding them.

INFORMATION SOURCES

There are several key sources for public health information. Two of the best sources are the World Health Organization (WHO) and the U.S. Centers for Disease Control and Prevention (CDC), which compile health information from around the world and regularly update the information presented on their websites. The various offices within the World Health Organization publish online versions of easy-to-read fact sheets and reports on global health issues ranging from aging to zoonoses. The CDC also has fact sheets about infectious diseases (often under the "travelers" tab) and other global issues like nutrition. (Quick access to the WHO, CDC, and other global health websites can be found on the website for this book.)

Most United Nations agencies put out annual updates like the World Health Report and Human Development Report that include health and development indicators for member nations and that often focus on a particular

Table 14-1. Selected Annual Publications with Global Public Health Information.

Report	Source
Human Development Report	United Nations Development Programme (UNDP)
State of World Population	UNFPA
State of the World's Children	UNICEF
World Development Report	World Bank
World Health Report	World Health Organization (WHO)

theme (Table 14-1). These reports provide a wealth of practical information and statistics about health concerns.

The U.S. National Institutes of Health and the CDC have online fact sheets, health glossaries, and image databanks. Several commercial websites also provide access to information about disease symptoms, diagnostic techniques, and treatments. In addition to using these reports to find public health information and statistics, you may find that they help you to understand and make better decisions about your own health. You might be surprised to find some of the misconceptions you may have about health. For example, a survey of women living in the United States conducted by the American Heart Association in 2003 found that although 46% of respondents correctly identified heart disease as the leading cause of death in women (up from 30% in 1997 and 34% in 2000), most women (51%) identified cancer as the health risk they were most concerned about for themselves.[1] Perceived risks do not always match up to actual risks.

Fact sheets, annual reports from UN agencies, news stories, and other summaries of research findings are called **secondary sources** because they provide "second-hand" information about a topic. The best place to find detailed information is by reading **primary sources**—original research reports that provide details about the research methods and results—in scientific and medical journals. Much of the scientific research that informs global public health is available online, and you may find it helpful to be able to understand, to interpret, and to critique these studies on your own.

PubMed is an online abstract database that allows users to read a one-paragraph summary of the methods, results, and discussion points from nearly all published journal articles that relate to medicine and public health. (PubMed is maintained by the National Library of Medicine and can be accessed from their website.) The articles from journals indexed in PubMed are all peer-reviewed, which means that before the paper was published the manuscript was sent to other experts in the field who scrutinized the methodology and reviewed the results to make sure they seem reasonable.

Reading an Abstract

Most abstracts provide several key pieces of information about the study that was conducted (Table 14-2). The first step is to identify: (1) the study population, (2) key exposures (often identified as risk factors or protective factors), and (3) the health outcome. This information is often in the title of the article. Ideally, the exposures and outcomes are based on measurements or laboratory testing. The results of interviews that ask people to recall events from the distant past or to comment on their feelings are less reliable than quantitative data. You should then find (4) the association between the exposure and outcome. Is the exposure associated with an increase or decrease in the disease outcome, or is there no association? Finally, find (5) the sample size. When it comes to the number of people participating in a study, bigger is always better. The results of a study that included only 15 or even 50 participants may be unreliable, but the results of a well designed study that included hundreds or even thousands of participants is likely to be fairly accurate and worth consideration by policy makers.

These five key pieces of information are also useful for interpreting news reports. The most common error in news reports is a failure to adequately describe the study population. The conclusions of a study that included only

Table 14-2. 5 Key Pieces of Information from an Abstract.

1	Study Population	Which people were studied? Note the distribution of age, sex, nationality, and other characteristics and remember that the conclusions of the study apply only to similar populations.
2	Exposure(s)	What were the exposures of interest? How were they measured?
3	Outcome(s)	What were the health outcomes of interest? How were they measured?
4	Association	Was the exposure a risk factor for disease, protective against disease, or did it have no association with the health outcome? Was the association strong?
5	Sample size	How many people participated in the study? A larger study will yield more accurate results.

male participants between 20 and 24 years of age should not be applied to women aged 80 to 89 and may not be generalizable to any other group. The conclusions of a study of women living in California probably do not apply to women living in Malawi. The conclusions of a study of non-smokers should not be applied to smokers. Results from tests done in rats do not apply to humans. Even health experts can become confused when they fail to keep in mind the particular groups that participate in a health study. In recent years there has been considerable confusion about the results of studies of the risks and benefits of hormone replacement therapy for peri-menopausal and post-menopausal women. Much of the confusion was due to muddled re-porting about the particular population groups at risk. Women in the study had been grouped by age, health history, and types of hormone pills taken, and the risks and benefits should have been reported as specific to these groups.

Finding Reliable Articles

Several characteristics of a good public health or medical report are listed in Table 14-3. A good article is peer-reviewed, has a large sample size, has a clearly defined population and an appropriate study design, explains its methodology, presents its results clearly, discusses its limitations and its re-lationship to previously published reports, draws reasonable conclusions, and follows ethical research practices.

Clinicians often use a systematic review process called **Evidence-Based Medicine (EBM)** to help them make patient-care decisions. After formulating a specific question related to patient care, the clinician searches the published literature to find information about the best current medical practices for a patient's specific condition. After considering which studies are valid, use the best methodology, and are the most applicable to the patient, the patient is treated and the outcomes evaluated. (Some people fear that EBM is used to limit patient access to new or expensive therapies, but the goal of EBM is to use facts rather than anecdotes or ideology to make clinical decisions.)

When you read a medical or public health article, be sure that you pay close attention to the population studied and the exact exposures and out-comes that were measured and analyzed. You should also keep in mind that it is rare for a "null results" study, one that does not find a significant as-sociation between the main exposure and outcome, to be published even if the study was designed well and conducted meticulously. As a result, if ten studies are conducted looking at a particular exposure (like living near

Table 14-3. Characteristics of Good Public Health and Medical Research Reports.

Good Report	*Poor Report*
• Peer-reviewed and published in a respected journal.	• Posted on a personal web site or printed in a newspaper or popular magazine.
• Large sample size.	• Only a few participants.
• The population studied is clearly defined and there are no obvious sources of bias.	• Few details about the population studied are given.
• Uses an epidemiological study design and has a control group if one is appropriate.	• Presents anecdotes of interactions with a few people who are ill or there are obvious flaws in the study design.
• The methods used to measure exposures and health outcomes are stated in detail and interventions are fully explained.	• Little information is given about interventions or the methods used to assess exposures and health outcomes.
• The study is conducted with humans.	• The experiment is conducted in a laboratory, on animals, or using a computer simulation.
• The results are statistically analyzed and presented using easy-to-read charts, graphs, and tables.	• Sound statistical practices are not followed and the results are not presented clearly.
• The results are reproducible.	• Other studies cannot repeat the findings of the original report.
• The limitations of the study are discussed.	• No limitations are mentioned in the report.
• The relationship of the study to previous studies is discussed and other articles are cited.	• The study is not compared to any other reports and there is no reference list or bibliography.
• The conclusions seem reasonable given the data.	• The conclusions do not logically follow from the data.
• The article is well written and follows a logical outline (usually Introduction, Methods, Results, Discussion).	• The article has grammatical and spelling errors and does not follow a sensible outline.
• The article states that the study was approved and overseen by an institutional review board (IRB) and there are no obvious conflicts of interest.	• There is no clear statement of ethical oversight by an IRB or there are obvious conflicts of interest (such as research on the benefits of a drug being sponsored by its manufacturer).

electric power lines) and a bad outcome (like brain cancer), the nine studies that find no association may not be published but the one study that
finds some level of statistical significance might be. Studies with findings
contrary to current medical and scientific beliefs are also less likely to be
published.

When a new medical report gets a lot of media hype, it may be wise to
wait for a second or third study to confirm the findings before making
changes in your lifestyle or medications. Good articles will always discuss
the limitations of their methodology and the relationship of their findings
to previously published studies. If the article finds new and unexpected results, attempts to explain these findings should be plausible and biologically
reasonable.

EPIDEMIOLOGIC STUDY DESIGNS

There are many different kinds of health research, each with a different
purpose and methodology. Some are designed to assess population health
status, to determine risk factors for disease, to test the effectiveness of interventions, or to find other health information. This section describes some
of the most common study types: ecological surveys, cross-sectional surveys, case-control studies, cohort studies, and clinical trials (Table 14-4).

Ecological Surveys

An **ecological survey** uses numeric data about a particular exposure and
a particular health outcome from several populations to look for trends
(Figure 14-1). The results of ecological surveys are often displayed using
a scatterplot. For each population, a point is placed on the graph by using
the value for the exposure as the x-coordinate and the value for the outcome as the y-coordinate.

After all the points are plotted, a line that represents the best fit to the
points is added to the graph to look at the **correlation** between the exposure and the outcome. The value of the correlation coefficient, r, which is
often reported as r^2, measures how well the line predicts the location of the
points (Figure 14-2). An r^2 of 0 is extremely weak and means that the line
has no predictive value. An r^2 of 1 means that all the points fall exactly on a
line and if you know the exposure level you can predict with high certainty of

Table 14-4. Epidemiologic Study Designs.

Study Design	How It Works	When It Is Used	Example
Ecological survey	Information about both the average level of exposure and the incidence or prevalence of disease are collected from several populations and plotted to look for trends.	Used when no individual data is available or when studying environmental characteristics (such as air quality and temperature) that affect an entire population.	Is the average number of days of rain in a city in one year (exposure) associated with an increase in clinical depression (outcome)?
Cross-sectional (prevalence) survey	Individuals in a population are asked a series of questions.	Used to quickly determine the prevalence of an exposure or outcome in a population.	What percent of teenagers who live in Bangkok use tobacco products?
Case-control study	Individuals with a particular disease and individuals without the disease are both asked about their exposure histories so that potential risk factors for the disease can be identified.	Used to study relatively uncommon diseases or to study multiple exposures that could be related to one health outcome.	How do the exposure histories of people with leprosy differ from people without leprosy in Andhra Pradesh, India? What are likely risk factors for leprosy in that region of India?
Cohort study	A large group of individuals is followed through time and disease incidence is measured. The incidence in individuals with a particular exposure may be compared to disease incidence in individuals without the exposure.	Used to study the time to disease incidence, to study relatively uncommon exposures, or to study multiple health outcomes related to one exposure.	Out of every 100,000 Bolivian women without breast cancer, how many will likely develop breast cancer in a ten-year period? Do Nigerian men who work with benzene have a higher incidence rate of leukemia than Nigerian men who do not work with benzene?
Clinical trial	Study participants are randomly assigned to receive a new intervention (such as a medication) or a placebo (such as a sugar pill) and their response to the therapy is measured.	Used to test the effectiveness of new interventions (preventive or therapeutic) by comparing them to existing treatment options.	Do children who sleep under insecticide-treated bednets have a lower incidence of malaria than children who sleep under bed-nets that have not been treated with insecticide?

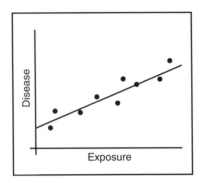

Figure 14-1. Ecological Survey.

Population data about a particular exposure and a particular disease are collected from many populations and plotted to look for a trend.

the outcome. An r^2 of 0.404 or 0.269 would be a moderately strong correlation. The slope of the line shows the direction of association. A positive slope (one that goes up from left to right), which is indicated by a positive value for r, means that an increase in the exposure is associated with an increase in the outcome. A negative slope, indicated by a negative value for r, means that an increase in exposure is associated with a decrease in the outcome.

Ecological surveys do not prove that there is a causal relationship between the exposure and the outcome, only that there is an association. Ecological surveys also do not say anything about the status of individuals within a population. For example, if an ecological survey that showed a strong positive correlation between the number of tanning beds in a town and number of cases of skin cancer diagnosed, that would not prove that the *individuals* who

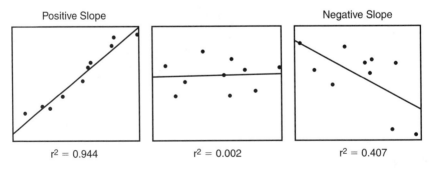

Figure 14-2. Correlation in an Ecological Study.

used tanning beds were the ones who were diagnosed with skin cancer. It would only show that towns with many tanning beds tend to have more people with skin cancer, and it could be possible that none of the individuals who use the tanning beds were among the individuals with cancer. It is called an **ecological fallacy** when incorrect conclusions about individuals are made from population data. Even so, ecological surveys can be a very helpful first step in testing a hypothesis about a possible risk factor for disease.

Cross-Sectional Surveys

A **cross-sectional survey**, also called a **prevalence survey**, can be used to get a "snapshot" of a population's health status at one point in time (Figure 14-3). Cross-sectional surveys are a very useful way to conduct a community assessment, especially when there are time or budget constraints. They are often used for rapid needs assessment during humanitarian crises. For example, public health workers in a refugee camp might use a survey to measure the prevalence of pregnancy among women in the camp or an urban health clinic might use a cross-sectional study design to assess the prevalence of HIV and TB infections in the community they serve.

Cross-sectional surveys divide the study population into groups based on exposure and disease status. For example, a cross-sectional survey measured body size (the exposure) and lung function (the disease outcome) in 1170 young adults in Chile.[2] Breathlessness after exercise was found in 446 of the participants, and the results were reported by exposure status. 36.4% of the normal

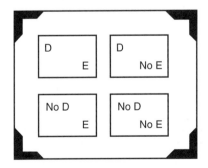

Figure 14-3. Cross-Sectional Survey.

A "snapshot" of the population is taken by measuring both exposure (E) and disease status (D) at the same time.

weight participants, 37.2% of the overweight participants, and 45.1% of the obese participants experienced breathlessness after exercise (Figure 14-4).

The limitation of cross-sectional surveys is that there is no time component to the data because all the questions are asked at the same time. For example, a cross-sectional survey of chewing tobacco use (the exposure) and dental cavities (the disease) among a group of 1000 high school students might find a significantly higher prevalence of cavities among people who use chew, but that would not prove that chew caused cavities nor would it prove that cavities cause people to chew.

Case-Control Studies

Case-control studies recruit people with a disease (**cases**) and similar people who do not have that disease (**controls**) so that their past exposures can be compared (Figure 14-5). After confirming their disease status, all participants provide information about topics like their history of environmental exposures, diet and health practices, and family and health history. Statistical analysis is then used to determine which exposures are most associated with developing the disease outcome.

A simple way to look at the association between an exposure and a disease outcome is to create a 2×2 table that has two rows for exposure status

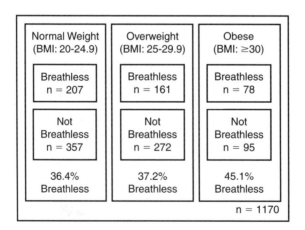

Figure 14-4. Example of a Cross-Sectional Study of Body Size and Breathlessness After Exercising.

Data Source: Bustos P, Amigo H, Oyarzún M, Rona RJ. Is there a causal relation between obesity and asthma? Evidence from Chile. *Int J Obes* 2005;29:804–809.

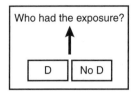

Figure 14-5. Case-Control Study.

People with a disease (cases) and without the disease (controls) are asked about their exposure history.

and two columns for disease status. Each individual in the study population is classified into one of the four groups created by the 2×2 table—exposed and diseased, exposed but not diseased, not exposed but diseased, and not exposed and not diseased. The count of the number of individuals in each of the four groups is tallied and placed in the 2×2 table, and various measures of association can then be calculated from those values.

The typical measure of association between an exposure and an outcome in a case-control study is the odds ratio (Figure 14-6). This is the same type of measurement used in betting. If someone thinks that a horse has a 25%

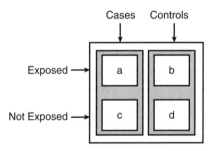

The 2×2 table (named because it has 2 rows and 2 columns) places every individual from a study into one box based on both exposure and disease status. There are four categories—exposed and diseased, exposed but not diseased, not exposed but diseased, and not exposed nor diseased.

The number of participants in each category is represented by *a* (exposed cases), *b* (exposed controls), *c* (unexposed cases), and *d* (unexposed controls). The total number of study participants = $a + b + c + d = N$.

Odds of Exposure for Cases = # of cases exposed / # of cases not exposed = a / c
Odds of Exposure for Controls = # of controls exposed / # of controls not exposed = b / d

$$\text{Odds Ratio (OR)} = \frac{a/c}{b/d} = \frac{ad}{bc}$$

Figure 14-6. Analysis for a Case-Control Study.

chance of winning a race (and a 75% chance of losing), then the odds on the horse are 25:75, which can be simplified to 1:3 or 1/3—one chance of winning compared to 3 chances of losing. The **odds ratio** (OR) compares the odds of a case (a person with a disease) having a history of a particular exposure to the odds of a control (a person without the disease) having been exposed to the potential risk factor. An odds ratio near 1 means that there is probably no association between the disease and the exposure. An odds ratio greater than 1 suggests that people with disease are more likely than people without disease to have a history of the exposure. An odds ratio less than 1 suggests that people with the disease are less likely than people without disease to have a history of the exposure.

For example, a case-control study of stomach cancer in Mumbai, India, studied the association between drinking tea (the exposure) and stomach cancer (the outcome).[3] Of the cases, who all had stomach cancer, 105 had a history of drinking tea daily and 14 had a history of drinking tea rarely or never. Of the controls, who did not have stomach cancer, 1513 had a history of drinking tea daily and 64 had a history of drinking tea rarely or never. The authors used a 2×2 table to calculate an odds ratio of OR = 0.32, which is less than 1, and concluded that drinking tea was protective against stomach cancer (Figure 14-7). The association was even stronger after statistically adjusting for other variables like age and sex. In this study, people with

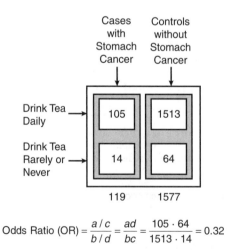

$$\text{Odds Ratio (OR)} = \frac{a/c}{b/d} = \frac{ad}{bc} = \frac{105 \cdot 64}{1513 \cdot 14} = 0.32$$

Figure 14-7. Example of a Case-Control Study of Stomach Cancer and Tea Drinking Habits.

Data Source: Rao DN, Ganesh B, Dinshaw KA, Mohandas KM. A case-control study of stomach cancer in Mumbai, India. *Int J Cancer* 2002;99:727–731.

stomach cancer were much less likely than people without stomach cancer to report a habit of drinking tea daily. This does not necessarily mean that you should start drinking tea daily. Remember that the results of studies only apply to certain populations and that the results of one study should be validated by other studies.

Because participants in a case-control study are selected based on their disease status, this type of study design cannot determine how common a disease is in a population. A different kind of study design—a cohort study—must be used to measure incidence of disease.

Cohort Studies

A **cohort** is a group of similar people, and **cohort studies** recruit a group of similar participants who can be followed through time. At the start of the study period no one enrolled in the study has the disease outcome of interest. The participants are followed, usually for several years or even decades, and researchers track the number of people who develop the disease or disability or die from a particular condition (Figure 14-8). Statistical analysis is then used to compare the rate of disease incidence for people with different exposure histories. The incidence rate is calculated by putting the number of cases diagnosed in the numerator and the total number of people in the exposure group in the denominator. (In some cohort studies, people are enrolled over a period of time rather than all at once at the start of the study. In this case, each participant contributes a certain number of years of observation to the study, and the denominator for the rate calculation would have "person-years" as the unit of measurement. For example, a person enrolled for the full 5 years of a five-year study would contribute 5 person-years and a person who joined 2 years into the five-year study would contribute 3 person-years.)

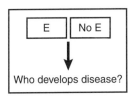

Figure 14-8. Cohort Study.

People with a particular exposure (the exposed cohort) and without that exposure (the unexposed cohort) are followed to see who develops disease.

There are two common measures of association for a cohort study (Figure 14-9), the rate ratio and the attributable risk. The **rate ratio** (also called the **risk ratio** or **relative risk**, or simply shortened to RR) is calculated by dividing the rate of disease incidence in the exposed cohort by the rate in the unexposed cohort. A rate ratio near 1 means that the exposure probably is not associated with the disease. A rate ratio greater than 1 suggests that the exposure is associated with increased risk of disease. A rate ratio less than 1 suggests that the exposure might be protective.

For example, a study in Uganda looked at the effect of domestic violence during pregnancy on the risk of delivering a low birthweight baby. 79 of 169 who reported domestic violence during pregnancy had low birthweight babies and 148 of 443 women who did not report domestic violence gave birth to low birthweight babies.[4] The authors calculated a rate ratio of RR = 1.40, which is greater than 1, and concluded that domestic violence during pregnancy was

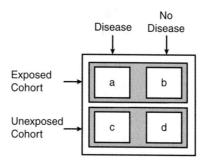

The number of participants in each category is represented by *a* (exposed and developed disease), *b* (exposed and healthy), *c* (unexposed and developed disease), and *d* (unexposed and healthy). The total number of study participants = $a + b + c + d$ = N.

$$\text{Incidence of Disease in Exposed} = \frac{a}{a+b}$$

$$\text{Incidence of Disease in Unexposed} = \frac{c}{c+d}$$

$$\text{Rate Ratio (RR)} = \frac{a/(a+b)}{c/(c+d)}$$

$$\text{Rate Difference} = \text{Attributable Risk} = \frac{a}{a+b} - \frac{c}{c+d}$$

$$\text{Odds of Disease in Exposed} = a/b$$

$$\text{Odds of Disease in Unexposed} = c/d$$

$$\text{Odds Ratio (OR)} = \frac{a/b}{c/d} = \frac{ad}{bc}$$

Figure 14-9. Analysis for a Cohort Study.

a risk factor for giving birth to a low birthweight baby (Figure 14-10). The association was even stronger after statistically adjusting for other variables like age, number of living children, and years of marriage.

The **rate difference** (also known as **excess risk** or **risk difference** or **attributable risk**) subtracts the rate of disease in the unexposed from the rate of disease in the exposed. The amount of risk left over represents the extra cases that developed in the exposed group because of their exposure. This conclusion is based on the assumption that the rate of disease in the unexposed group is the baseline rate for the population. If that is true, then any diseases in the exposed group that are above the baseline rate can be attributed to the extra risk of the exposure (Figure 14-11). For example, the Women's Health Initiative, a 15-year study of postmenopausal women's health sponsored by the National Heart, Lung, and Blood Institute (NHLBI) of the U.S. National Institutes of Health, found that women who took an estrogen plus progestin hormone combination were more likely to develop breast cancer than women taking a placebo. The authors reported that there were eight excess cases of breast cancer every year for every 10,000 women taking a combination hormone. The attributable risk in this study was 8/10,000, which corresponded to a 24% increase in the risk of breast cancer for women who took estrogen plus progestin.[5]

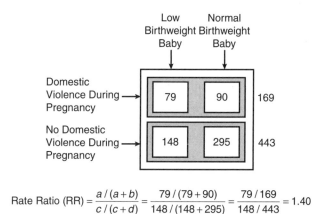

$$\text{Rate Ratio (RR)} = \frac{a/(a+b)}{c/(c+d)} = \frac{79/(79+90)}{148/(148+295)} = \frac{79/169}{148/443} = 1.40$$

Figure 14-10. Example of a Cohort Study of Domestic Violence Against Pregnant Women and Low Birthweight (LBW) Babies.

Data Source: Kaye DK, Mirembe FM, Bantebya G, Johansson A, Ekstrom AM. Domestic violence during pregnancy and risk of low birthweight and maternal complications: a prospective cohort study at Mulago Hospital, Uganda. *Trop Med Int Health* 2006;11: 1576–1584.

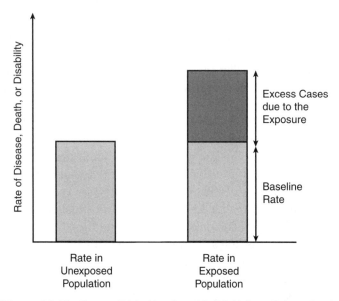

Figure 14-11. Excess Risk (Attributable Risk) in a Cohort Study.

Cohort studies are often used in occupational health research because it is relatively easy to establish exposed and unexposed cohorts. For example, a study of the health effect of benzene could compare workers at a plant that produces or uses benzene to workers at a plant that has never had benzene on the premises. Cohort studies are particularly useful for studying rare exposures.

A few cohort studies have followed whole communities over time. One of the most famous cohort studies is the Framingham Heart Study, which has followed the residents of one town in Massachusetts for more than 50 years. The Framingham study has identified many of the key risk factors for cardiovascular disease: high blood pressure, high blood cholesterol, smoking, obesity, diabetes, and physical inactivity. Because people who have the disease at the start of the study period are not eligible to participate in a cohort study, cohort studies can be used to determine the incidence rate (rate of new cases) of disease in a particular population.

Clinical Trials

Clinical trials are similar to cohort studies, except that the exposure is assigned by the researchers (Figure 14-12). **Randomized trials** (or randomized controlled trials) use a random process to allocate some participants to the new

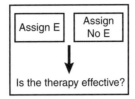

Figure 14-12. Clinical Trial.
Participants are either assigned to an exposure group or a control group and outcomes related to the exposure are assessed.

therapy and some to a comparison therapy like a placebo (pill with no active
ingredient) or the drug regimen that is considered to be the current "standard
of care." (For example, a study of a new analgesic would not be compared to
a sugar pill but to an existing drug known to be at least somewhat effective
in treating the type of pain the new pill is supposed to alleviate.)

Most clinical trials are also **double-blind**, which means that neither the
patient nor the doctor assessing the participant's health outcomes know
whether the participant is receiving the trial drug or a placebo. That way neither the participants nor the examiners will be tempted, even subcon-
sciously, to find a better outcome in a patient who they know is taking the
new drug. Researchers then measure the safety and **efficacy** of the therapy,
which is the ability of the therapy to produce the desired effect. The efficacy
is calculated by determining the difference in the rate of disease, death, or
disability between the placebo group and the intervention group and then
dividing by the rate in the placebo group.

$$Efficacy = \frac{(Rate\ in\ the\ placebo\ group) - (Rate\ in\ the\ intervention\ group)}{(Rate\ in\ the\ placebo\ group)}$$

Clinical trials are most commonly used to study new pharmaceutical agents
or medical products. Pharmaceutical clinical trials undergo several stages of
testing. In Phase I, a small group of human volunteers take the drug and are
observed to be sure that there is no toxicity. Phase II trials are conducted in larger
groups and test efficacy while continuing to look for toxicity. Phase III is a large
double-blind randomized controlled trial which tests how well the new drug
works in comparison to currently available alternatives. In Phase IV the drug
is available to the public but reports of negative side effects are monitored.

Clinical trials are considered to be the "best" epidemiologic study design,
the "gold standard," because similar people can be randomly assigned to an

intervention. However, it is not always possible or ethical to do this kind of study. In some cases, there is no reasonable comparison therapy to which people can be assigned. In other cases it is not ethical to continue a study when preliminary results indicate that one of the therapies being used, either the trial therapy or the control, could be harmful. For example, the Women's Health Initiative (WHI) study stopped a study of a particular type of hormone replacement therapy (HRT) when analysis of data collected in the early stages of the study showed a marked increase in risk of breast cancer, heart disease, blood clots, and stroke.[6]

RESEARCH ETHICS

Clinical trials and nearly all other types of epidemiological studies are supervised by ethics committees, commonly called **Institutional Review Boards** or IRBs. IRBs will not approve studies that do not meet the four main ethical considerations in medical and public health research: beneficence, respect for autonomy, nonmaleficence, and distributive justice.

Beneficence means that the study should be good ("beneficial") for the individual participants and for society-at-large. Researchers need to be able to explain why their research projects are important and how they will contribute to the common good. For example, IRB applications often require applicants to clearly state how collecting population data or conducting an intervention trial will be beneficial. Beneficence is a goal of all public health practice. Public health practitioners seek to maximize the benefit to both individuals and society, and the principle of beneficence supports choosing the option that does the greatest good for the greatest number of people. (Sometimes these decisions are ethically difficult, as when what is good for an individual, such as doctor-patient confidentiality, is not good for society. For example, when a person has a highly contagious disease and wants to forgo treatment it might be more important to respect the public's right to safety than the individual's right to privacy.)

Respect for autonomy means respecting the ability of all individuals to make decisions about themselves for themselves. It is the opposite of paternalism. All research participants must be informed about the risks and benefits of participation in a study and must give their **informed consent** before participating. Respect for autonomy means that even though, for example, parents are the legal decision-makers for their children and have the final say over whether children will be enrolled in a clinical trial, the project will be explained to children in a way they can understand and the concerns of the children will be addressed. No participant should feel pressured to participate in a study because of coercion or intimidation, and all people who choose to participate in a study need to know that they can choose to drop out of the study at any time with no penalty.

Nonmaleficence (literally "non-badness") means that the study does not cause harm. This means, for example, that any drug being used in a clinical trial, whether it is an active drug or a placebo, needs to have been adequately tested before it is administered to humans. Even if a researcher does not intend to cause harm, the researcher and sponsoring institution can be found negligent if any negative outcomes occur during the course of their study.

Distributive justice requires that the benefits and risks of research should be equally distributed among people. For example, this means that the population in which a new drug or therapy is tested should be a population that will be able to afford the drug once it is approved and marketed.

An IRB will not give approval for studies that it deems to be potentially dangerous, poorly planned, or unnecessarily targeting members of a special population. Researchers who wish to study people from vulnerable population groups, such as children, pregnant women, people with developmental disabilities, and prisoners, must demonstrate that it is necessary to conduct the research in these populations, that study participants will be able to understand the risks and benefits of participation, and that no one will feel pressured to participate. (An example of pressure to participate is when prisoners think that participation in a research study will yield special benefits even if the informed consent statement states that no rewards will be given for participation.)

For all approved research projects, the researchers must inform the IRB of the steps they will take to guarantee that they will be able to maintain the privacy and confidentiality of health data and other personally-identifiable information. After approval, the IRB monitors on-going studies to be sure that the approved protocols are followed. Any changes to the protocol and all adverse events must be immediately reported to the IRB.

The rules for studying vulnerable populations also apply to international research. International research must be approved by both the IRB from the researcher's institution and the appropriate IRBs in the country where the research will be conducted. An IRB may require that certain conditions be met before a study is approved. For example, an IRB may require that the researchers provide participants with health care beyond the standard available in their home communities, that free medical exams and treatment be provided, and that informed consent be obtained both orally and in writing.

Recent debates about the ethics of international research have focused on how to guarantee that the benefits of research are available to members of the communities where studies are conducted and on what constitutes fair compensation for research participants. While there have been some concerns expressed about exploitation of research subjects in low-income countries (including those raised by the movie *The Constant Gardener*, a fictional story about abuses by a drug company testing a new TB drug in Kenya), most international research is conducted by researchers who do their best to meet or exceed the standards of medical ethics.

INTERPRETING MEASURES OF ASSOCIATION

Epidemiologic reports often list both an estimate of the relative risk (RR) or other statistic and a **95% confidence interval (CI)** for the estimate. The only way to truly know a risk in a population is to collect data from every individual, but this is rarely able to be accomplished because of time and money constraints. Instead, statistical methods are used to make an estimate of the true value of a parameter in a population from a small sample of the population. While a sample of a small proportion of the population might not give the exact value of the relative risk in the population, it does provide an estimate (Figure 14-13).

The 95% confidence interval indicates how certain a researcher is about a particular estimate. A range of possible values for the true population

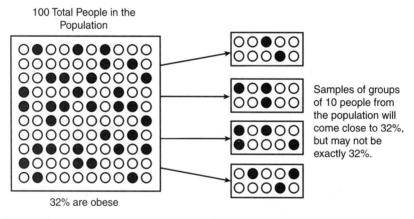

Figure 14-13. Sampling from a Population.

parameter (the value that would be found if every individual was studied instead of just a sample drawn from the larger population) is calculated using methods that capture the true parameter 95% of the time. If thousands of different samples of the same number of people were drawn from the population, each capturing a slightly different set of participants, we would expect 95% of the resulting confidence intervals for the risk ratio to include the true parameter.

Say a reported risk ratio is RR = 1.28 [1.13, 1.44]. In this example, 1.28 is the value of the rate ratio calculated from the sample data, and the 95% confidence interval range is from 1.13 to 1.44. This means that we are 95% confident that the true risk ratio is between 1.13 and 1.44. Because this range does not include the number 1, this is fairly strong evidence that the exposure being analyzed is a risk factor for the disease being studied. If a confidence interval for a risk ratio or odds ratio is less than 1, like RR = 0.65 [0.61, 0.69], then there is evidence that the risk factor is protective. If the number 1 falls within the given 95% confidence interval, like RR = 1.03 [0.89, 1.17], then there is not strong evidence that the exposure is risky or that it is protective. These 95% confidence intervals are graphically displayed in Figure 14-14.

As sample size increases (and a higher percent of the total population is included in the study) the confidence interval will get narrower (a smaller difference between the lower estimate and the higher estimate) because researchers will be closer to finding the true value of the parameter. Statistical **power** is the ability to detect a difference between two groups when they really are different. Increasing sample size is the easiest way to improve the power of a test because larger numbers of participants make it possible to identify very small differences in means, proportions, risks, and other measures.

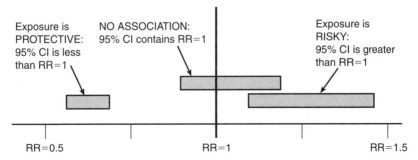

Figure 14-14. Interpreting 95% Confidence Intervals.

Some studies report **p-values** (probability values) for their statistics, especially when a statistical test has been conducted, such as a t-test for comparing the means (averages) of two populations or a chi-squared (χ^2) test for comparing the distribution of responses in different populations. The p-value gives the estimated probability that, given the number of people in the sample, an even bigger difference between the two groups than the one calculated from the sample would be found by chance even if there really was no difference at all between the groups. A small p-value (usually less than .05, or 5%) means that a statistical test says that it is unlikely that such a large difference between groups would occur by chance. Tests that produce p-values less than 0.05 are said to have "statistically significant" results. For example, say that a researcher tests whether the mean age of men in a study population is different than the mean age of women in the study population. If the t-test has a p-value of 0.02, then the researcher would say that because the p-value is less than 0.05 the test is significant and would conclude that the mean ages for men and women were different. Other examples are shown in Table 14-5. Knowing the meaning of confidence intervals and p-values will allow you to interpret almost all statistical results. Just remember that the findings are considered to be statistically significant if the confidence interval does not include 1 or the p-value is less than 0.05.

Table 14-5. Examples of p-value Interpretation.

Test	p-value	Conclusion
Compare mean age	0.13	No difference in mean age between the populations.
Compare mean score on a test	0.002	The mean test scores are significantly different in different populations.
Compare distribution of responses about language spoken at home	0.43	No difference in the distribution of responses by the various groups.
Compare prevalence of diabetes in City A and City B	0.03	The proportions of people with diabetes in the two cities are different.
Compare incidence rates (which is the same as calculating an RR)	0.0001	The incidence rates are different (and the 95% CI for the RR will not include 1).

BIAS AND CONFOUNDING

Bias is a systematic error in study design, data collection, or data analysis that creates a difference between what the study intended to measure and what it actually measured. It can lead to an overestimation or to an underestimation of the association between an exposure and an outcome. The discussion section of an article should include an explanation of the limitations of the study and the possible sources of bias. The two most common types are selection bias and information bias.

Selection bias occurs when the people who participate in a study are not representative of the intended sample population. One example of selection bias is **volunteer bias**, which occurs when people who volunteer to be part of an experiment turn out to be different than the desired sample population. For example, volunteers may participate in a study because they had a family member die of the disease being studied. However, if the volunteers are supposed to be the "control" population and they have an unusually high risk of genetic vulnerability to the disease, then the study results are likely to be less significant than if the volunteers had been more representative of the true population.

Information bias occurs when incorrect information is given to researchers. For example, **recall bias** may happen when participants do not accurately recall past events. When there is differential recall—say, when people with cancer strain to recall any potentially harmful past exposure but people in the control group are not similarly motivated to remember past exposures—the results of a study may be skewed and inaccurate. Information bias can also cause **misclassification**, which is when participants are assigned to the wrong exposure or disease category.

Bias can be avoided or minimized when a study is carefully designed, conducted, and analyzed.

Confounding occurs when exposed and unexposed cohorts have different associations with some "third variable" (which is why confounding is sometimes called a "third variable" effect). A confounder is associated with both the exposure and the outcome of interest, and adjusting for the effect of the confounder may change or eliminate the association between the exposure and outcome. For example, because most people who use tobacco also consume alcohol and both smoking and drinking are associated with an increased risk for many disease outcomes, smoking may confound the effect of drinking in a study where alcohol use is the primary exposure of interest. This means that a finding that alcohol increases the risk of lung cancer may be misleading because it could be that smoking increases the risk of lung cancer or that smoking increases the likelihood of alcohol use and there really is no direct association between alcohol and lung cancer. By including both smoking and drinking in the statistical analysis, the independent effect of alcohol on a lung cancer can be assessed. Another example of a common confounder is age in studies of women's health. Because pre-menopausal and post-menopausal women have different health risks, age (or menopausal status) usually must be controlled for in studies that include a wide age range of women.

Confounding is different than **effect modification**, which is when two risk factors interact and the strength of the effect of one predictor variable is dependent on the exposure level of the other predictor variable. Statistical analysis can adjust for both confounding and effect modification. Epidemiology articles will often mention that the statistical analysis was "adjusted for potential confounders" like age, sex, education, or tobacco use, and this means that the reported measure of association (like an RR or OR) has been adjusted to remove the effect of possible confounders.

VALIDITY

Validity asks how well a test measures what it is supposed to measure (internal validity) or how well a study measures the "truth" in a population (external validity or **generalizability**). You want a test to be **accurate** (valid), which means that it gives the actual values of height, blood pressure, or some other measure. You also want a test to be **precise** (**reliable**), which means that when the test is given several times the results are consistent. Figure 14-15 illustrates the relationship between accuracy and precision. The results of a reliable study can be reproduced.

As an example of accuracy in health research, imagine that as part of a community survey you are measuring the heights of all children under 5 years of age in a village. You want to be sure that you have the correct height to within 1 cm. One way to make sure that the people taking the measurements are being accurate and precise is to have two people measure each child and compare their results. If both measurements are accurate, then the two heights recorded for the same child should be within 1 cm. Another example of checking the validity (accuracy) of a test would be to have two radiologists look at the same X-ray and see if they agree whether a fracture is visible.

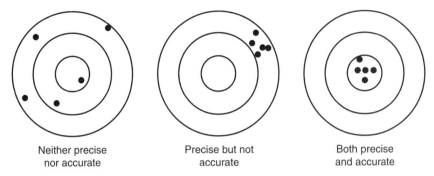

| Neither precise nor accurate | Precise but not accurate | Both precise and accurate |

Figure 14-15. Example of Accuracy and Precision.

Say that a dart thrower tosses 5 darts and aims for the bulls-eye. The target on the left shows results that are neither precise nor accurate. The center target has results that are precise but not accurate. The target on the right shows results that are both precise and accurate.

How do you know if the tests or measurements or observers are agreeing? One way to statistically test inter-rater reliability is to calculate the **kappa coefficient** (Figure 14-16). The kappa coefficient compares the frequency of agreement between two observers and calculates how different that percentage is from the amount of agreement that would be expected by chance. For example, say that two radiologists independently look at the same set of 100 X-rays and indicate whether or not they see a fracture. If the two radiologists come to the same conclusion regarding every X-ray, then $\kappa = 1$. If they agree no more or less than chance, then $\kappa = 0$. If they agree less than would be expected by chance, then the kappa coefficient is negative. A kappa coefficient that is positive and close to 1 indicates that the test is probably precise.

A similar kind of validity test can be used to compare the results of a lab test with the actual disease status of the person being tested (Figure 14-17). When the test gives the correct answer the result is called a true positive if the test says a person with the disease has the disease. It is called a true negative if the test says a person without the disease does not have the disease. A false positive results when the test wrongly indicates that a person has the disease when the truth is that the person is healthy. The probability of getting a false positive is sometimes called a Type I error or an α error. A false negative wrongly indicates that a person does not have the disease when the person actually does have the disease. The probability of getting a false negative is sometimes called a Type II error or a β error.

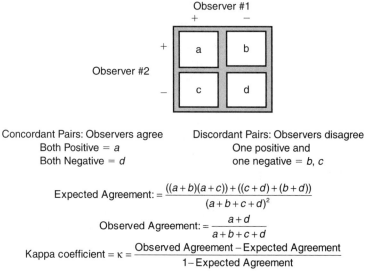

Concordant Pairs: Observers agree
Both Positive $= a$
Both Negative $= d$

Discordant Pairs: Observers disagree
One positive and
one negative $= b, c$

$$\text{Expected Agreement:} = \frac{((a+b)(a+c)) + ((c+d) + (b+d))}{(a+b+c+d)^2}$$

$$\text{Observed Agreement:} = \frac{a+d}{a+b+c+d}$$

$$\text{Kappa coefficient} = \kappa = \frac{\text{Observed Agreement} - \text{Expected Agreement}}{1 - \text{Expected Agreement}}$$

Figure 14-16. Analysis for Inter-rater Agreement.

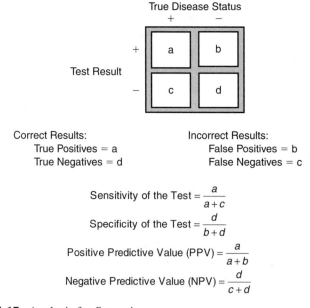

Correct Results:
True Positives = a
True Negatives = d

Incorrect Results:
False Positives = b
False Negatives = c

$$\text{Sensitivity of the Test} = \frac{a}{a+c}$$

$$\text{Specificity of the Test} = \frac{d}{b+d}$$

$$\text{Positive Predictive Value (PPV)} = \frac{a}{a+b}$$

$$\text{Negative Predictive Value (NPV)} = \frac{d}{c+d}$$

Figure 14-17. Analysis for Screening.

The **sensitivity** of a test is the percent of people who truly have disease who test positive for the disease condition. The **specificity** of a test is the percent of people who are truly free of the disease who test negative for the disease condition. A test is usually considered to be a relatively reliable tool, one that makes a correct diagnosis most of the time, if it has a sensitivity of at least 95% and a specificity of at least 80%. The **positive predictive value** is the percent of people who truly have disease among those who test positive for the disease condition and the **negative predictive value** is the percent of people who truly do not have disease among those who test negative for the disease condition.

What do sensitivity and specificity have to do with international health? Say you are running a supplemental feeding program at a refugee camp and want to know which children are at risk of severe consequences of undernutrition. You weighed and measured each child and calculated the weight-for-height ratio for each one. (Height-for-age and weight-for-age would give additional helpful information, but in many low-resource settings parents do not know the birthdates of their children.) You then listed all of the weight-for-height ratios from least to greatest. Now you have to determine where the cut-off point is that will distinguish between children whose growth is stunted and children who do not have stunted growth. (The statistical way to do this is to calculate a z-score for each child based on the distribution of all the values for the children. The z-score is the number of standard deviations an individual child's value is above or below the mean value.) How will you decide where the cut point should be? You do not want to make the value so low that children whose growth is truly stunted are not included in your supplemental feeding program, but you only have the resources to include the most seriously undernourished children in your program. This is the same kind of problem discussed above; you are trying to maximize your sensitivity and positive predictive value by using your test result (the weight-for-height ratio) to estimate true disease status (extreme undernutrition).

For many screening tests, like the weight-for-height test, there is not an obvious cut-off point to distinguish between a person with disease and a person without disease (Figure 14-18). This is true for the relationship between blood sugar and diabetes, blood pressure and hypertension, and weight and obesity. The people who design and use the tests do their best to determine the level at which the risk is sufficient to declare that the person has the disease. For some diseases, especially those with no treatment or treatment that is expensive and potentially harmful, it is better to have a high

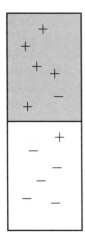 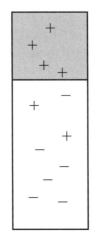 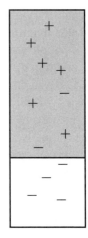

The initial cut-off point misclassifies some people.	Raising the cut-off point will increase the specificity (% of negatives classified as negative) and decrease the sensitivity.	Lowering the cut-off point will increase the sensitivity (% of positives classified as positive) and decrease the specificity.
There are some false positives and some false negatives.	There will be few false positives, but some people with the disease will think they are healthy.	There will be few false negatives, but some people who are healthy will think they have the disease.

Figure 14-18. The Effect of Selecting Different Cut-off Points for Classifying Disease Status.

Note: A "+" sign indicates a person who truly has the disease and a "−" sign indicates a person who truly does not have the disease. The shaded area shows the population that is classified as diseased based on selecting a cut-off point for a test for the disease condition. If sensitivity increases, specificity decreases. If sensitivity decreases, specificity increases.

threshold for declaring that a person has the condition. For others, especially when early intervention can prevent serious complications, it is better to have a low threshold.

The research articles and public health reports that are the primary means of communication within the field of global health often refer to concepts like validity, bias, statistical significance, and study design. A basic familiarity with these terms will allow you to better understand the work that is being done around the world to improve health, and will allow you to more easily communicate with other people working in global health.

REFERENCES

1. Mosca L, Ferris A, Fabunmi R, Robertson RM. Tracking women's awareness of heart disease: an American Heart Association National Study. *Circulation.* 2004; 109: 573–379.
2. Bustos P, Amigo H, Oyarzún M, Rona RJ. Is there a causal relation between obesity and asthma? Evidence from Chile. *Int J Obes.* 2005; 29: 804–809.
3. Rao DN, Ganesh B, Dinshaw KA, Mohandas KM. A case-control study of stomach cancer in Mumbai, India. *Int J Cancer.* 2002;99:727–731.
4. Kaye DK, Mirembe FM, Bantebya G, Johansson A, Ekstrom AM. Domestic violence during pregnancy and risk of low birthweight and maternal complications: a prospective cohort study at Mulago Hospital, Uganda. *Trop Med Int Health.* 2006;11:1576–1584.
5. Chlebowski RT, Hendrix SL, Langer RD, et al, for the WHI Investigators. Influence of estrogen plus progestin on breast cancer and mammography in healthy postmenopausal women. *JAMA.* 2003;289:3243–3253.
6. The first results from the WHI study were reported in July 2002, shortly after the trial was stopped. Rossouw JE, Anderson GL, Prentice RL, LaCroix AZ, Kooperberg C, Sterfanick ML, Jackson RD, Beresford SA, Howard BV, Johnson KC, Kotchen JM, Ockene J, and the Writing Group for the Women's Health Initiative Investigators. Risks and benefits of estrogen plus progestin in health postmenopausal women: principle results from the Women's Health Initiative randomized controlled trial. *JAMA.* 2002;288;321–333.

APPENDIX I

Countries of the World by WHO Region

The World Health Organization is subdivided into six regional offices.

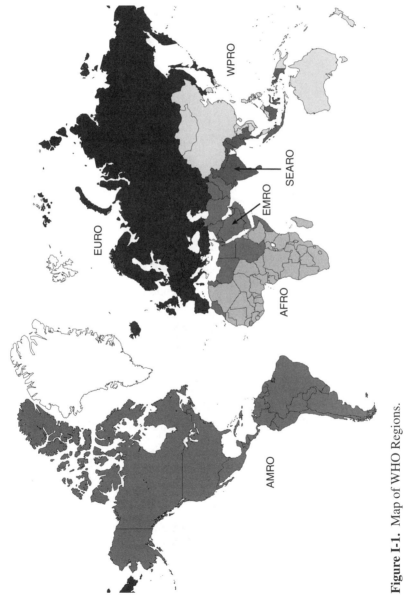

Figure I-1. Map of WHO Regions.

AFRICA

Sub-Saharan Africa
(AFRO: Regional Office for Africa)

Algeria
Angola
Benin
Botswana
Burkina Faso
Burundi
Cameroon
Cape Verde
Central African Republic
Chad
Comoros
Congo
Côte d'Ivoire
Democratic Republic of the Congo
  (formerly Zaire)
Equatorial Guinea
Eritrea
Ethiopia
Gabon
Gambia
Ghana
Guinea
Guinea-Bissau
Kenya

Lesotho
Liberia
Madagascar
Malawi
Mali
Mauritania
Mauritius
Mozambique
Namibia
Niger
Nigeria
Rwanda
Sao Tome and Principe
Senegal
Seychelles
Sierra Leone
South Africa
Swaziland
Togo
Uganda
United Republic of Tanzania
  (Tanzania)
Zambia
Zimbabwe

THE AMERICAS

(AMRO: Regional Office for the Americas
= PAHO: Pan American Health Organization)

Antigua and Barbuda
Argentina
Bahamas
Barbados
Belize
Bolivia
Brazil
Canada
Chile
Colombia

Costa Rica
Cuba
Dominica
Dominican Republic
Ecuador
El Salvador
Grenada
Guatemala
Guyana
Haiti

THE AMERICAS—cont'd

Honduras
Jamaica
Mexico
Nicaragua
Panama
Paraguay
Peru
Saint Kitts and Nevis

Saint Lucia
Saint Vincent and the Grenadines
Suriname
Trinidad and Tobago
United States of America
Uruguay
Venezuela

EASTERN MEDITERRANEAN

North Africa and the Middle East
(EMRO: Regional Office for the Eastern Mediterranean)

Afghanistan
Bahrain
Djibouti
Egypt
Iran
Iraq
Jordan
Kuwait
Lebanon
Libyan Arab Jamahiriya (Libya)
Morocco

Oman
Pakistan
Qatar
Saudi Arabia
Somalia
Sudan
Syrian Arab Republic (Syria)
Tunisia
United Arab Emirates
Yemen

EUROPE

Includes the nations formerly part of the U.S.S.R.
(EURO: Regional Office for Europe)

Albania
Andorra
Armenia
Austria
Azerbaijan
Belarus
Belgium
Bosnia and Herzegovina
Bulgaria
Croatia
Cyprus
Czech Republic

Denmark
Estonia
Finland
France
Georgia
Germany
Greece
Hungary
Iceland
Ireland
Israel
Italy

(Continued)

EUROPE—cont'd

Kazakhstan
Krygyzstan
Latvia
Liechtenstein
Lithuania
Luxembourg
Malta
Monaco
Montenegro
Netherlands
Norway
Poland
Portugal
Republic of Moldova
Romania
Russian Federation (Russia)

San Marino
Serbia
Slovakia
Slovenia
Spain
Sweden
Switzerland
Tajikistan
The former Yugoslav Republic of
    Macedonia
Turkey
Turkmenistan
Ukraine
United Kingdom
Uzebekistan

SOUTH-EAST ASIA

(SEARO: Regional Office for South-East Asia)

Bangladesh
Bhutan
Democratic People's Republic of
    Korea (North Korea)
India
Indonesia

Maldives
Myanmar
Nepal
Sri Lanka
Thailand
Timor-Leste

WESTERN PACIFIC

East Asia and Oceania
(WPRO: Regional Office for the Western Pacific)

Australia
Brunei Darussalam
Cambodia
China
Cook Islands
Fiji
Japan
Kiribati
Lao People's Democratic Republic

Malaysia
Marshall Islands
Federated States of Micronesia
Mongolia
Nauru
New Zealand
Niue
Palau
Papua New Guinea

WESTERN PACIFIC—*cont'd*

Philippines
Republic of Korea (South Korea)
Samoa
Singapore
Solomon Islands

Tonga
Tuvalu
Vanuatu
Viet Nam

APPENDIX **II**

Selected Articles from the Constitution of the World Health Organization

The States parties to this Constitution declare, in conformity with the Charter of the United Nations, that the following principles are basic to the happiness, harmonious relations, and security of all peoples:

- Health is a state of complete physical, mental, and social well-being and not merely the absence of disease or infirmity.
- The enjoyment of the highest attainable standard of health is one of the fundamental rights of every human being without distinction of race, religion, political belief, economic, or social condition.
- The health of all peoples is fundamental to the attainment of peace and security and is dependent upon the fullest cooperation of individuals and States.
- The achievement of any State in the promotion and protection of health is of value to all.
- Unequal development in different countries in the promotion of health and control of disease, especially communicable disease, is a common danger.
- Healthy development of the child is of basic importance; the ability to live harmoniously in a changing total environment is essential to such development.
- The extension to all peoples of the benefits of medical, psychological, and related knowledge is essential to the fullest attainment of health.
- Informed opinion and active cooperation on the part of the public are of the utmost importance in the improvement of the health of the people.
- Governments have a responsibility for the health of their peoples which can be fulfilled only by the provision of adequate health and social measures.

Accepting these principles, and for the purpose of co-operation among themselves and with others to promote and protect the health of all peoples, the contracting parties agree to the present Constitution and hereby establish the World Health Organization as a specialized agency within the terms of Article 57 of The Charter of the United Nations.

Chapter I: Objective

Article 1.   The objective of the World Health Organization (hereinafter called the Organization) shall be the attainment by all peoples of the highest possible level of health.

Chapter II: Functions

Article 2.   In order to achieve its objective, the functions of the Organization shall be:

(a) to act as the directing and coordinating authority on international health work;

(b) to establish and maintain effective collaboration with the United Nations, specialized agencies, governmental health administrations, professional groups, and other organizations as may be deemed appropriate;

(c) to assist governments, upon request, in strengthening health services;

(d) to furnish appropriate technical assistance and, in emergencies, necessary aid upon the request or acceptance of governments;

(e) to provide or assist in providing, upon the request of the United Nations, health services and facilities to special groups, such as the peoples of trust territories;

(f) to establish and maintain such administrative and technical services as may be required, including epidemiological and statistical services;

(g) to stimulate and advance work to eradicate epidemic, endemic, and other diseases;

(h) to promote, in cooperation with other specialized agencies where necessary, the prevention of accidental injuries;

(i) to promote, in cooperation with other specialized agencies where necessary, the improvement of nutrition, housing, sanitation, recreation, economic, or working conditions and other aspects of environmental hygiene;

(j) to promote cooperation among scientific and professional groups which contribute to the advancement of health;

(k) to propose conventions, agreements, and regulations, and make recommendations with respect to international health matters and to perform such duties as may be assigned thereby to the Organization and are consistent with its objective;

(l) to promote maternal and child health and welfare and to foster the ability to live harmoniously in a changing total environment;

(m) to foster activities in the field of mental health, especially those affecting the harmony of human relations;

(n) to promote and conduct research in the field of health;

(o) to promote improved standard of teaching and training in the health, medical, and related professions;

(p) to study and report on, in cooperation with other specialized agencies where necessary, administrative and social techniques affecting public health and medical care from preventive and curative points of view, including hospital services and social security;

(q) to provide information, counsel, and assistance in the field of health;

(r) to assist in developing an informed public opinion among all peoples on matters of health;

(s) to establish and revise as necessary international nomenclature of diseases, of causes of death, and of public health practices;

(t) to standardize diagnostic procedures as necessary;

(u) to develop, establish, and promote international standards with respect to food, biological, pharmaceutical, and similar products;

(v) generally to take all necessary action to attain the objective of the Organization.

Chapter XVI: Relations With Other Organizations

Article 69.   The Organization shall be brought into relation with the United Nations as one of the specialized agencies referred to in Article 57 of the Charter of the United Nations. The agreement or agreements bringing the Organization into relation with the United Nations shall be subject to approval by a two-thirds vote of the Health Assembly.

Article 70.   The Organization shall establish effective relations and cooperate closely with such other inter-governmental organizations as may be desirable.

Article 71.   The Organization may, on matter within its competence, make suitable arrangements for consultation and cooperation with non-governmental international organizations and, with the consent of the government concerned, with national organizations, governmental or non-governmental.

APPENDIX III

Selected Articles from the Convention on the Rights of the Child

(6) States Parties recognize that every child has the inherent right to life and shall ensure to the maximum extent possible the survival and development of the child.

(17) States Parties recognize the important function performed by the mass media and shall ensure that the child has access to information . . . especially those aimed at the promotion of his or her social, spiritual and moral well-being and physical and mental health.

(19) States Parties shall take all appropriate . . . measures to protect the child from all forms of physical or mental violence, injury or abuse, neglect or negligent treatment, maltreatment or exploitation, including sexual abuse.

(23) States Parties recognize that a mentally or physically disabled child should enjoy a full and decent life, in conditions which ensure dignity, promote self-reliance and facilitate the child's active participation in the community.

(24) States Parties recognize the right of the child to the enjoyment of the highest attainable standard of health and to facilities for the treatment of illness and rehabilitation of health. States Parties shall pursue full implementation of this right and, in particular, shall take appropriate measures:

(a) To diminish infant and child mortality;

(b) To ensure the provision of necessary medical assistance and health care to all children with emphasis on the development of primary health care;

(c) To combat disease and malnutrition, including within the framework of primary health care, through, inter alia, the application of readily available technology and through the provision of adequate nutritious foods and clean drinking-water, taking into consideration the dangers and risks of environmental pollution;

(d) To ensure appropriate pre-natal and post-natal health care for mothers;

(e) To ensure that all segments of society, in particular parents and children, are informed, have access to education and are supported in the use of basic knowledge of child health and nutrition, the advantages of breastfeeding, hygiene and environmental sanitation and the prevention of accidents;

(f) To develop preventive health care, guidance for parents and family planning education and services.

(27)   States Parties recognize the right of every child to a standard of living adequate for the child's physical, mental, spiritual, moral and social development.

(28)   States Parties recognize the right of the child to education . . . and on the basis of equal opportunity, they shall, in particular make primary education compulsory and available free to all.

(31)   States Parties recognize the right of the child to rest and leisure, to engage in play . . .

(32)   States Parties recognize the right of the child to be protected from economic exploitation and from performing any work that is likely to be hazardous . . .

(34)   States Parties undertake to protect the child from all forms of sexual exploitation and sexual abuse.

(39)   States Parties shall take all appropriate measures to promote physical and psychological recovery and social reintegration of a child victim of: any form of neglect, exploitation, or abuse; torture or any other form of cruel, inhuman or degrading treatment or punishment; or armed conflicts.

Universal Declaration of Human Rights

Whereas recognition of the inherent dignity and of the equal and inalienable rights of all members of the human family is the foundation of freedom, justice and peace in the world,

Whereas disregard and contempt for human rights have resulted in barbarous acts which have outraged the conscience of mankind, and the advent of a world in which human beings shall enjoy freedom of speech and belief and freedom from fear and want has been proclaimed as the highest aspiration of the common people,

Whereas it is essential, if man is not to be compelled to have recourse, as a last resort, to rebellion against tyranny and oppression, that human rights should be protected by the rule of law,

Whereas it is essential to promote the development of friendly relations between nations,

Whereas the peoples of the United Nations have in the Charter reaffirmed their faith in fundamental human rights, in the dignity and worth of the human person and in the equal rights of men and women and have determined to promote social progress and better standards of life in larger freedom,

Whereas Member States have pledged themselves to achieve, in co-operation with the United Nations, the promotion of universal respect for and observance of human rights and fundamental freedoms,

Whereas a common understanding of these rights and freedoms is of the greatest importance for the full realization of this pledge,

Now, Therefore THE GENERAL ASSEMBLY proclaims THIS UNIVERSAL DECLARATION OF HUMAN RIGHTS as a common standard of achievement for all peoples and all nations, to the end that every individual and every organ of society, keeping this Declaration constantly in mind, shall strive by teaching and education to promote respect for these rights and freedoms and by progressive measures, national and international, to secure their universal and effective recognition and observance, both among the peoples of Member States themselves and among the peoples of territories under their jurisdiction.

Article 1.   All human beings are born free and equal in dignity and rights. They are endowed with reason and conscience and should act towards one another in a spirit of brotherhood.

Article 2.   Everyone is entitled to all the rights and freedoms set forth in this Declaration, without distinction of any kind, such as race, color, sex, language, religion, political or other opinion, national or social origin, property, birth or other status. Furthermore, no distinction shall be made on the basis of the political, jurisdictional or international status of the country or territory to which a person belongs, whether it be independent, trust, non-self-governing or under any other limitation of sovereignty.

Article 3.   Everyone has the right to life, liberty and security of person.

Article 4.   No one shall be held in slavery or servitude; slavery and the slave trade shall be prohibited in all their forms.

Article 5.   No one shall be subjected to torture or to cruel, inhuman or degrading treatment or punishment.

Article 6.   Everyone has the right to recognition everywhere as a person before the law.

Article 7.   All are equal before the law and are entitled without any discrimination to equal protection of the law. All are entitled to equal protection against any discrimination in violation of this Declaration and against any incitement to such discrimination.

Article 8.   Everyone has the right to an effective remedy by the competent national tribunals for acts violating the fundamental rights granted him by the constitution or by law.

Article 9.   No one shall be subjected to arbitrary arrest, detention or exile.

Article 10.   Everyone is entitled in full equality to a fair and public hearing by an independent and impartial tribunal, in the determination of his rights and obligations and of any criminal charge against him.

Article 11.   (1) Everyone charged with a penal offence has the right to be presumed innocent until proved guilty according to law in a public trial at which he has had all the guarantees necessary for his defense. (2) No one shall be held guilty of any penal offence on account of any act or omission which did not constitute a penal offence, under national or international law, at the time when it was committed. Nor shall a heavier penalty be imposed than the one that was applicable at the time the penal offence was committed.

Article 12. No one shall be subjected to arbitrary interference with his privacy, family, home or correspondence, nor to attacks upon his honor and reputation. Everyone has the right to the protection of the law against such interference or attacks.

Article 13. (1) Everyone has the right to freedom of movement and residence within the borders of each state. (2) Everyone has the right to leave any country, including his own, and to return to his country.

Article 14. (1) Everyone has the right to seek and to enjoy in other countries asylum from persecution. (2) This right may not be invoked in the case of prosecutions genuinely arising from non-political crimes or from acts contrary to the purposes and principles of the United Nations.

Article 15. (1) Everyone has the right to a nationality. (2) No one shall be arbitrarily deprived of his nationality nor denied the right to change his nationality.

Article 16. (1) Men and women of full age, without any limitation due to race, nationality or religion, have the right to marry and to found a family. They are entitled to equal rights as to marriage, during marriage and at its dissolution. (2) Marriage shall be entered into only with the free and full consent of the intending spouses. (3) The family is the natural and fundamental group unit of society and is entitled to protection by society and the State.

Article 17. (1) Everyone has the right to own property alone as well as in association with others. (2) No one shall be arbitrarily deprived of his property.

Article 18. Everyone has the right to freedom of thought, conscience and religion; this right includes freedom to change his religion or belief, and freedom, either alone or in community with others and in public or private, to manifest his religion or belief in teaching, practice, worship and observance.

Article 19. Everyone has the right to freedom of opinion and expression; this right includes freedom to hold opinions without interference and to seek, receive and impart information and ideas through any media and regardless of frontiers.

Article 20. (1) Everyone has the right to freedom of peaceful assembly and association. (2) No one may be compelled to belong to an association.

Article 21. (1) Everyone has the right to take part in the government of his country, directly or through freely chosen representatives. (2) Everyone has the right of equal access to public service in his country. (3) The will of the people shall be the basis of the authority of government; this will shall be expressed in periodic and genuine elections which shall be by universal and equal suffrage and shall be held by secret vote or by equivalent free voting procedures.

Article 22.   Everyone, as a member of society, has the right to social security and is entitled to realization, through national effort and international co-operation and in accordance with the organization and resources of each State, of the economic, social and cultural rights indispensable for his dignity and the free development of his personality.

Article 23.   (1) Everyone has the right to work, to free choice of employment, to just and favorable conditions of work and to protection against unemployment. (2) Everyone, without any discrimination, has the right to equal pay for equal work. (3) Everyone who works has the right to just and favorable remuneration ensuring for himself and his family an existence worthy of human dignity, and supplemented, if necessary, by other means of social protection. (4) Everyone has the right to form and to join trade unions for the protection of his interests.

Article 24.   Everyone has the right to rest and leisure, including reasonable limitation of working hours and periodic holidays with pay.

Article 25.   (1) Everyone has the right to a standard of living adequate for the health and well-being of himself and of his family, including food, clothing, housing, and medical care and necessary social services, and the right to security in the event of unemployment, sickness, disability, widowhood, old age or other lack of livelihood in circumstances beyond his control. (2) Motherhood and childhood are entitled to special care and assistance. All children, whether born in or out of wedlock, shall enjoy the same social protection.

Article 26.   (1) Everyone has the right to education. Education shall be free, at least in the elementary and fundamental stages. Elementary education shall be compulsory. Technical and professional education shall be made generally available and higher education shall be equally accessible to all on the basis of merit. (2) Education shall be directed to the full development of the human personality and to the strengthening of respect for human rights and fundamental freedoms. It shall promote understanding, tolerance and friendship among all nations, racial or religious groups, and shall further the activities of the United Nations for the maintenance of peace. (3) Parents have a prior right to choose the kind of education that shall be given to their children.

Article 27.   (1) Everyone has the right freely to participate in the cultural life of the community, to enjoy the arts and to share in scientific advancement and its benefits. (2) Everyone has the right to the protection of the moral and material interests resulting from any scientific, literary or artistic production of which he is the author.

Article 28.   Everyone is entitled to a social and international order in which the rights and freedoms set forth in this Declaration can be fully realized.

Article 29.   (1) Everyone has duties to the community in which alone the free and full development of his personality is possible. (2) In the exercise of his rights and freedoms, everyone shall be subject only to such limitations as are determined by law solely for the purpose of securing due recognition and respect for the rights and freedoms of others and of meeting the just requirements of morality, public order and the general welfare in a democratic society. (3) These rights and freedoms may in no case be exercised contrary to the purposes and principles of the United Nations.

Article 30.   Nothing in this Declaration may be interpreted as implying for any State, group or person any right to engage in any activity or to perform any act aimed at the destruction of any of the rights and freedoms set forth herein.

Millennium Development Goals, Targets, and Selected Indicators

The Millennium Development Goals (MDGs), adopted by the United Nations in 2000, aim to reduce world poverty significantly by 2015. 18 quantifiable targets and 48 indicators are used to measure progress toward the achievement of the 8 MDGs.

The United Nations agency listed in parentheses next to each indicator is the agency that has been designated as the official data source for that indicator.

Goal 1: Eradicate extreme poverty and hunger.

- Target 1: Reduce by half the proportion of people living on less than a dollar a day.
  - Indicator 1: Proportion of population below $1 (PPP) per day (World Bank)
  - Indicator 2: Poverty gap ratio [incidence x depth of poverty] (World Bank)
  - Indicator 3: Share of poorest quintile in national consumption (World Bank)
- Target 2: Reduce by half the proportion of people who suffer from hunger.
  - Indicator 4: Prevalence of underweight children under five years of age (UNICEF-WHO)
  - Indicator 5: Proportion of population below minimum level of dietary energy consumption (FAO)

Goal 2: Achieve universal primary education.

- Target 3: Ensure that all boys and girls complete a cull course of primary schooling.
  - Indicator 6: Net enrollment in primary education (UNESCO)
  - Indicator 7: Proportion of pupils starting grade 1 who reach grade 5 (UNESCO)
  - Indicator 8: Literacy rate of 15 to 24-year-olds (UNESCO)

Goal 3: Promote gender equality and empower women.

- Target 4: Eliminate gender disparity in primary and secondary education by 2005, and at all levels by 2015.
    - Indicator 9: Ratios of girls to boys in primary, secondary, and tertiary education (UNESCO)
    - Indicator 10: Ratio of literate women to men, 15 to 24 years old (UNESCO)
    - Indicator 11: Share of women in wage employment in the non-agricultural sector (ILO)
    - Indicator 12: Proportion of seats held by women in national parliament (IPU)

Goal 4: Reduce child mortality.

- Target 5: Reduce by two-thirds the mortality rate among children under five.
    - Indicator 13: Under-five mortality rate (UNICEF-WHO)
    - Indicator 14: Infant mortality rate (UNICEF-WHO)
    - Indicator 15: Proportion of 1-year-old children immunized against measles (UNICEF-WHO)

Goal 5: Improve maternal health.

- Target 6: Reduce by three-quarters the maternal mortality ratio.
    - Indicator 16: Maternal mortality ratio (UNICEF-WHO)
    - Indicator 17: Proportion of births attended by skilled health personnel (UNICEF-WHO)

Goal 6: Combat HIV/AIDS, malaria, and other diseases.

- Target 7: Halt and begin to reverse the spread of HIV/AIDS.
    - Indicator 18: HIV prevalence among pregnant women aged 15–24 years (UNAIDS-WHO-UNICEF)
    - Indicator 19: Condom use rate of the contraceptive prevalence rate (UNPF)
        - Indicator 19a: Condom use at last high-risk sex (UNICEF-WHO)

- – Indicator 19b: Percentage of population aged 15-24 years with comprehensive correct knowledge of HIV/AIDS (UNICEF-WHO)
- – Indicator 20c: Contraceptive prevalence rate (UNPF)
  - ○ Indicator 20: Ratio of school attendance of orphans to school attendance of non-orphans aged 10–14 years (UNICEF-UNAIDS-WHO)
- • Target 8: Halt and begin to reverse the incidence of malaria and other major diseases.
  - ○ Indicator 21: Prevalence and death rates associated with malaria (WHO)
  - ○ Indicator 22: Proportion of population in malaria-risk areas using effective malaria prevention and treatment measures (UNICEF-WHO)
  - ○ Indicator 23: Prevalence and death rates associated with tuberculosis (WHO)
  - ○ Indicator 24: Proportion of tuberculosis cases detected and cured under directly observed treatment short course DOTS (internationally recommended TB control strategy) (WHO)

Goal 7: Ensure environmental sustainability.

- • Target 9: Integrate the principles of sustainable development into country policies and programs; reverse loss of environmental resources.
  - ○ Indicator 25: Proportion of land area covered by forest (FAO)
  - ○ Indicator 26: Ratio of area protected to maintain biological diversity to surface area (UNEP-WCMC)
  - ○ Indicator 27: Energy use (kg oil equivalent) per $1 GDP (PPP) (IEA, World Bank)
  - ○ Indicator 28: Carbon dioxide emissions per capita and consumption of ozone-depleting CFCs (ODP tons) (UNEP-Ozone Secretariat)
  - ○ Indicator 29: Proportion of population using solid fuels (WHO)
- • Target 10: Reduce by half the proportion of people without sustainable access to safe drinking water.
  - ○ Indicator 30: Proportion of population with sustainable access to an improved water source, urban and rural (UNICEF-WHO)
  - ○ Indicator 31: Proportion of population with access to improved sanitation, urban and rural (UNICEF-WHO)

- Target 11: Achieve significant improvement in the lives of at least 100 million slum dwellers by 2020.
  - Indicator 32: Proportion of households with access to secure tenure (UN-HABITAT)

Goal 8: Develop a global partnership for development.

- Target 12: Develop further an open, rule-based, predictable, non-discriminatory trading and financial system.
- Target 13: Address the special needs of the least developed countries.
- Target 14. Address the special needs of landlocked countries and small island developing States.
- Target 15. Deal comprehensively with the debt problems of developing countries through national and international measures in order to make debt sustainable in the long term.
  - Indicator 44: Debt service as a percentage of exports of goods and services (IMF-World Bank)
- Target 16: In cooperation with developing countries, develop and implement strategies for decent and productive work for youth.
  - Indicator 45: Unemployment rate of young people aged 15–24 years, each sex and total (ILO)
- Target 17: In cooperation with pharmaceutical companies, provide access to affordable essential drugs in developing countries.
  - Indicator 46: Proportion of population with access to affordable essential drugs on a sustainable basis (WHO)
- Target 18: In cooperation with the private sector, make available the benefits of new technologies, especially information and communications.
  - Indicator 47: Telephone lines and cellular subscribers per 1000 population (ITU)
  - Indicator 48: Personal computers in use per 100 population and internet users per 100 population (ITU)

Preventive and Treatment Interventions for Major Health Issues

Area	Preventive Interventions (Primary Prevention)	Treatment Interventions (Secondary Prevention)
Child mortality	• Breastfeeding • Hand-washing • Safe disposal of stool • Latrine use • Safe preparation of weaning food • Use of insecticide-treated bednets (ITNs) • Complementary feeding • Immunization • Micronutrient supplementation (zinc and vitamin A) • Prenatal care, including steroids and tetanus toxoid • Antimalarial intermittent preventive treatment in pregnancy • Newborn temperature management • Nevirapine and replacement feeding for babies born to mothers with HIV infection • Antibiotics for premature rupture of membranes • Clean delivery	• Oral rehydration therapy (ORT) for diarrhea • Antibiotics for dysentery, pneumonia, and sepsis • Antimalarials for malaria • Newborn resuscitation • Breastfeeding • Complementary feeding during illness • Micronutrient supplementation (zinc and vitamin A)
Maternal mortality	• Family planning • Intermittent malaria prophylaxis • Use of insecticide treated bednets (ITNs) • Micronutrient supplementation (iron, folic acid, calcium) for those who are deficient	• Antibiotics for preterm rupture of membranes • Skilled attendants during labor and delivery • Basic and emergency obstetric care

Area	Preventive Interventions (Primary Prevention)	Treatment Interventions (Secondary Prevention)
Nutrition	<ul><li>Exclusive breastfeeding for 6 months</li><li>Appropriate complementary child feeding for 6 to 24 month-olds</li><li>Iron and folic acid supplementation for children</li><li>Improved hygiene and sanitation</li><li>Improved dietary intake of pregnant and lactating women</li><li>Micronutrient supplementation for prevention of anemia and vitamin A deficiency for mothers and children</li><li>Antihelminthic treatment in school-age children</li></ul>	<ul><li>Appropriate feeding of sick children</li><li>Oral rehydration therapy (ORT)</li><li>Control and timely treatment of infectious and parasitic diseases</li><li>Treatment and monitoring of severely malnourished children</li><li>High-dose treatment of clinical signs of vitamin A deficiency</li></ul>
HIV/AIDS	<ul><li>Safe sex, including condom use</li><li>Unused needles for drug users</li><li>Treatment of other sexually transmitted infections (STIs)</li><li>Safe, screened blood supplies</li><li>Antiretrovirals (ARVs) in pregnancy to prevent maternal-to-child (MTC) transmission and after occupational exposure</li><li>Health education on abstinence, condom use, STI treatment, ARV use to prevent MTC transmission, feeding substitutions for mothers with HIV</li><li>Use of universal precautions for safety when handling blood and other body fluids</li></ul>	<ul><li>Treatment of opportunistic infections (OIs)</li><li>Co-trimoxazole prophylaxis</li><li>Highly active antiretroviral therapy (HAART)</li><li>Palliative care (pain management)</li></ul>

(Continued)

Area	Preventive Interventions (Primary Prevention)	Treatment Interventions (Secondary Prevention)
Tuberculosis	• Directly observed treatment (DOTS) of infectious cases to prevent transmission and emergence of drug-resistant strains • Treatment of contacts • BCG immunization	• Directly observed treatment (DOTS) from diagnosis until cure • Early identification of cases with active TB disease
Malaria	• Use of insecticide-treated bednets (ITNs) • Indoor residual spraying of insecticide in epidemic-prone areas • Intermittent presumptive treatment of pregnant women	• Rapid detection and early treatment of uncomplicated cases • Treatment of complicated cases such as cerebral malaria and severe anemia

Source: Interventions adapted from Table 9.1 of Wagstaff A, Claeson M, Hecht RM, Gottret P, Fang Q. Chapter 9: Millennium Development Goals for Health: What Will It Take to Accelerate Progress? In: Jamison DT, Breman JG, Measham AR, Alleyne G, Claeson M, Evans DB, Jha P, Mills A, Musgrove P, eds. Disease Control Priorities in Developing Countries, 2nd edition. Washington, DC: Oxford University Press and The World Bank, 2006, p. 184.

APPENDIX VII

Recommended Childhood Immunizations

The UNICEF schedule is for most children worldwide.
The CDC schedule is for children in the United States.

Agent	Agent Type	UNICEF Schedule	CDC Schedule
Chickenpox (varicella)	Virus		●
Diphtheria	Bacterium	●	●
Hepatitis A virus	Virus		●
Hepatitis B virus	Virus	○	●
Haemophilus influenzae type b (Hib)	Bacterium	○	●
Human Papillomavirus	Virus		●
Influenza	Virus		●
Measles	Virus	●	●
Meningococcus	Bacterium		●
Mumps	Virus	○	●
Pertussis ("whooping cough")	Bacterium	●	●
Pneumococcus	Bacterium		●
Polio (poliomyelitis)	Virus	●	●
Rotavirus	Virus		●
Rubella ("German measles")	Virus	○	●
Tetanus	Bacterium	●	●
Tuberculosis (BCG: Bacille Calmette-Guérin)	Bacterium	●	
Yellow fever	Virus	○	

● recommended for all children
○ recommended for children in some countries

Sources: UNICEF, WHO, UNESCO, UNFPA, UNDP, UNAIDS, WFP, and the World Bank. Facts for Life. New York, NY: UNICEF, 2002.

CDC, 2007 Childhood & Adolescent Immunization Schedule.

Index

A

ABCs of AIDS prevention, 157
Abortion, 73–74, 76, 77, 88–89
Abstinence, 76, 78, 157
Abstracts, 293
Access to health care (*see* Health care access)
Accuracy, 314–315
Acid rain, 243
ActionAid, 267
Active immunity, 144
Activities of Daily Living, 110
Acupuncture, 16–17
Acute, 121, 142
Acute Respiratory Infection (ARI), 14, 58–61 (*see also* Pneumonia)
Adventist Development and Relief Agency (ADRA), 266, 268
Advocacy organizations, 267
Aedes aegypti mosquitoes, 128, 172, 232
Afghanistan, 75
African-Americans, 20, 92, 93–94
African Development Fund, 256
African sleeping sickness (*see* Trypanosomiasis, *Trypanosoma brucei*), 73, 117, 131, 132, 278
Aga Khan Foundation, 265
Age adjustment, 142
Agent, 122–139
Agent-Host-Environment, 122–142

Aging
  Health effects, 30, 72, 108–110, 174, 243
  Population planning, 86, 110–111
Aging Index, 85
Agriculture, 6, 208, 235, 243–245
AIDS (Acquired Immunodeficiency Syndrome), (*see also* HIV/AIDS) 149–152
AIDS orphans, 155, 338
Air filters, 117
Air pollution (indoors), (*see* Indoor air pollution)
Air pollution (outdoors), 213, 226, 230, 235, 240, 242, 244
Air quality, 6, 212–213, 235 (*see also* Air pollution)
Airborne transmission, 116–117
Alcohol use, 140, 213, 313–314
Alcoholism, 26, 28, 98–99
Aldehydes, 226
Allele, 37
Allergies, 28, 233, 244
Alma-Ata Conference, 65
Alpha (α) error, 315
Alternative energy sources, 227, 245
Alveoli, 58–59
Alzheimer's Disease, 28, 71, 73, 98–99, 140
American Cancer Society, 12, 18
American Heart Association, 292

American sleeping sickness (Chagas Disease, *Trypanosoma cruzi*), 131, 132, 230–231, 278
Amino acids, 182
Amish, 92
Amnesty International, 267
Amoeba, 130
Amoebiasis, 130–131
Amoebic dysentery, 130–131
Analytic epidemiology, 7, 8, 122
Anemia, 29, 73
  Causes, 133, 186, 209, 240
  Iron deficiency, 188, 194–195
  Malarial, 158–160
Anencephaly, 185
Annan, Kofi, 19, 40
Anopheles mosquitoes, 130, 131, 158–159
Anorexia nervosa, 99, 207
Antenatal (prenatal) care, 55, 67, 76
Anthrax (*Bacillus anthracis*), 125, 176–177
Anthropometry, 196–197
Anthroponosis, 118
Antibiotics, 31, 59–60, 127, 130, 176
Antibiotic misuse, 127, 174
Antibiotic resistance (*see* Antimicrobial resistance)
Antibodies, 121, 182, 199
Antigenic drift, 175
Antigenic shift, 175
Antihelminthic drugs, 59, 137, 223–224
Antimicrobial resistance, 127, 130, 132, 160–162, 173–174, 282
Antioxidants, 185–186
Antiretroviral drugs (ARVs), 152, 155, 157, 277–278, 287
Antiviral drugs, 130 (*see also* Antiretroviral drugs)
Anxiety disorders, 98–99
Appendicitis, 29
Appropriate technology, 216
Arbovirus, 117
Argentina, 42, 237
Arm circumference, 197
Arsenic, 239, 241
Arsenicosis, 241
Arsenopyrites, 241

Artemisia (artemisinin), 16, 160
Arthritis (osteoarthritis), 29, 73, 103, 108, 110, 203
Arthropods, 117
Arusha Conference (Second African Population Conference), 90
Asbestos, 214, 238
Ascariasis, 133–134, 136
Ascaris lumbricoides, 133–134
Aspergillosis (*Aspergillus*), 139
Association, 9, 293
Asthma, 29, 203, 233, 238, 240, 242, 244
Atherosclerosis, 11, 185
Athlete's foot, 138–139
Attention Deficit Hyperactivity Disorder (ADHD), 99
Attributable Risk, 304–306
Australia, 93, 263
Austria, 263
Autism, 28, 98–99
Autoimmune disorders, 24, 28–29, 73
Autonomy, 308–309
Avian influenza (*see* Influenza)
Ayurvedic medicine, 17
AZT (*see* Zidovudine)

B

Babesiosis (*Babesia*), 131
Bacilli, 123
Back pain, 203, 238
Bacteria/bacterial infections, 123–127
  (*see also* specific infections)
The Bahamas, 222
Bahrain, 222
Bangladesh, 44, 51, 189, 241, 267
Bartering, 42
Bartonellosis (*Bartonella bacilliformis*), 124
BCG (Bacillus Calmette-Guerin), 166
Beauty, 206–207
Bednets (*see* Insecticide-treated bednets)
Behavior disorders, 99
Behavioral risk factors, 6, 140, 171–172
Beijing Declaration on Women, 70
Belgium, 263

Beneficence, 308
Benin, 42, 53
Benzene, 239
Beriberi (thiamine deficiency), 186, 193
"Best buys" in global health, 280–281
Beta-carotene (*see* Vitamin A)
Beta (β) error, 315
Bhopal, India, 240
Bias, 313
Bidil, 92
Bifidus factor, 199
"Big Mac Index", 45
Bilateral aid, 252
Bilharzia (*see* Schistosomiasis)
Bill & Melinda Gates Foundation, 252–253, 280
Binge-purge cycles, 207
Bioavailability, 192
Biodiversity, 243, 338
Biomass, 225–226, 245
Biostatistics, 4
Bioterrorism, 176–177, 179
Bipolar Disorder, 28, 98–99
Bird flu (*see* Influenza)
Birth asphyxia, 55, 58
Birth control pills (*see* Oral contraceptives)
Birth defects, 30, 59, 104–105, 185
Birth rate, 84
Birth spacing, 59, 81, 89
Birth trauma, 55–59, 74–76
Black death (*see* Plague)
Black (*Simulium*) flies, 135, 137
Bladder cancer, 28, 73, 121, 137, 241
Blindness, 28, 71, 105, 190
    Infectious causes, 103, 125–126, 137
    Vitamin A deficiency, 101–102, 186, 193–194
Blood, 187
Blood disorders, 37 (*see also* Anemia)
Blood pressure, 15–16, 61, 187 (*see also* Hypertension)
Bloodborne transmission, 116, 128
Body image, 206–207
Body Mass Index (BMI), 196
Bolivia, 51, 52, 220–221
Borehole, 216

Botswana, 21, 97, 155, 251–252, 284
Botulism (*Clostridium botulinum*), 125, 126, 176–177
Bovine spongiform encephalopathy (BSE), 138, 174, 202
Brazil, 44, 84, 85, 96, 237, 277
BRCA1 gene, 12
Breakbone fever (*see* Dengue fever)
Breast cancer, 12, 15, 28, 34–36, 73, 93–94
Breastfeeding, 59, 64, 66, 157, 189, 199–201
Breastmilk, 144, 157, 199
Breastmilk substitutes (*see* Infant formula)
Breech births, 59
Broad Street pump, 8
Bronchitis, 29, 58–61, 226
Brucellosis (*Brucella*), 125, 126, 177
Bubonic plague, 123
Bulgaria, 53
Bulimia nervosa, 99, 207
Bulls-eye rash, 172
Burkina Faso, 51, 53
Burns, 25–27, 73, 226
Buruli ulcer (*Mycobacterium ulcerans*), 125
Businesses and health, 6, 269–270

C

Cadmium, 238, 239
Cairo Conference on Population and Development, 88
Calcium, 11, 186, 187–188, 193
Cambodia, 251–252
Cameroon, 47, 51, 52, 53
Campaign for Access to Essential Medicines, 278
Campylobacteriosis (*Campylobacter jejuni*), 123, 124
Canada, 75, 93, 248, 251–252, 259, 263
Canadian Institutes of Health Research (CIHR), 259, 280
Canadian International Development Agency (CIDA), 263
Cancer, 27–28, 30, 33–36, 108, 109, 121–122, 169–170, 213 (*see also* specific cancers by site)

Infectious causes, 121–122
Incidence rates, 33–34
Mortality rates, 33–35
Survival rates, 34–36
Candidiasis (*Candida albicans*), 138, 139, 150–151
Candles, 225–226
Capsid, 128
Carbohydrates, 181–182
Carbon dioxide, 58–60, 240, 338
Carbon monoxide, 226, 240
Carcinogens, 30, 237, 238
Carcinogenesis, 30
Cardiovascular disease, 29, 33, 71, 169–170, 280–281, 287
    Risk factors, 11, 48, 108–109, 185, 203, 206, 240
CARE, 265, 266, 267, 268
Careers related to global health, 3–7, 16, 212–214
Carotene (*see* Vitamin A)
Carpal tunnel syndrome, 238
Carrier, 120
Carrying capacity, 82
Carson, Rachel, 242
Carter Center, 253, 266
Carter, Jimmy, 253
Case, 300
Case-control study, 297, 300–303
Case fatality rate, 121, 174
Caste system, 48–49
Cataracts, 28, 73, 103, 244
Catholic Agency for Overseas Development (CAFOD), 267
Catholic Medical Mission Board, 266
Catholic Relief Services, 265, 266
Causal web, 11–12
Causation, 9–13
Causes of death by world region, 31–36
CD4 cells, 149–152
CDC (U.S. Centers for Disease Control and Prevention), 259, 291–292
Cellular respiration, 181
Central African Republic, 155
Cerebral malaria, 62–63, 159

Cerebral palsy, 28, 104–105, 190
Cerebrovascular disease (*see* Stroke)
Cervical cancer, 15, 28, 34–36, 122
Cesarean section, 59, 74–76
Chad, 51, 52
Chagas Disease (American Sleeping Sickness, *Trypanosoma cruzi*), 131–132, 230–231, 278
Chancre, 126
Charcoal, 225–226
Chernobyl, Ukraine, 240
Chickenpox (varicella), 128, 129, 343
Chikungunya fever, 129
Child abuse, 25, 67, 69–70
Child growth, 50, 65–66, 196–197
Child health, 3, 50–51, 55–70
    Infectious disease, 55–64, 126, 128, 133, 138, 157, 158–162
    Injury, 58, 67, 226
    Mortality, 21, 51, 55–64, 167, 284, 337, 340
    Neonatal conditions, 55–58, 59, 337
    Nutrition, 64, 189–197, 199–201
    Programs, 65–70, 280–281
Child labor, 69–70, 330
Child spacing, 59, 81, 89
Childbirth (*see* Pregnancy)
Children International, 266
Chile, 299–300
China, 84, 85, 111, 120, 138, 155, 170, 221, 237
    Population planning policies, 88
Chiropracty, 17
Chi-squared (χ^2) test, 312
Chlamydia (*Chlamydia trachomatis*), 124, 126
Chloride, 187
Cholera (*Vibrio cholerae*), 8–9, 61, 117, 118, 123, 124, 174, 177, 212, 232, 244
Chloroquine, 132, 160
Cholesterol, 185
Christian Aid, 267
Christian Children's Fund, 266
Chromosomes, 37, 70
Chronic, 121, 142

Chronic conditions, 27–30 (*see also* Non-communicable conditions and specific chronic conditions)

Chronic Obstructive Pulmonary Disease (COPD), 29, 73, 108, 109, 238, 240

Church World Service, 265, 266, 268

Circumcision–Female (*see* Female genital mutilation)

Circumcision–Male, 157

Cirrhosis, 26, 29, 73

Cleft lip/cleft palate, 104

Climate, 141, 213–214, 242–245

Climate change, 242–245

Clinical trial, 297, 306–308

Clonorchiasis (*Clonorchis sinensis*), 134

Clusters, 143

Coal, 225–226

Coca-colonization, 206

Cocci, 123

Coccidioidomycosis (*Coccidioides immitis*), 139

Cochabamba, Bolivia, 220–221

Cohort, 303

Cohort study, 10, 297, 303–306

Colds (viral), 60, 121, 128, 129

Collapse: How Societies Choose to Fail or Succeed, 230–231

Collective violence, 25

Colombia, 53, 100, 174

Colorectal cancer (colon cancer), 28, 34–36

Colostrum, 199

Commercial sex workers (CSWs), 155–156

Communicable (infectious) diseases, 30–33, 115–177 (*see also* specific diseases)

Communication technologies, 43, 227, 234, 339

Community development organizations, 265–267

Community health, 4–7, 240–242 (*see also* Public health)

Compassion International, 266

Complementary/Alternative Medicine (CAM), 16–17

Complementary feeding, 64, 66, 199

Complementary protein, 182

Complete protein, 182

Condoms, 76, 77, 79, 156–157, 337

95% Confidence interval (95% CI), 310–311

Confounding, 313–314

Congestive heart failure (CHF), 29

The Constant Gardener, 310

Contraception, 52, 76–79, 88

Control (of disease in a population), 118–119, 144–146 (*see also* Vector control)

Control (in epidemiological research), 300

Convention on the Prohibition of the Use, Stockpiling, Production, and Transfer of Anti-Personnel Mines and on Their Destruction, 106

Convention on the Rights of the Child, 69, 329–330

COPD (*see* Chronic Obstructive Pulmonary Disease)

Copper, 187

Copyrights, 278–279

Corneal ulceration, 193

Correlation, 296–298

Cost-effectiveness, 283, 286–287

Côte d'Ivoire, 155

Cretinism, 188, 194

Creutzfeldt-Jakob Disease (CJD), 138

Cri du Chat Syndrome, 38

Crimean-Congo hemorrhagic fever, 129

Crop rotation, 208

Cross-sectional survey, 297, 299–300

Crowding, 42, 141, 163, 233, 234

Cryptococcosis (*Cryptococcus neoformans*), 139, 150–151

Cryptosporidiosis (*Cryptosporidium*), 130, 131, 177, 232

Culture, 2, 16–17, 64, 92–93, 170, 206–207, 274

Culture of dependency, 269

Cutaneous leishmaniasis, 132

Cut-off point, 317–318

Cutting, 25

Cycle of displacement, 95–96

Cycle of disease and poverty, 285–286 (*see also* Poverty and health)

Cycle of infection, 118
Cystic fibrosis (CF), 29, 37

D

DALY (disability-adjusted life year), 101–102, 286–287
Dams, 137–138, 171–172, 232
DDT (dichloro-diphenyl-trichyloroethane), 238, 241–242
Deafness, 28, 101–102, 105
Death rate, 84
Debt repayment, 253–256, 339
Deer flies (*Chrysops*), 135
Deer tick (*Ixodes scapularis*), 124, 172
Deforestation, 171–172, 226, 230–232, 243
Dehydration, 61, 187, 189
Delusional disorders, 99
Delusions, 98–99
Dementia, 28, 73, 98–99, 108, 110
Democratic Republic of the Congo, 84, 85
Demographic transition, 86–87, 169
Demography, 83–87
Denatured proteins, 138–139
Dengue fever, 117, 129, 144–145, 172, 231–232, 244
Denmark, 47, 252, 263
Dental health, 3–4, 29, 188, 248
Dependency ratio, 85
Depression and depressive disorders, 28, 73, 98–99, 108
Dermatomycoses, 138–139
Descriptive epidemiology, 7, 122
Desertification, 208, 243
Development organizations (*see* Community development organizations)
Developmental disorders, 30, 98–99
DFID (U.K. Department for International Development), 263, 264
Diabetes, 9–11, 28, 73, 108, 109, 203, 206, 317
Diamond, Jared, 230–231
Diaper rash, 138, 139
Diaphragm, 76, 79

Diarrhea
  Causes, 11–12, 117, 123, 124, 129, 130, 150–151, 193, 231–232, 244
  Children, 55–57, 58, 61–63, 157, 189
  Prevention, 66, 223–225
Diet (*see* Nutrition)
Digitalis, 16
Dioxins, 238
Diphtheria (*Corynebacterium diphtheriae*), 125, 126, 343
Direct transmission, 116–117, 123
Directed donation, 267–268
Disability, 13, 14, 30, 98, 101–106
Disaccharide, 182
Disasters (*see* Natural disasters)
Disasters Emergency Committee, 267
Disease, 119–120
Disease Control Priorities Project, 279–281
Diseases of affluence, 206 (*see also* Non-communicable conditions)
Diseases of Workers, 237, 245
Disparities (*see* Health inequalities)
Distributive justice, 309–311
DNA (deoxyribonucleic acid), 37
Doctors (*see* Medicine)
Doctors Without Borders (Médecins Sans Frontières, MSF), 265, 278
Domains of activity and participation, 104
Domestic violence (*see* Interpersonal violence)
Dominant genes, 37
Dominican Republic, 53
Donor countries, 252, 256, 259–264
Donor-driven aid, 267–268
Dose-response effect, 10
DOTS (Directly-Observed Therapy, Short-course), 163–166, 338
DOTS Plus, 166
Double-blind studies, 307
Down Syndrome (Trisomy, 21), 37
Dracunculiasis (Guinea worm disease, *Dracunculus medinensis*), 133–137, 145, 253
Drought, 208, 244
Drowning, 24–27, 73, 231, 244
Drug abuse, 28, 73, 98–99

Drug companies, 277–278
Drug resistance (*see* Antimicrobial resistance)
Drug sales (*see* Pharmaceutical sales)
Dry eye, 193
Duchenne muscular dystrophy, 38
Dung, 225–226
Durban Declaration, 39–40

E

Easter Island, 230
Eastern Equine Encephalitis, 129, 177
Eating disorders, 99, 207
Eating practices, 64, 207
Ebola, 129, 174, 176–177
Echinococcosis (*Echinococcus granulosus*), 134
Eclampsia, 73–74
E. coli, 61, 123, 124, 173, 177, 201–202
E. coli O157:H7, 123, 173, 177, 201–202
Ecological fallacy, 298–299
Ecological footprint, 82
Ecological survey, 296–299
Economic indicators, 43–47
Ectoparasite, 133
Ecuador, 174
Edema, 189
Education and educational level, 6, 11, 50–54, 140, 336
Effect modification, 314
Efficacy, 307
Egypt, 44, 138, 173, 222
Ehrlichiosis (*Ehrlichia*), 124
Elder abuse, 25, 72
Elderly support ratio, 85
Electricity, 12, 43, 225–227, 234, 235
Electrolytes, 61–62, 187
Elephatiasis (*see* Lymphatic filariasis)
Elimination, 145, 160
Emergency response, 95–96
Emerging infectious diseases, 171–175, 177 (*see also* specific diseases)
Emphysema, 29
Employee benefits, 48, 249–250
Employment, 6, 48–49

Encephalitis, 124, 129, 151
Endemic, 143
Endoparasite, 133
Endotoxin, 126
Energy, 225–227, 338
Enterobiasis (*Enterobius vermicularis*), 134
Enrichment of food, 192
Environment, 105, 140–141
    Risk factors, 25–26, 110, 140–141, 213–214, 230, 231
Environmental change, 158, 229–237, 242–245
Environmental Health, 4, 144–145, 211–227, 229–245
    History, 211–212
    Indoor air quality, 225–227
    Industrial/occupational health, 214, 237–240
    Laws, regulations, and policies, 6
    Sanitation, 222–225
    Water, 215–222
EPI (Expanded Programme on Immunization), 65–66
Epidemic, 8, 143
Epidemiologic transition, 169–170
Epidemiology, 4–5, 7
    Study designs, 296–308
Epilepsy, 24, 28, 98
Equilibrium theory of health, 17
Eradication, 128, 145–146
Ergonomics, 214
Escherichia coli (*see E. coli*)
Esophageal cancer, 28, 34–35, 73
Essential amino acids, 182
Ethics (*see* Research ethics and Health as a human right)
Ethics committee (*see* Institutional Review Board)
Ethnic minorities, 92–94
Ethnicity, 92
Etiology, 23
Evidence-Based Medicine (EBM), 294
Excess risk (RD), 304–306
Exclusive breastfeeding, 64, 66, 199–200
Exotoxin, 126

Expanded Programme on Immunization (EPI), 65–66
Expatriates ("expats"), 268
Exposure, 8, 119–120, 293
External validity, 314
Extinction, 145
Eukaryote, 132–133

F

Faith-based organizations (FBOs), 265
Falls, 11, 25–27, 73
False negative, 315–316
False positive, 315–316
Family planning, 66, 76–81
Family planning pill (*see* Oral contraceptives)
Famine, 207–208
FAO (Food and Agriculture Organization of the United Nations), 260, 262, 336, 338
Farmer, Paul, 275–276, 286
Farr, William, 9
Fascioliasis (*Fasciola hepatica*), 134
Fasciolopsiasis (*Fasciolopsis buski*), 134
Fats, 182–185
Fat-soluble vitamins, 189, 193–194
Fatty acids, 182–185
FDA (U.S. Food and Drug Administration), 92
Fecal-oral transmission, 11, 123, 134, 223, 232
Feed the Children, 266
Female education, 50–53, 66, 81, 234
Female genital mutilation (FGM), 69, 72, 76
Female literacy, 50–53
Fertility, 77, 80, 81, 84, 86, 110–111, 169
Fiber, 182
Fiji, 207
Filariasis, 134–137
Filters (*see* Air filters, Water filters)
Finland, 263
Fistula (*see* Obstetric fistula)
Flagellates, 131
Flatworms, 133–137

Fleas, 123–125
Flies, 135, 137, 223
Floods, 243–244
Flour, 192, 195
Fluoride, 187–188
Fluorosis, 187
Flying toilet, 223
Fogarty International Center, 279
Folate/Folate deficiency, 59, 185, 186, 192
Folic acid (*see* Folate)
Fomite, 117
Food and Agriculture Organization of the United Nations (FAO), 260, 262
Food and Drug Administration (FDA), 92
Food production, 66, 201–203, 208
Food safety, 201–203, 212–213
Food security, 207
Foodborne transmission, 116–117, 123
Fortification of food, 192, 193–196, 203
Fracture, 7, 11, 24
Framework Convention on Tobacco Control, 240, 258–259
Framingham Heart Study, 306
France, 248, 252, 263
Free radicals, 185
Freedom from Hunger, 265
Freshwater resources, 217, 221, 243
Fructose, 181–182
Fuel, 6, 43, 225–227, 235, 284, 338
Functional impairment, 102
Functional literacy, 50
Fungi/fungal infections, 138–139, 150–151

G

G8 nations, 256
Gallstones, 29, 203
Gang violence, 25
Garbage (*see* Waste)
Gates, Bill, 19, 285, 288
Gates Foundation (*see* Bill & Melinda Gates Foundation)
Gates, Melinda, 285
Gender, 70–72
Gender roles, 70–72, 337

General Agreement on Tariffs and Trade (GATT), 279

General Agreement on Trade in Services (GATS), 279

General Assembly of the United Nations, 258, 260

Generalizability, 314

Generic drugs, 277–279

Genes, 37

Genetic mutations, 30

Genetics/Genetic disorders, 12, 29–30, 37–38, 92, 206

Genetically modified organism (GMO), 194, 203

Geneva Convention, 269

Genocide, 92

Genotype, 37

Geology, 141, 213

German measles (*see* Rubella)

Germany, 111, 248, 251–252, 263

Ghana, 53

Giardiasis (*Giardia*), 130, 131

Gini Index, 45–47

Glanders (*Burkholderia mallei*), 177

Glaucoma, 28, 73

Global Alliance for Improved Nutrition (GAIN), 253

Global Alliance for Vaccines and Immunizations (GAVI), 253

Global environmental change, 242–245

Global Fund to Fight AIDS, Malaria, and Tuberculosis (GFATM), 253

Global health, 1–2

Global health priorities, 279–283

Global Plan to Stop TB, 285

Global warming (*see* Climate change)

Globalization, 170–171, 201–203, 244–245

Glucose, 181–182

GOBI (Growth monitoring, ORT, Breastfeeding, Immunizations), 65–66

GOBI/FFF, 65–66

Goiter, 188, 194

Golden rice, 194

Gonorrhea (*Neisseria gonorrhoeae*), 124, 126, 127

Government-sponsored health care systems, 247–251, 256–257

Governmental responsibilities for health, 3, 208, 256–257, 276–277

Gram-negative bacteria, 123, 126

Gram-positive bacteria, 123

Grameen Bank, 267

Grand Challenges in Global Health, 280, 282

Gravidity, 77

Greece, 263

Gross domestic product (GDP), 41, 44–45, 47

Gross national income (GNI), 44–46

Gross national product (GNP), 44–45

Group A *Strep* (*Streptococcus*), 125, 126

Growth monitoring, 65–66, 197

Growth standards, 196–197

GTZ (Germany's Deutsche Gesellschaft für Technische Zusammenarbeit), 263

Guinea, 251–252

Guinea worm disease (dracunculiasis, *Dracunculus medinensis*), 133–137, 145, 253

H

H5N1 influenza (*see* Influenza)

HAART (Highly Active Anti-Retroviral Therapy), 152, 155, 157

Habitat for Humanity, 265

Haemophilus influenzae type B (Hib), 61, 125, 343

Haiti, 17, 275

Hallucinations, 98

Hand-washing (*see* Hygiene)

Hansen's Disease (leprosy, *Mycobacterium leprae*), 119, 125, 126

Hantavirus, 129, 172, 177, 244

HDL (high-density lipoprotein) cholesterol, 185

Health, 2, 3, 326

Health as a human right, 273–277

Health behavior, 6, 13–14, 17, 110, 198

Health beliefs, 16–17

Health care access, 3, 5–6, 14, 20, 50, 52, 235, 277
Health care costs, 43, 247–253, 285–288
Health disparities (*see* Health inequalities)
Health economics, 4, 40–47, 247–253
Health education, 3, 4, 5, 13, 62, 68
"Health for All by 2000," 65
Health inequalities, 1–3, 20–23, 43, 74
    By country, 20–22, 42, 44, 47, 51–53, 56, 75, 80, 84–85, 100, 111, 153, 161, 164, 191, 204–205, 219, 224, 251–252, 284
    By income level, 30, 33–36, 41–43, 48–49, 64, 103, 116 (*see also* Poverty and health)
    By sex, 26–27, 70–72, 73, 156
    By world region, 23, 24, 31–36, 39–40, 53–57, 61, 63, 74, 102, 108–109, 154, 162, 165, 190, 195, 200, 220, 225, 226
Health inequities, 20–21
Health insurance, 6, 17, 48, 247–251
Health policy, 3, 4, 5–7
Health services administration, 4–5, 256–257
Hearing impairment/hearing loss, 28, 105, 108, 212, 214, 237–238 (*see also* Deafness)
Heart attack (myocardial infarction), 71, 185, 287 (*see also* Cardiovascular disease)
Heart disease (*see* Cardiovascular disease)
Heat waves, 243–244
Heifer Project International, 265
Height-for-age, 189, 196
Helen Keller International, 265
Helicobacter pylori, 121, 125
Helminths/Helminth infections, 132–138, 223–225, 231–232 (*see also* specific agents)
Hemagglutinin, 175
Heme iron, 188, 195
Hemochromatosis, 29
Hemoglobin, 182, 188, 194–195

Hemophilia, 29, 38
Hemorrhagic fevers, 129, 174, 176–177 (*see also* specific types)
Hepatitis A virus, 12, 117, 119, 129, 202, 343
Hepatitis B virus, 73, 128–129, 130, 343
Hepatitis C virus, 73, 121, 129, 130
Herbal remedies, 16–17
Herd immunity, 144
Herpes (Herpes simplex virus, HSV-2), 129, 130, 151
Hinduism, 48–49
Hippocrates, 17, 211
Histoplasmosis (*Histoplasma capsulatum*), 138, 139
HIV/AIDS, 129–130, 149–157, 280–281
    Africa, 152–155, 156
    AIDS (Acquired Immunodeficiency Syndrome), 149–152
    Asia, 155–156
    Cause of, 39–40
    Children, 58, 157, 167, 199
    Drugs, 152, 155, 157, 277–278, 287
    HIV-1 (Human Immunodeficiency Virus type, 1), 149, 168
    HIV-2 (Human Immunodeficiency Virus type, 2), 149
    Incidence/Prevalence, 152–155, 284, 285, 337
    Opportunistic infections, 138, 149–152
    Orphans, 155, 338
    Prevention, 156, 157, 341
    Risk Factors, 155–157, 167
    Stages, 150–152
    TB co-infection, 150, 151, 163
    Treatment, 152, 155, 157, 167
    Women, 154, 156–157
Holistic approaches to health, 17
Homeopathic remedies, 17
Honduras, 53, 111, 251–252
Hookworm, 118, 133, 135, 136, 195
Hormone replacement therapy (HRT), 294, 308
Host, 118, 139–140

Household size (*see* Crowding)
Housing construction, 42, 214–215, 231, 234
Human Development Index (HDI), 40–41
Human Development Report (HDR), 291–292
Human Immunodeficiency Virus (*see* HIV)
Human papillomavirus (HPV), 122, 129, 130, 343
Human rights, 221, 273–276
Human trafficking, 69, 72
Human Rights Watch, 267
Humanitarian aid, 262–270
Hunger, 207–208 (*see also* Undernutrition)
Huntington Disease, 12, 28, 37
Hydatid cyst (*see* Echinococcosis)
Hygiene, 11–12, 62, 66, 198, 215, 223–225, 286
Hymenolepiasis (*Hymenolepsis nana*), 135
Hypertension (high blood pressure), 29, 108, 187–188, 203, 206, 317
Hypoglycemia, 189
Hypothermia, 59, 189
Hypothyroidism, 188
Hypovolemic shock, 187
Hypoxia, 59

I

IBRD (International Bank for Reconstruction and Development), 253–254
IDA (International Development Association), 253–254
Idiopathic, 24
ILO (International Labor Organization), 239, 260, 337, 339
IMCI (Integrated Management of Childhood Illness), 65–68
IMF (International Monetary Fund), 252–256, 260, 339
Immigrants, 94–96
Immune system, 28–29, 121, 144, 175, 233

Immunization, 13, 66, 121, 128, 129, 144, 147, 281–282, 286, 287
Childhood recommendations, 343
Immunoglobulin (Ig), 144, 199
Immunosuppression, 138, 149–152
Impairment, 101–103
Impetigo, 125
Impulse control disorders, 98–99
Inactivity (*see* Physical inactivity)
Incidence, 142–143
Incidence rate, 303–304
Income, 6, 42, 50, 140
Incubation period, 119–120
India, 48–49, 84, 85, 96, 111, 155, 170, 189, 237, 240, 251–252, 277, 284, 302–303
Indian Health Service (IHS), 249
Indigenous peoples, 93, 95–96, 170, 176, 206
Indonesia, 44, 237
Indoor air pollution, 213, 225–227, 230–231, 233, 235
Induced abortion (*see* Abortion)
Industrial accidents, 240
Industrial health, 214, 237–240
Inequalities (*see* Health inequalities)
Inequities (*see* Health Inequities)
Infant formula, 157, 199–201
Infant mortality, 44, 55–57, 58, 59, 75, 169
Infection, 119–120
Infectious diseases, 30–33, 115–177 (*see also* specific diseases)
Infectivity, 119–120
Infertility, 126
Inflammation, 28–29
Influenza, 117, 118, 121, 128, 129, 171, 174–175, 343
Information bias, 313
Information sources, 291–293
Informed consent, 94, 308–309
Injecting drug use (IDU), 155–156
Injury, 24–27, 32, 33, 58, 67, 102, 108, 226, 238, 280–281 (*see also* specific types of injury)

Insect-borne transmission (*see* Vectorborne transmission)
Insecticide, 160, 232, 238, 241–242
Insecticide-treated bednets (ITNs), 59, 63, 66, 162, 286
Institute of Medicine, 171
Institutional Review Board (IRB), 94, 257, 308–310
Insulin, 9–11
Insurance (*see* Health insurance)
Integrated Management of Childhood Illness (IMCI), 65–68
Intentional injury, 24–27, 71
Interferon, 130
Intergovernmental Panel on Climate Change (IPCC), 243
Intermediate hosts, 118
Internal validity, 314
Internally displaced person (IDP), 94–96
International Bank for Reconstruction and Development (IBRD), 253–254
International Classification of Functioning, Disability, and Health (ICF), 104–105, 112
International Code of Marketing of Breast-milk Substitutes, 200–201
International Committee of the Red Cross (*see* Red Cross)
International Court of Justice, 258, 260
International development and cooperation agencies, 262–265
International Development Association (IDA), 253–254
International health, 1–2
International Labor Organization (ILO), 238, 260, 337, 339
International Medical Corps, 266
International Monetary Fund (IMF), 252–256, 260, 339
International Rescue Committee, 265, 266
Interpersonal violence, 25–27, 71–72, 304–305
Inter-rater agreement, 315–316
Intervention, 16–17 (*see also* specific interventions)
Intrauterine device (IUD), 77

Iodine/Iodine deficiency disorders (IDD), 59, 188, 194
Iran, 53
Ireland, 263
Iron/Iron deficiency anemia (IDA), 59, 73, 186, 187, 188, 192, 194–195
Irrigation, 208, 232
Islamic Relief, 265, 267
Isolation, 117
Israel, 222
Italy, 111, 248, 263
IUD (intrauterine device), 77
Ivermectin, 137
IVF (*in vitro* fertilization), 275

J

Jacob Syndrome, 37
Japan, 20, 21, 24, 111, 201, 208, 237, 248–249, 252, 263, 264
Japanese encephalitis, 129, 231–232
Jaundice, 128
JICA (Japan International Cooperation Agency), 263, 264
Job security, 48, 239
Jordan, 222

K

Kala azar (visceral leishmaniasis), 131, 132, 278
Kangaroo mother care, 59
KAP (knowledge, attitude, practice), 198
Kaposi's Sarcoma, 150, 151
Kappa (κ) coefficient, 315–316
Kenya, 51, 75, 155
Kerosene lamps, 225–226
Kidney disease, 29, 241
Kilimanjaro Programme of Action, 90
Kissing bugs, 131, 132
Klinefelter Syndrome, 37
Knock knees (*see* Rickets)
Kuru, 139
Kuwait, 222
Kwashiorkor, 189
Kyoto Protocol, 240

L

Lactobacillus bifidus, 199
Lactose, 181
Lactose intolerance, 61–62
Landmine Monitor, 106
Landmines, 106–108
Lassa fever, 129, 177
"Late, long, few" policy in China, 88
Latent stage, 119–120, 150
Latrine, 222–223
LDL (low-density lipoprotein) cholesterol,
    185
Lead, 214, 238, 239
Lebanon, 100
Legionnaire's Disease (legionellosis,
    Legionellae), 124, 173
Leishmaniasis (*Leishmania*), 73, 131, 132,
    232, 278
Leprosy (Hansen's Disease, *Mycobac-
    terium leprae*), 119, 125, 126
Leptospirosis (*Leptospira interrogans*), 124
Lesotho, 21, 155
Leukemia, 28, 36, 238
Libya, 222
Lice, 133
Life expectancy, 20–23, 35, 40–41, 47, 71,
    110, 155, 169
Lifestyle disease, 170 (*see also*
    Non-communicable conditions)
Lind, James, 237
Lipids, 182–185
Listeriosis (*Listeria monocytogenes*), 124,
    202
Literacy, 6, 41, 50–54, 336
Liver cancer (hepatocellular carcinoma
    and others), 28, 34–35, 121
Loans, 253–256
Logistic organizations, 267
Loiasis (*Loa loa*), 135
Low birthweight (LBW), 59, 63, 159, 190,
    304–305
Lower respiratory infections
    (*see* Pneumonia)
Lung cancer, 7, 28, 34–35, 48, 73, 213,
    214, 226, 238, 241

Lupus (Sytemic Lupus Erythematosus,
    SLE), 28, 73
Lutheran World Relief, 265
Luxembourg, 252, 263
Lyme Disease (*Borrelia burgdorferi*), 117,
    124, 172, 232
Lymphatic filariasis (LF), 73, 134, 137, 231
Lymphoma, 28

M

Machupo virus, 177
Macroeconomic indicators, 43–47
Macronutrients, 181–185
"Mad cow" disease (*see* Bovine
    spongiform encephalopathy)
Madagascar, 51, 53, 97
Magnesium, 187
Malaria, 131, 158–162, 280–282, 285, 287
    Agent (*Plasmodium*), 130–131, 158, 159
    Anemia, 158–160
    Cerebral malaria, 62–63, 169
    Children, 57–58, 62–63, 68, 159–160,
        167, 190, 193
    Combination therapy, 160, 287
    Drug resistance, 132, 160–162
    Incidence/Prevalence, 63, 158, 160, 161,
        162, 167, 284, 338
    Pregnancy, 59, 63, 158–159
    Prevention, 59, 63, 66, 160–162, 241–
        242, 286, 338, 342
    Risk Factors, 158, 160, 190, 193, 195,
        214, 230–232, 244
    Transmission, 117, 118, 130–131, 141,
        158
    Treatment, 132, 160
Malaysia, 221
Malawi, 44, 155
Maldives, 222
Malnutrition, 12, 31, 57, 62, 64, 189–196,
    203–206, 231, 244
Malta, 222
Malta fever (Brucellosis, *Brucella*), 125,
    126, 177
Malthus, Thomas, 82–83
Malthusian catastrophes, 83

Mammograms, 15
Manganese, 187
Mantoux test for TB, 166
Manual laborers, 48–49
MAP International, 267
Marasmus, 189
Marburg virus, 129, 174, 176–177
Marie Stopes International, 267
Marriage/marital status, 20, 140, 156–157
Massage, 17
Maternal and child health (MCH), 55 (see also Child health, Pregnancy, and other related topics)
Maternal literacy, 50–53
Maternal mortality (death), 72–75, 284, 337, 340
Mauritania, 222
Mbeki, Thabo, 39–40, 54
MDGs (Millennium Development Goals), 282–284, 285
MDR-TB (Multidrug-resistant TB), 97, 127, 166
Measles, 57, 58, 63–64, 118, 119, 128, 129, 146, 190, 193, 343
Mechanistic theory of health, 17
Medicaid, 249
Medical research (see Research)
Medical Research Council (MRC), 259
Medical technology, 275–276, 282, 286
Medicare, 248, 249
Medicine, 3–5, 16
Medicines for Malaria Venture (MMV), 285
Médecins Sans Frontières (MSF, Doctors Without Borders), 265, 278
Mefloquine (Lariam), 160
Meliodosis (Burkholderia pseudomallei), 177
Memory loss, 2
Meningitis, 124, 129, 151, 244
Meningococcus, 124, 343
Men's health, 26–27, 70–73
Mental health/mental illness, 28, 95, 98–101, 108, 232
Mental retardation, 98–99, 190
Mercury, 202, 238, 239

Mercy Corps, 266
Merozoites, 159
Metabolism, 186, 193
Methicillin-resistant Staphylococcus aureus (MRSA), 126–127
Methyl isocyanate, 240
Mexico, 174, 202, 206, 237, 284
Miasma, 212
Microcredit programs, 265–267
Microfilariae, 137
Microloans, 265–267
Micronutrients, 181, 185–188, 190–196
Mid-upper arm circumference (MUAC), 197
Migraine headaches, 28, 73
Migration, 94–96, 142, 232
Millennium Development Goals (MDGs), 282–284, 285, 336–339
Mine Ban Treaty, 106
Minerals, 187–188, 194–196
Ministry of Health, 256–257
Miscarriage (spontaneous abortion), 77, 202
Misclassification, 313
MMWR (Morbidity and Mortality Weekly Report), 18
Modes of transmission, 116–118
Modifiable risk factors, 6, 140
Mold, 138, 214
Mole checks, 15
Molluscicides, 137, 145
Mongol expansion, 170
Mononucleosis, 129
Monounsaturated fatty acids, 185
Mood disorders, 98–99
Morbidity, 4
Morocco, 51, 53
Mortality, 4
Mortality rate, 84
Mosquito nets, 59, 63, 66, 162, 286
Mosquitoes, 117, 128, 130, 131, 141, 145, 158–159, 172, 173, 214, 232, 244
Mother-to-child (MTC) transmission, 59, 116, 118, 149, 157, 287
Mouth cancer, 28, 73
Mozambique, 51, 52, 53

MRSA (Methicillin-resistant *Staphylococcus aureus*), 126
MSF (Médecins Sans Frontières, Doctors Without Borders), 265, 278
Mucocutaneous leishmaniasis, 132
Multidrug-resistant TB (MDR-TB), 97, 127, 166
Multifactorial conditions, 9–11
Multilateral aid, 252
Multiple sclerosis (MS), 11, 28
Multivitamins (*see* Supplementation)
Mumps, 128–129, 343
Muscular dystrophy (MD), 29, 38
Mutations, 30
Mycobacterium tuberculosis (*see* Tuberculosis)

N

Namibia, 47, 155
National Health Service, 249
National health systems, 248–251
National Institutes of Health (NIH), 259, 279, 280, 292
Natural disasters, 94–96, 141, 172, 208, 243–244
Natural history of disease, 15, 119–120
Necessary, 11–12
Negative predictive value (NPV), 316–317
Neglected diseases, 278
Neisseria meningitides (*see* Meningitis)
Nematodes, 134–135
Neonatal conditions, 55–57, 58, 59, 75, 287
Neoplasms (*see* Cancer)
Nepal, 42
Nestlé, 200–201
The Netherlands, 252, 263
Neural tube defects, 59, 185–186
Neuraminidase, 175
New World Syndrome, 206
New Zealand, 93, 263
NGOs (Non-governmental organizations), 265–269
Niacin, 186, 193
Niger, 84, 85
Nigeria, 42, 51, 52, 53, 84, 85, 251–252

Night blindness, 186, 193
NIH (U.S. National Institutes of Health), 259, 279, 280, 305
Nipah virus, 129, 177
Nitrogen, 123
Nitrogen oxide, 226, 240
Noise/Noise control, 213, 214, 230
Non-communicable conditions, 27–30, 31–36, 101, 102, 108, 169–170
Non-governmental organizations (NGOs), 265–269
Non-heme iron, 188, 195
Nonmaleficence, 309
Norovirus, 129
Norplant, 77–78
Norway, 252, 263
Norwegian Agency for Development Cooperation (NORAD), 263
Nosocomial (hospital-acquired) infections, 173
Null results, 294–295
Nurses (*see* Medicine)
Nutrition, 13, 31, 181–209, 235, 280, 341
  Child, 64, 189–197, 199–201
  Macronutrients, 181–185
  Micronutrients (Vitamins and Minerals), 181, 185–188, 190–196
  Overnutrition, 203–206
  Undernutrition, 64, 189–196
Nutrition behavior, 198
Nutrition transition, 206

O

Obesity, 170, 196, 203–206, 213, 317
Obsessive-compulsive disorder, 28, 99
Obstetric fistula, 76
Obstructed labor, 73, 74–76
Occupation, 48–49, 140 (*see also* Employment)
Occupational hazards, 26, 106, 128, 214, 233, 235, 237–240
Occupational health, 214, 237–240
Occupational therapy, 106
Odds, 301–302
Odds Ratio (OR), 301–302, 304

Official development assistance (ODA), 252

OHCHR (Office of the UN High Commissioner for Human Rights), 258, 261, 276

Oils, 182–185

Older adults (*see* Aging)

Omega-3 fatty acids, 185

Onchocerciasis (River Blindness), 103, 135, 137, 232

One child policy in China, 88

Opportunistic Infections (OIs), 150–152

Oral contraceptives, 77–78

Oral Rehydration Solution (ORS)/Oral Rehydration Therapy (ORT), 14, 51, 62, 63, 66, 67, 68

Organ transplantation, 173, 275–276

Organic food, 245

Orphan drugs, 278

Osteoarthritis (Arthritis), 29, 73, 103, 108, 110, 203

Osteomalacia, 186, 193

Osteoporosis, 7, 11, 29, 108, 188, 193

Outbreak, 142, 143

Outcome, 8, 293

Outhouse, 222–223

Out-of-pocket health payments, 248–251

Ovarian cancer, 12, 28

Overgrazing, 208

Overhunting/overfishing, 230–231

Overnutrition, 203–206 (*see also* Obesity, Overweight)

Overweight, 196, 203, 206, 213

Ovulation, 76–77

Oxfam, 265, 267

Oxygen, 58–60, 194–195

Ozone depletion, 243–244, 338

P

Paid sex, 155–156

Pakistan, 84, 85, 189

Palliative care, 13–14

Pancreatic cancer, 28

Pandemic, 143

Panic Disorder, 29, 73, 99

Pap smear, 15

Paragonimiasis (*Paragonimus*), 135

Paralysis, 101

Paramecium, 130

Parasite, 132–133

Paratyphoid fever (*Salmonella* Paratyphi), 123, 124

Parity, 77

Parkinson's Disease, 11, 24, 28, 110

Particulate matter, 226, 240

Parvovirus, 129

Passive immunity, 144

Pasteurization, 126

Patents, 278–279

PATH, 266

Pathogenesis, 23

Pathogenicity, 119–120, 146

Pathologies of Power, 275

PCBs (polychlorinated biphenyls), 239

Peace, 3

Peer review, 292–293

Pellagra (niacin deficiency), 186, 193

Pelvic Inflammatory Disease (PID), 29, 126

Penicillin, 31, 94

Pension plans, 111

Peptidoglycan, 123

Percussion therapy, 29

Perinatal conditions, 31, 55–57, 58, 59, 75

Periodic abstinence, 76, 79

Person-Place-Time, 7–8, 122

Person years, 303

Person-to-person transmission (*see* Direct transmission)

Personalistic theory of health, 17

Pertussis (whooping cough, *Bordatella pertussis*), 125, 126, 343

Peru, 75, 174

Pesticides, 160, 232, 235, 238, 241–242

Pharmaceutical sales, 21, 24, 277–279, 339

Phases of drug trials, 307

Phenylalanine, 30

Phenylketonuria (PKU), 29–30

Phenotype, 37

Philippines, 51, 52, 53, 75

Phosphorus, 186, 187

PhRMA (Pharmaceutical Research and Manufacturers of America), 278, 288–289

Physical impairment, 101–106

Physical inactivity, 11, 170, 213, 235
Physical therapy, 104–106
Pima Indians, 206
Pinworm, 133, 134
Pit latrine, 222–223
Placebo, 305, 307
Plague (*Yersinia pestis*), 117, 123, 125, 176–177, 232
Plan International, 267
Planned Parenthood, 88, 267
Planned urbanization, 233–235
Plasmodium, 130, 131, 141, 158–159, 162
Play, 66, 69, 330
Pneumococcal pneumonia (*Streptococcus pneumoniae*), 124, 343
Pneumocystis carinii pneumonia (PCP), 138, 150, 151
Pneumonia, 55–57, 58–61, 109, 124, 150–151, 174, 226, 231–232
Pneumonic plague, 123
Poisoning, 25–27, 73, 231–232
Poland, 84, 85
Policy (*see* Health policy)
Polio (poliomyelitis), 101, 128, 129, 145, 343
Polyaromatic compounds, 226
Polycyclic aromatic hydrocarbons (PAHs), 239, 240
Polysaccharides, 181–182
Polyunsaturated fatty acids, 182, 185
Poly-X Syndrome, 37
Pooled risk, 248, 249
Population Council, 267
Population density, 82, 141, 230–231
Population growth, 82–83, 84, 230–231
Population planning, 86, 88–89
Population pyramid, 85–87
Population Reference Bureau, 279
Portal of entry, 117, 171
Portugal, 263
Positive predictive value (PPV), 316–317
Positive pressure room, 117
Post-Exposure Prophylaxis, 130, 152, 177
Postpartum hemorrhage (bleeding), 73–74
Post-Traumatic Stress Disorder (PTSD), 28, 73, 96, 99
Potassium, 61, 62, 187–188

Pott, Percival, 237
Poverty and health, 11–12, 20–21, 25–26, 30, 39–40, 41–47, 103, 189–190, 192, 243–244, 251, 336
Power (social), 91
Power (statistical), 311
PPD test for TB, 166
Praziquantel, 137
Precision, 314–315
Pre-eclampsia, 73
Pregnancy, 11, 31, 59, 63, 72–76, 132, 189, 234
Prenatal (antenatal) care, 59, 67, 76
Preterm (premature) birth, 55, 58, 59, 275
Prevalence, 142–143
Prevalence survey (*see* Cross-sectional survey)
Prevention, 13–14, 340–342
    Methods, 20, 27, 32, 43, 62, 103, 118–119
    (*see also* specific prevention methods)
Primary Health Care (PHC), 65, 100
Primary prevention, 13–14, 340–342
Primary sources, 292
Prions, 138–139
Prisoners, 96–98, 141, 156, 309
Private health insurance, 248–251
Private voluntary organization (PVO), 265–269
Professional workers, 48–49
Project HOPE, 266
Prospective study (*see* Cohort study)
Prostate cancer, 15, 28, 34–36
Prosthetics, 106
Protease inhibitors, 152
Proteins, 138–139, 182, 183
Protein-Energy Malnutrition (PEM), 189
Protozoa/Protozoal infections, 130–132, 133 (*see also* specific agents)
PSA (prostate-specific antigen) test, 15
Psittacosis (*Chlamydia psittaci*), 124, 177
Psychiatry, 100, 112
Psychology, 112
Public health, 4–7, 247, 252–253
Public health careers (*see* Careers)
Public health laws and regulations, 5, 166
Public-private partnerships, 253
PubMed, 292–293

Pulmonary TB (*see* Tuberculosis)
Purchasing power parity (PPP), 45
Pterygium, 28, 214
P-value (probability-value), 312
Pyrethroid insecticide, 162

Q

Q fever (*Coxiella burnetii*), 124, 125, 177
Qatar, 222
Quality of life (*see* Standard of living)
Quarantine, 120

R

r², 296, 298
Rabies, 117, 118, 121, 129, 130
Race, 92
Radiation, 26, 212–213, 230, 238, 240
Radio (*see* Communication technologies)
Radon, 214
Ramazzini, Bernadino, 237
Randomized Controlled Trials, 306–308
Randomized Trials, 306–308
Rapanui, 230
Rape (*see* Sex abuse)
Rate difference (RD), 304–306
Rate ratio (RR), 304–306
Reading global health reports, 293–297
Recall bias, 313
Recessive genes, 37
Recovery rate, 120–121
Red blood cells (RBCs), 158–159, 185,
    186, 188, 194–195
Red Crescent (*see* Red Cross)
Red Cross, 267, 269
Re emerging infectious diseases, 171
Reforestation, 171–172, 232
Refrigeration, 43, 227
Refugees, 94–96, 141
Registered trademarks, 278–279
Rehabilitation, 13–14, 100, 106
Relative risk (RR), 304
Reliability, 314–315
Relief organizations, 265
Religion and health practices, 17

Religious minorities, 92
Repetitive motion injury, 214, 238
Replacement population, 84
Reproductive health, 55, 70–81
Reproductive history, 77
Reproductive rights, 88
Research, 5, 94, 293–318
Research ethics, 94, 308–310
Reservoir, 118, 146
Respect for autonomy, 308–309
Respiratory system, 58–60
Retinol (*see* Vitamin A)
Reverse transcriptase inhibitors, 152
Rheumatic fever, 125, 126
Rheumatoid arthritis, 28–29, 73, 140
Rhinovirus, 121, 129
Riboflavin, 186, 193
Ricin, 177
Rickettsia, 124–125
Rickets, 186, 193
Rift Valley fever, 244
Right to health (*see* Health as a human right)
Rights of the girl-child, 69–70
Ringworm, 138, 139
Risk difference (RD), 304–305
Risk factor, 6, 8–13 (*see also* specific risk
    factors)
Risk ratio (RR), 304
Road traffic injuries (*see* Traffic accidents)
Rocky Mountain spotted fever (*Rickettsia
    rickettsii*), 124, 125
Rodents, 117, 232, 244
Roman Catholic Church, 88
Rotary International, 265, 266
Rotavirus, 61, 129, 343
Roundworm, 133–136
Rubella (German measles), 128, 129, 343
Rural health, 43, 190, 217, 220, 225, 226,
    234–237
Russia, 96, 111, 163

S

Safe motherhood programs, 76
Salmonellosis (*Salmonella*), 123, 124, 177,
    202

Salt, 62, 187–188, 192, 194–195
Samaritan's Purse, 266
Samoa, 207
Sample size, 293, 311
Sampling, 310–311
Sandflies, 117, 124, 131, 132
Sanitation, 6, 12, 62, 222–225, 230, 231, 233–235, 284, 338
SARS (Severe Acute Respiratory Syndrome), 117, 120, 170–171, 173
Saturated fatty acids, 185
Saudi Arabia, 53, 222
Save the Children, 265, 266, 267
Scabies, 133
Scarlet fever, 125, 126
Scatterplot, 296, 298
Schistosomiasis (*Schistosoma*), 73, 118, 121, 135, 137–138, 145, 195, 231, 232
Schizophrenia, 28, 98–99
Screening, 14–16, 142, 316–318
Scrotal cancer, 237
Scurvy (vitamin C deficiency), 186, 193, 237
Secondary attack rate, 119
Secondary contacts, 120
Secondary prevention, 13–14, 340–342
Secondary sources, 292
Second-hand smoke, 212, 213
Security, 3
Selection (biological process), 127
Selection bias, 313
Selenium, 187
Self-directed violence, 25–27, 98
Sen, Amartya, 208
Senegal, 75
Sensitivity, 316–318
Sentinel surveillance, 143–144
Septic tank, 222–223
SES (*see* Socioeconomic status)
Sewage system, 222–223, 235
Sex, 70
 Differences in health status, 26–27, 70–72, 73, 156
Sex abuse, 69, 71–72, 99
Sex-linked genetic disorders, 38
Sex-selective abortions, 72, 88

Sex workers, 155–156
Sexually-transmitted infections (STIs), 73, 116, 118, 124, 126, 129, 130, 131 (*see also* specific infections)
Shelter, 214–215
Shigellosis (*Shigella dysentariae*), 123, 124, 177
Shingles, 128, 129
Sickle cell anemia, 29, 37, 92
Sickness funds, 248–251
Sierra Leone, 20, 21, 284
Sight Savers International, 267
Silent Spring, 242
Silk Road, 170
Singapore, 208, 222
Slope (on a graph), 298
Skilled birth attendant, 59, 67, 73, 75–76, 284
Skilled workers, 48–49
Skin cancer, 15, 28, 213, 242, 244
Smallpox, 95–96, 118, 128, 145, 176–177, 258
Snails, 118, 135, 137, 145, 232
"Snail fever" (*see* Schistosomiasis)
Snow, John, 8–9
Social insurance systems, 248–251
Social security systems, 248–251
Socioeconomic status (SES), 40–41, 54, 140
Sodium, 61, 187–188
Soil-transmitted helminth (STH), 133, 136
South Africa, 53, 111, 155, 259, 277
South Korea, 84, 85, 111
Spain, 100, 263
Spatial clustering, 143
Specificity, 316–318
Spice Route, 170
Spina bifida, 104–105, 185
Spirilla, 123
Spirochetes, 123
Spontaneous abortion (*see* Miscarriage)
Spores, 125, 126
Sporozoa, 131
Sporozoites, 159
Spousal abuse, 25, 72
St. Louis Encephalitis, 129, 232

"Standard of health", 2–3
Standard of living, 45, 69, 82, 234, 273–275
Standardized mortality ratio (SMR), 49
Standpipe (standpost), 216
Staphylococus aureus, 125, 126–127, 173, 177
State of the World's Children, 292
State of World Population, 292
Statistical significance, 312
Sterilization, 77, 78
Stomach cancer, 28, 34–35, 73, 302–303
Stomach ulcers, 29, 121, 125
Strep throat (*Streptococcus pyogenes*), 125, 126
Stroke (cerebrovascular accident, CVA), 29, 48, 72, 106, 108, 109, 185, 203, 287
Strongyloidiasis (*Strongyloides stercoralis*), 135
Structural Adjustment Programs (SAPs), 254
Stove, 225, 227
Study designs, 296–308
Study population, 293–294
Stunting, 189
Subclinical infections, 120
Subsistence farming, 41, 159
Substance abuse (*see* Drug abuse, Alcoholism)
Sucrose, 182
Sudan, 173
Sufficient, 12
Sugar, 62, 181–182, 192, 194
Suicide, 25–27, 48, 73, 98
Sulfadoxone/pyrimethamine (SP, Fansidar), 160
Sulfer, 187
Sulfer oxides, 226, 240
Sun vitamin (*see* Vitamin D)
"Superbugs" (*see* Antimicrobial resistance)
Supernatural theory of health, 17
Supplementation, 59, 66, 192
Surveillance, 5, 143–144
Susceptibility, 118–119, 121
Sustainability, 45, 283, 338–339
Swaziland, 21, 155

Swedish International Development Cooperation Agency (SIDA), 263
Sweden, 252, 263
Swimming pools, 123, 173
Switzerland, 263
Syndrome, 149
Syphilis (*Treponema pallidum*), 59, 124, 126

T

Taeniasis (*Taenia*), 135
Tajikistan, 42
Tampons, 173
Tanzania, 51, 53, 155
Tapeworm, 133–135
Tartar siege of Kaffa, 176
Taxol, 16
Tay-Sachs Disease, 92
TB (*see* Tuberculosis)
Tea, 302–303
Tearfund, 267
Technical aid, 262
Telephone (*see* Communication technologies)
Temporal (time) clustering, 143
Teratogen, 238
Terrorist acts, 25, 176–177
Tertiary prevention, 13–14
Tetanus (*Clostridium tetani*), 14, 55, 59, 125, 126, 144, 176, 211, 343
Thailand, 97, 156, 277, 284
Thalassemia, 29, 37
Thiamine, 186, 193
Third variable effect (*see* Confounding)
Thrush, 138, 139
Thyroid, 194
Thyroid cancer, 240
Thyroid hormones, 188, 194
Tic disorders, 99
Ticks, 117, 124, 125, 131
Tinea, 139
Tobacco use, 140, 174, 212, 258–259, 280–281, 287, 313–314
    Lung cancer, 7, 212, 213
Toilet, 222–223

Tonga, 207
Tourette Syndrome, 28, 99
Toxic Shock Syndrome (TSS), 125, 173
Toxicology, 238–239
Toxoplasmosis (*Toxoplasma gondii*), 131, 132, 151
Trachoma (*Chlamydia trachomatis*), 73, 103, 125, 126, 231
Trade agreements, 170, 277–279
Trade-Related Aspects of Intellectual Property Rights (TRIPS), 279
Traditional medicine (TM), 16–17
Traffic accidents, 25–27, 73, 231
Trafficking (*see* Human trafficking)
Trained birth attendant (TBA), 58, 67, 73, 75–76, 284, 337
Trans fats, 185
Transmission modes (*see* Modes of transmission)
Trash (*see* Waste)
Triatominae bugs (*see* Kissing bugs)
Transportation, 6, 20, 170, 173
Transmissibility, 171
Transnational health (*see* Global health)
Travel, 171, 173, 175
Trematodes, 134–135
Triage, 276
Tribal minorities, 92–93
Trichinosis (trichinellosis, *Trichinella spiralis*), 133, 135
Trichomoniasis (*Trichomonas vaginalis*), 131
Trichuriasis (*Trichuris trichiura*), 133, 135
TRIPS Plus, 278–279
True negative, 315–316
True positive, 315–316
Trypanosomiasis (*see* African Sleeping Sickness and American Sleeping Sickness)
Tsetse fly, 117, 131, 132
T-test, 312
Tubal ligation, 77–78
Tuberculosis (TB), 73, 125, 163–167, 211, 232, 280, 281
   Disease (active TB), 119, 163

DOTS (directly-observed therapy), 163–166, 338
HIV co-infection, 150, 151, 163, 165
Incidence/Prevalence, 127, 164–165, 167, 284, 338
Infection (latent TB), 119, 163
MDR-TB, 97, 127, 166
Prevention, 342
Prisons, 96–98
Tests, 166
Transmission, 117, 118
Treatment, 163–166
Vaccine, 166, 343
Tube wells, 241
Tularemia (*Francisella tularensis*), 125
Turkey, 42
Turner Syndrome, 37
Tuskegee syphilis experiment, 94
2, 3, 2 tables, 300–301
Type, 2 diabetes (*see* Diabetes)
Type I error, 315
Type II error, 315
Typhoid fever (*Salmonella* Typhi), 123, 124, 125
Typhoid Mary, 120
Typhus fever (*Rickettsia prowazekii*), 117, 124–125, 177, 211, 232

U

Uganda, 44, 111, 157, 173, 304–305
Ukraine, 96, 100, 163, 176, 240
Ulcers (*see* Stomach ulcers)
Ultraviolet (UV) radiation, 213, 214, 243, 244
UN (*see* United Nations)
UNAIDS (Joint United Nations Programme on AIDS), 258, 261, 262, 337–338
Unani, 17
Under-5 clinics, 65, 197
Under-5 mortality (*see* Child mortality)
Undernutrition, 31, 64, 159, 189–196
Underweight, 189–190, 196–197, 284, 336
Undulant fever (brucellosis, *Brucella*), 125, 126, 177

Unemployment, 48–49, 339
UNESCO, 260, 336–338
UN-HABITAT, 260, 339
UNICEF (United Nations Children's Fund), 70, 258, 261, 262, 266, 267, 292, 336–338
Unintentional injury, 24–27, 73, 226, 231–232, 244 (*see also* specific types of injury)
United Arab Emirates, 222
United Kingdom (UK), 20, 48–49, 111, 249, 251–252, 259, 263, 264, 267
United Nations (UN), 252, 257–262
United Nations Development Programme (UNDP), 258, 260, 262, 292
United Nations Drug Control Programme (UNDCP), 258, 261
United Nations Environment Programme (UNEP), 242, 258, 261, 262, 338
United Nations Population Fund (UNFPA), 88–89, 90, 260, 262, 292, 337–338
United Nations High Commissioner for Refugees (UNHCR), 95, 258, 260, 262
United States of America (USA)
    Infectious diseases, 97, 172, 173, 174, 176, 177, 202, 284
    Maternal and child health and population issues, 75, 84, 85, 89, 111, 207, 237, 284
    Non-communicable diseases, 12, 20, 71, 93–94, 100, 206
    Policies and economics, 47, 89, 249, 251, 252, 259, 262–264, 266, 277–278, 285
Universal Declaration of Human Rights, 273–275, 331–335
Universal health care, 248–250
Universal precautions, 156
Unmodifiable risk factors, 6, 140
Unplanned urbanization, 215, 233–235, 339
Unsafe sex, 76, 77–79, 126, 155–156, 213
Unsaturated fatty acids, 182, 185
Unskilled workers, 48–49
Untouchables, 48–49

Upper respiratory infections, 60–61
Urban health, 170, 217, 220, 225, 226, 235
Urbanization, 111, 172, 203, 232–237
USAID (United States Agency for International Development), 262–264
USDA (United States Department of Agriculture), 202, 207
Uterine cancer, 28

V

Vaccination (*see* Immunization)
Vaginal yeast infection (*see* Yeast infection)
Validity, 15, 314–315
Varicella, 128, 129
Vasectomy, 77–78
Vector, 117, 141–142
    Vector control, 144–145, 213, 230, 242, 282
    Vectorborne transmission, 116–117, 118, 124–125
Vehicle-borne transmission, 117
Venezuelan equine encephalitis (VEE), 117, 129, 177, 232
Ventilation, 117, 227
Ventilation-improved latrine, 222–223
Vertical transmission, 118 (*see also* Mother-to-child transmission)
Veterans Administration (VA), 249
Vibrios, 123
Vinyl chloride, 239
Violence, 25–27, 73, 232 (*see also* specific types)
Virulence, 120–121, 171
Viruses/viral infections, 127–130 (*see also* specific agents)
Visceral leishmaniasis (*see* Kala azar)
Visual impairment, 73, 105, 108 (*see also* Blindness)
Vital Statistics, 83–85
Vitamins, 185–187, 193–194
Vitamin A/Vitamin A deficiency (VAD), 182, 185–186

Prevention, 14, 59, 64, 66, 192, 193–194, 286–288
Symptoms, 102, 186, 193–194
Vitamin B1 (thiamine), 186, 193
Vitamin B2 (riboflavin), 186, 193
Vitamin C, 185–187, 192, 193, 237
Vitamin D, 182, 186, 187, 193
Vitamin E, 182, 185
Vitamin K, 182, 187
Voluntary organization (*see* Non-governmental organization)
Voluntary Service Overseas (VSO), 267
Volunteer bias, 313
Voodoo, 17

W

Waist circumference, 196
War, 25–27, 73
Warts, 129
Waste/Waste management, 6, 213, 214, 234, 235
Wasting, 189
Water, 6, 8–9, 12, 62, 187, 215–222, 230, 231, 233, 235
Access, 215–221, 284, 338
Cost, 217
Filters, 137, 145, 216, 241
Fleas, 133, 145
Ownership, 217–221
Privatization, 217–221
Proximity, 216, 218
Quality, 213, 215–216, 218
Quantity, 216, 218
Reliability, 216
Resources management, 144–145, 217–222, 230, 231
Rights, 221
Scarcity, 217, 221
Sources, 215–216
Transmission, 116–117, 123
Wealth, 42, 140
Weather extremes, 242–244
Weekly Epidemiological Record, 18
Weight-for-age, 196

Weight-for-height, 196, 189, 317
Wellcome Trust, 280
Wells, 216, 217, 220, 241
West Bank/Gaza, 222
West Nile virus, 118, 129, 173, 232
Western equine encephalitis, 129, 177, 232
Whipworm, 133, 135
WHO (*see* World Health Organization)
Whooping cough (pertussis), 125, 126, 343
Wolfensohn, James, 285
Women's health, 26, 52, 70–81, 156, 292, 314
Women's Health Initiative (WHI), 305, 308
Wood, 225–226
World Bank, 252, 253–256, 260, 279, 292, 336–339
World Development Report, 292
World Emergency Relief, 267
World Food Program (WFP), 258, 260, 262
World Health Assembly, 258
World Health Organization (WHO), 258–259, 260, 262, 279, 291–292, 336–339
Constitution, 2–3, 20, 326–328
Regions, 21, 23, 31–33, 109, 321–325
World Health Report (WHR), 258, 291–292
World Intellectual Property Organization (WIPO), 260, 278
World maps, 22, 46, 56, 80, 107, 136, 153, 161, 164, 183, 184, 191, 204, 205, 219, 224, 236, 255, 321
World Trade Organization (WTO), 261, 278
World Vision, 265, 266, 267
Worms (*see* Helminths)
Wound healing, 186, 187, 188

X

Xerosis (dry eye), 193

Y

Yeast, 138
Yeast infection, 138, 139
Yellow fever, 117, 128, 129, 232, 343
Yin and yang, 17
Yunus, Muhammad, 267

Z

Zambia, 21, 42, 155
Zimbabwe, 21, 155
Zidovudine (AZT), 157
Zinc, 59, 64, 187, 188, 196
Zoonosis, 118
Z-score, 317